FUNDAMENTAL RHEUMATOLOGICAL KNOWLEDGE OF ARTHRITIS IMAGES OF THE HAND AND CASE STUDIES FOR GENERAL PHYSICIANS

MEDICAL PROCEDURES, TESTING AND TECHNOLOGY

Additional books in this series can be found on Nova's website under the Series tab.

Additional e-books in this series can be found on Nova's website under the e-book tab.

MEDICAL PROCEDURES, TESTING AND TECHNOLOGY

FUNDAMENTAL RHEUMATOLOGICAL KNOWLEDGE OF ARTHRITIS IMAGES OF THE HAND AND CASE STUDIES FOR GENERAL PHYSICIANS

SYUICHI KOARADA
AND
YOSHIFUMI TADA
EDITOR

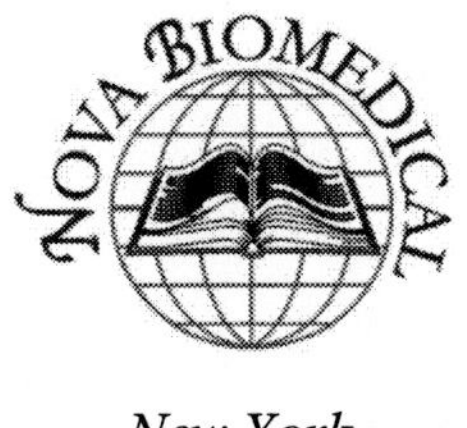

NOVA BIOMEDICAL

New York

Library of Congress Cataloging-in-Publication Data

ISBN: 978-1-62417-925-9

Published by Nova Science Publishers, Inc. † New York

CONTENTS

PREFACE

This work provides a simplified but high-quality diagnostic interpretation of hand radiography for residents in training and even experienced physicians who wish to improve their knowledge in contemporary rheumatology, according to the rapid progress of treatment using biologic agents and various new diagnostic tools, including MRI and ultrasound. The contents of this monograph are based on my own lectures that have been approved by our medical students and residents in Saga University. The diagnostic approach to make decision by conventional hand radiography is originated from my experience of research and education in the division of Rheumatology in the University of Pittsburgh. However, the presented all cases and radiographs in the book are our original. In addition, to make accurate diagnosis from hand radiographs, the methodology has been uniquely developed and improved by experience of more than 4,000 cases with rheumatic diseases in our institute in Japan.

In our experienced various cases, there are many interesting and rare diseases. For examples, there are a numbers of patients with Behcet's disease that are rare in the US. It also includes the cases of adult onset Still's disease (AOSD) with severe arthritis and are treated with various biologics and immunosuppressive drugs. Because we have established the diagnostic criteria of AOSD that has been approved world-widely, our hospital is a central institute of AOSD in Japan and also the world. We have proposed the method to prevent aseptic osteonecrosis of femoral head (AONF) induced by corticosteroid therapy in SLE patients. We reported the second case of RS3PE (Remitting Seronegative Symmetrical Synovitis with Pitting Edema) syndrome associated with malignancy. Several cases of IgG4-related disease are presented. We also investigate new therapy for SLE and B cell target therapy. These original findings are included in this article and it may be interesting for specialists of rheumatology.

Syuichi Koarada
2012/9/30
In Saga, Japan

Chapter 1

INTRODUCTION

Plain Film of hands provides basic information and a systematic approach for the diagnosis of rheumatic diseases.

Proper radiographs of the hands are probably the most informative among various methods for evaluating arthritis including CT, MRI, ultrasound, and so on.

The information from the film may help to make differential diagnosis of various disorders.

The following method to read films of hands can support the final decision and diagnosis of rheumatic diseases.

A: alignment
B: bone
C: cartilage
D: distribution
E: extra-bone
F: further information
G: goal (final diagnosis)

Because we are physicians working in clinic (not radiologists), it is difficult to make absolute and accurate diagnosis at any time only by a plain film. We emphasize the importance of item of "F" (further information; basic patient's information including age, sex and race, history, physical examination, laboratory data). The items from "A" to "E" (radiographic findings) work concert with the item "F" supporting each together in physicians' diagnosis.

Radiographs of the hands play important and basic roles in rheumatology such as ECG (electrocardiogram) in cardiology, chest radiographs in respiratory systems.

PLAIN HAND RADIOGRAPHS

Usually a plain hand radiograph is the posterroanterior view (PA view) and oblique view. Especially, the PA view provides basic information of the item "A"to "E".

Plain Hand Radiographs

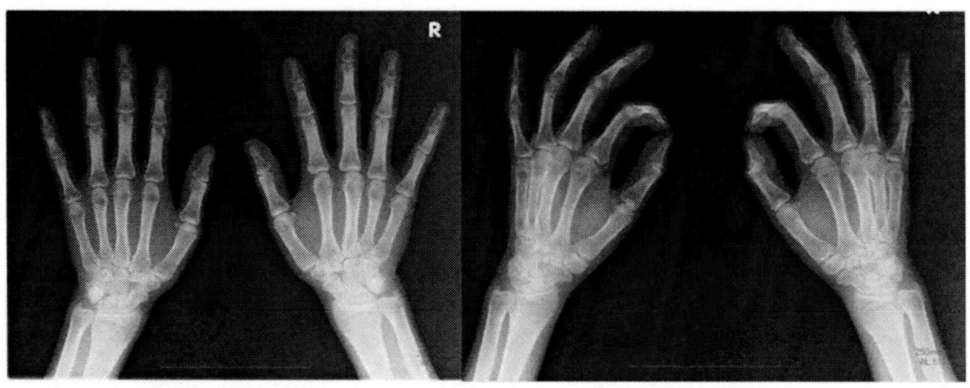

posteroanterior hand radiograph
Dorsopalmar radiograph
(PA view)

oblique hand radiograph
(oblique view)

Figure 1. An anterior-posterior oblique view, opposite view (Nørgaard view) or lateral view are also available.

The Nørgaard view, or semisupinated oblique view of the hands may present earlier erosive changes effectively in some cases, and lateral view show a fracture easier than PA and oblique views. However, in lateral view, to find signs of arthritis is difficult and the value of Norgaard view may be controversial.

PA view   Lateral view   Nørgaard view
semisupinated oblique view of the hands

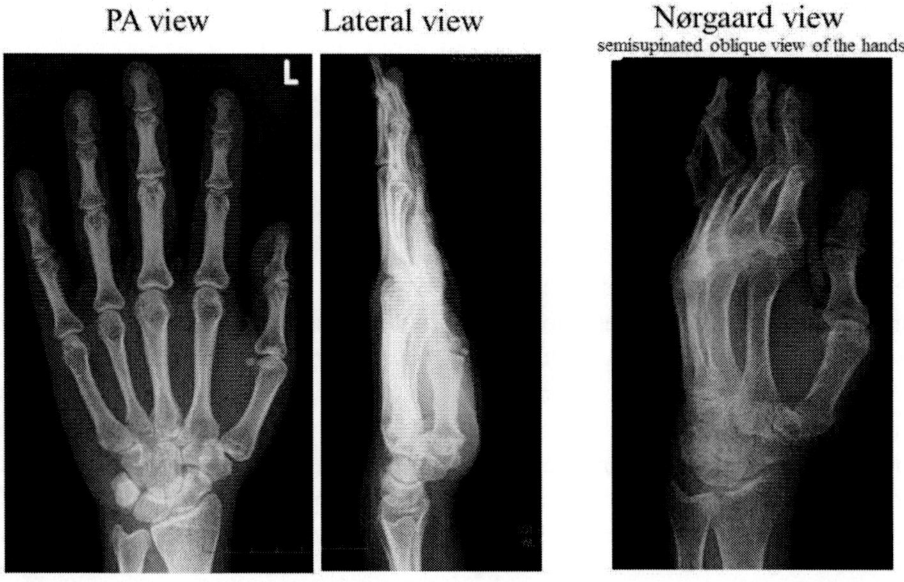

Figure 2. (A A De Smet, Radiographic projections for the diagnosis of arthritis of the hands and wrists. Radiology, 139, 577-581, 1981).

4 VIEWS OF THE HAND

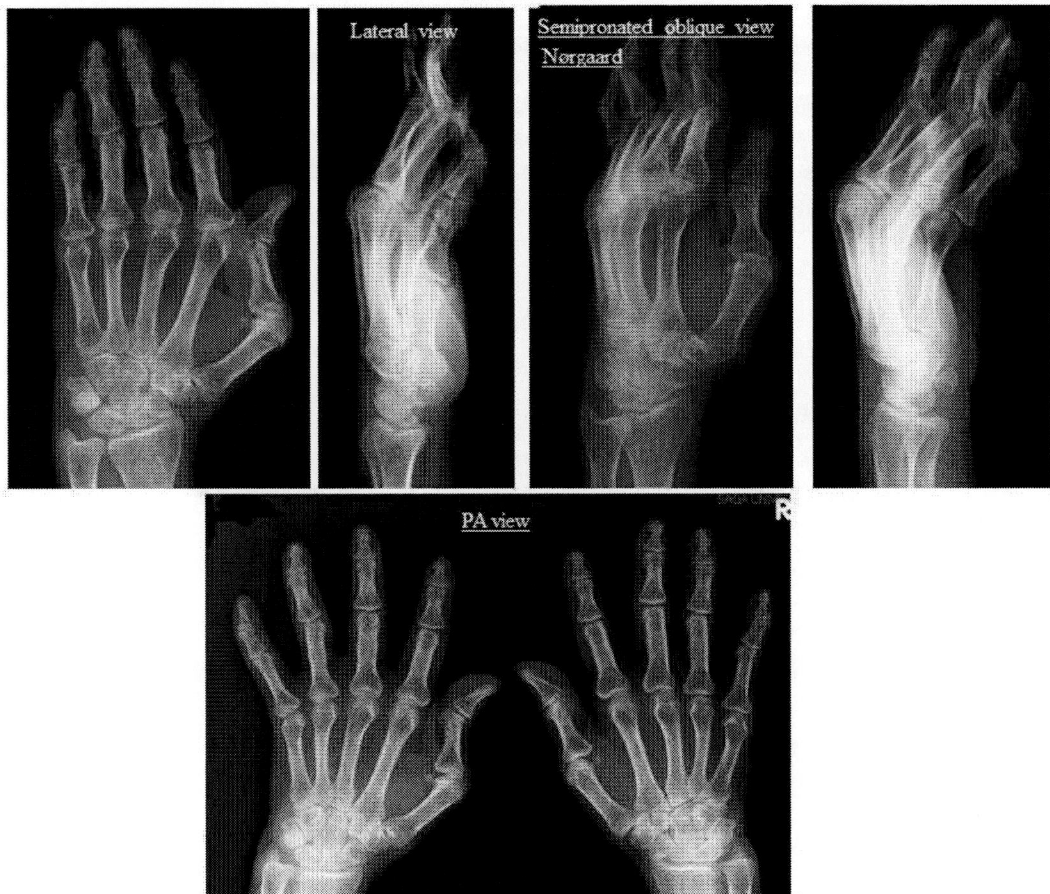

Figure 3. Deformity of fingers and deviation at the joints may be found easier in the 4 views than in the PA view.

ABCDEFG READING FOR HAND FILM

A. alignment
    Position of bones (axis, height of carpals, deformity, (sub)-luxation, fracture)
B. bone mineralization
    bone density, juxta-articular osteoporosis, osteosclerosis
C. cartilage
    JSN（joint space narrowing）· erosion · osteophyte · calcification
D. distribution
    Position of radiographic findings within the joints, hands, body and time
E. external bone lesion
    Soft tissue and calcification
F. further information

History, signs and symptoms, physical examination, blood tests, Chest X-ray, MRI, echogram, nuclear medicine and so on

G. goal
Comprehensive diagnosis based on A to F information

ALIGNMENT

The alignment is the positioning of the bones in the hand.

1) In the 2nd, 3rd, 4th fingers, the bones from metacarpal to distal phalangeal position in the straight lines. (except in the 1st and 5th finders)
2) The line between the scaphoid and the lunate (dot line) runs at the center of radius. More than 50% of width of the lunate overlaps RC joint.
3) Height of carpal bones: B/A (the 3rd metacarpal)> 0.54

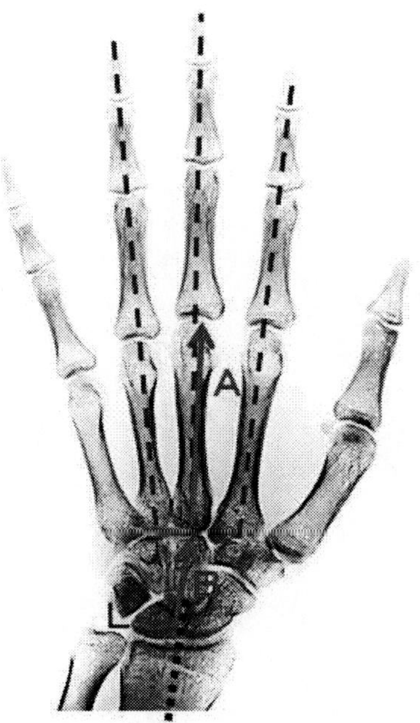

Figure 4. Alignment.

FINGERS

Fingers in Normal Hands

Even in normal persons, the first and the 5th fingers can open so widely that the alignment does not look well. We consider "the alignment" except in these fingers.

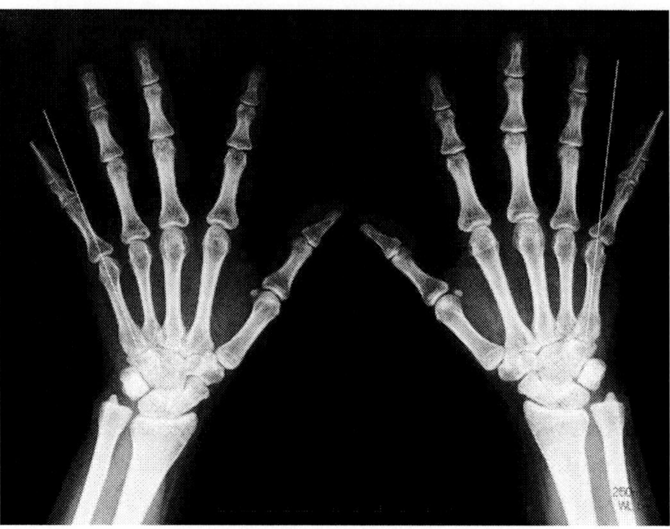

Figure 5. Even in normal persons, the first and the 5th fingers can open so widely that the alignment does not look well. We consider the alignment except in these finders.

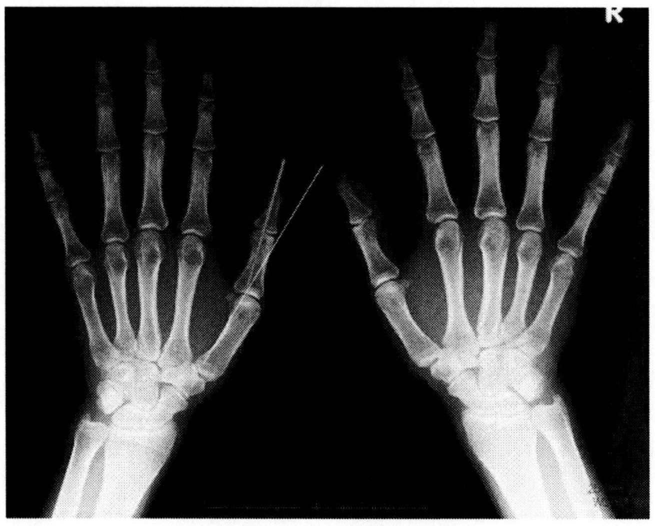

Figure 6. Flexion at MCP joint of the 1st finger occurs easily by the positioning.

Out of Alignment of Bones

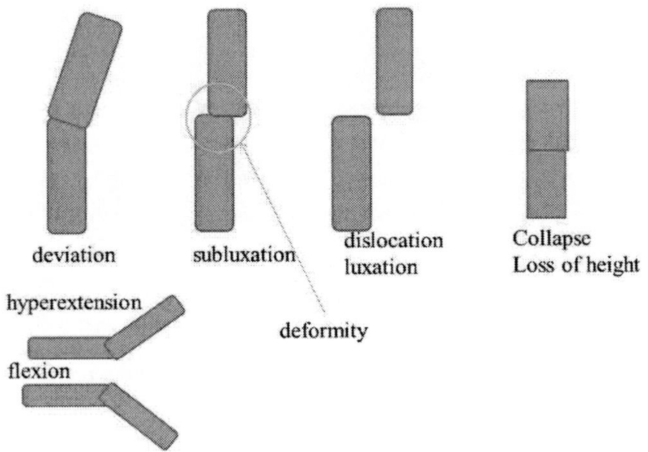

Figure 7. These findings include deviation, subluxation, dislocation, and collapse (loss of height), deformity.

Ulnar Deviation of the Fingers in the MCPs in Early RA

Usually, when the subluxations occur, the inflammatory arthritis at MCP joints presents, especially in RA.

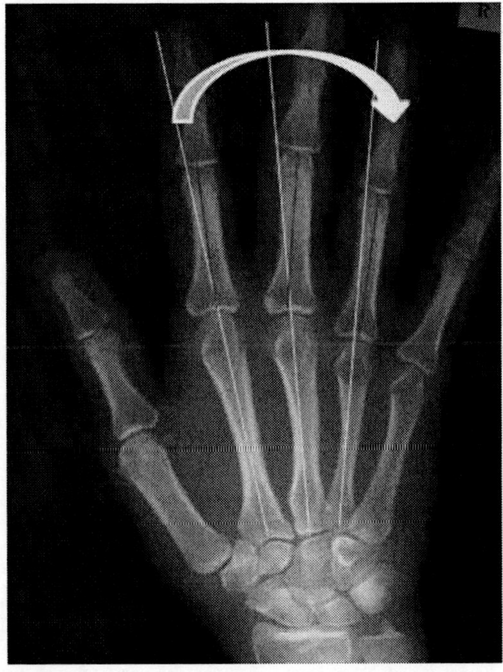

Figure 8. Deviation is found at the MCP joints: The proximal phalanges ulnarly (ulnar) and palmarly(volar) shift.

Jaccoud's Arthritis

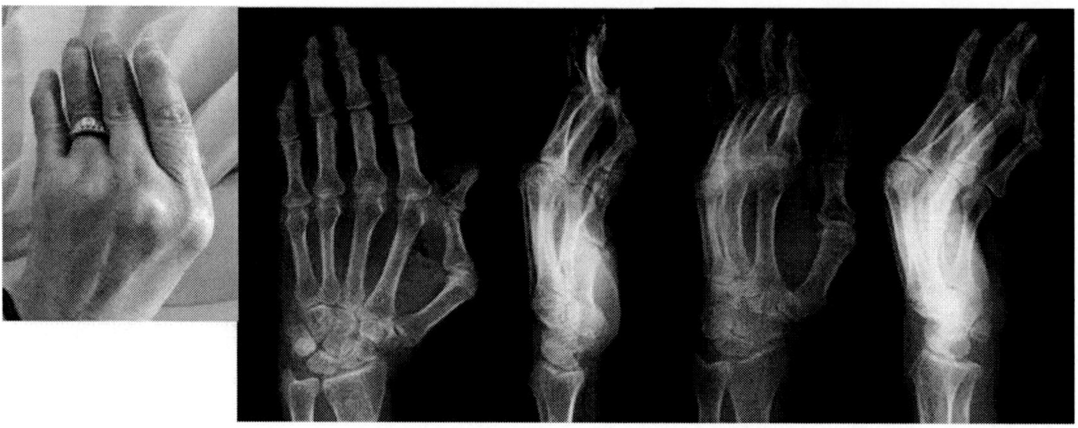

Figure 9. Four views of the hand show subluxation of the MCP joints in SLE patients. To know the deformity and deviation of fingers, these views are helpful. There is no evidence of erosion.

Subluxation; Laterally at 2nd DIP in OA

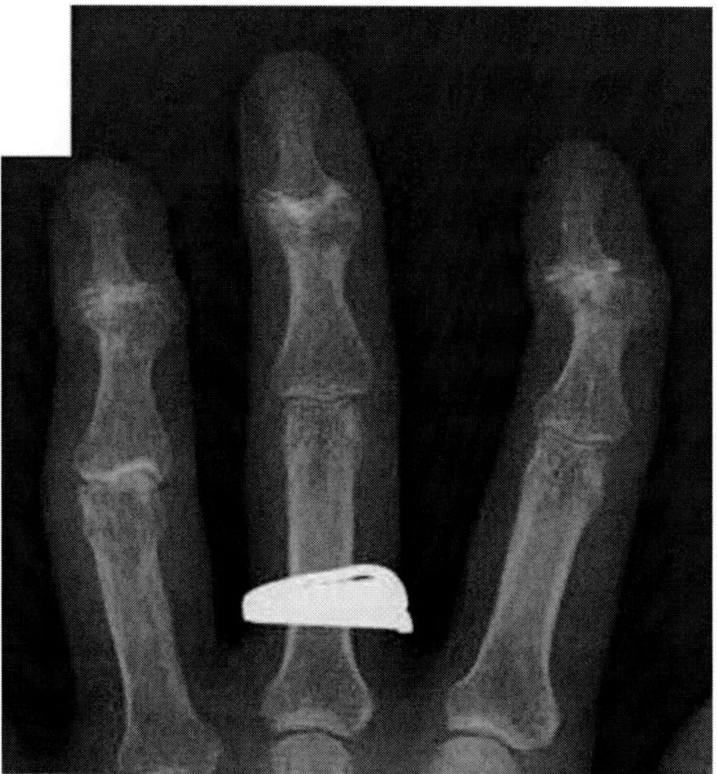

Figure 10. PA view of fingers shows lateral subluxation of the 2nd distal phalanx in relationship to the middle phalanx of the second digit in patient with osteoarthritis.

PA View of the Hand in a Patient with SLE

Posteroanterior (PA) view of both hands in a patient with SLE shows osteoporosis. Because the subluxations are reducible, plain PA view do not illustrate the deformity, Jaccoud's arthritis, clearly even in the same patient.

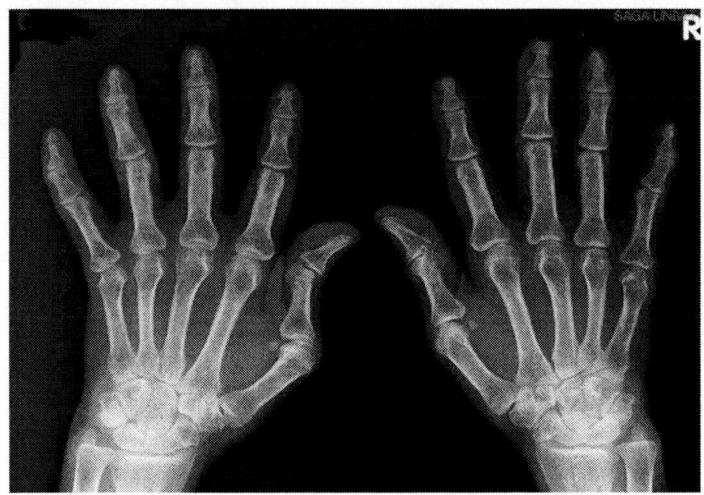

Figure 11. Plain PA view positions the digits properly, then it does not show evident deformity.

Pitfall of PA View in SLE

The PA view of the same hand shows very small mal-alignment of fingers, especially at MCP joint of the second finger (arrow), because the fingers are rigidly positioned.

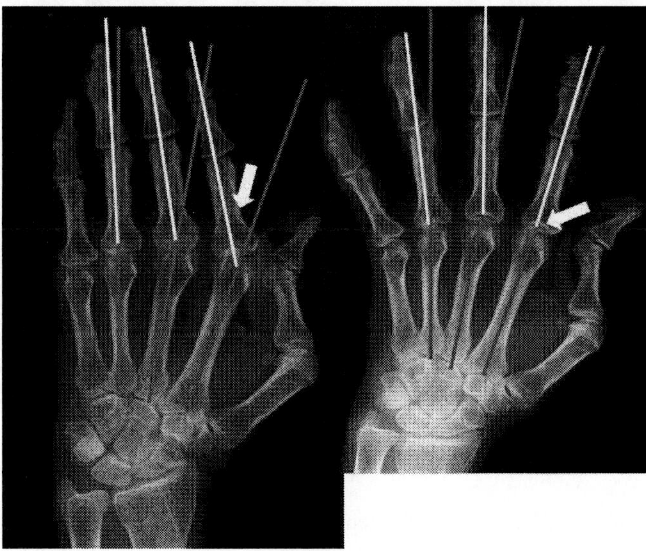

Figure 12. PA view of the same hand shows very small mal-alignment of fingers.

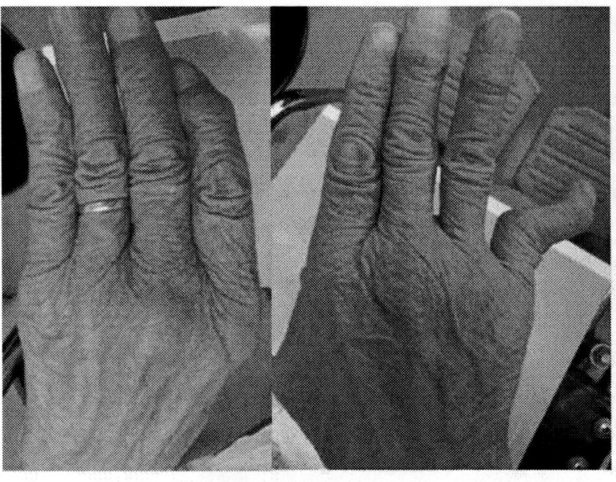
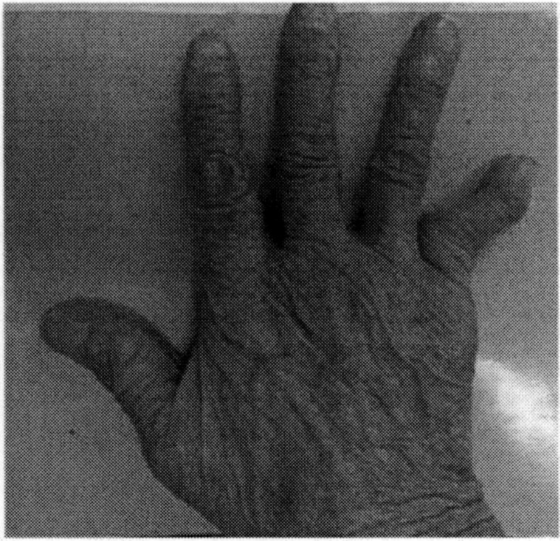

Figure 13. Urnal and reversible deviation.

CARPAL BONES

Not overlapping each other and detect outline of each carpal bone are found in normal hands. The line between scaphoid and lunate runs the center of the radius.

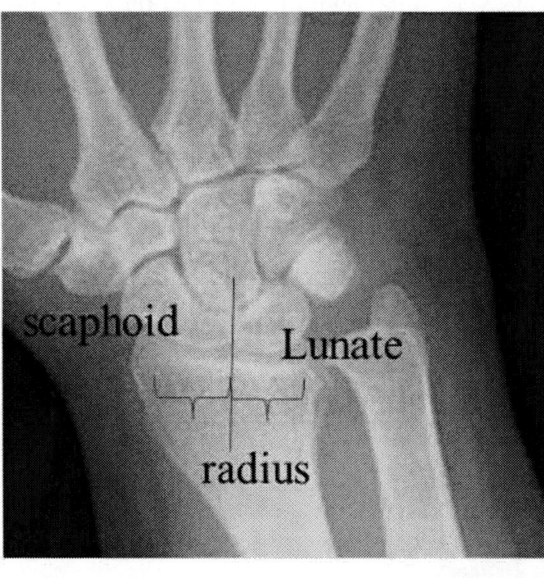

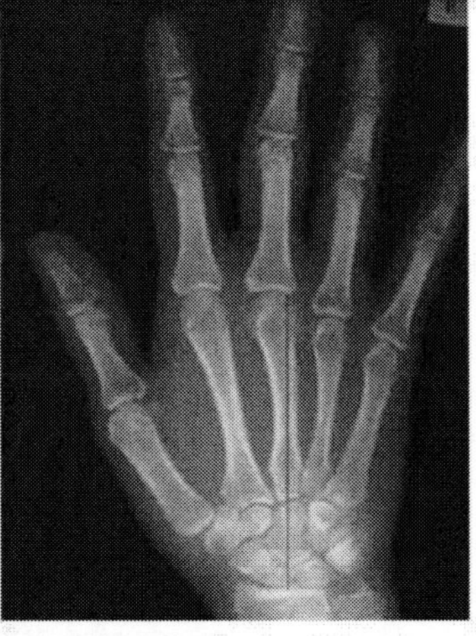

Figure 14. The height of carpals are half of the length of the 3rd metacarpal bone (ratio is more than 0.54).

The line between the scaphoid and the lunate deviates from the center of the radius to ulnar side.

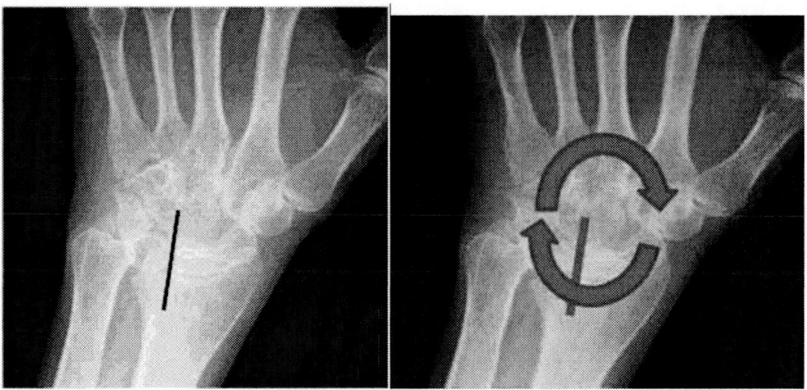

Figure 15. Radial Deviation. A 32-year-old Female Rheumatoid Arthritis.

Radial deviation of the carpus

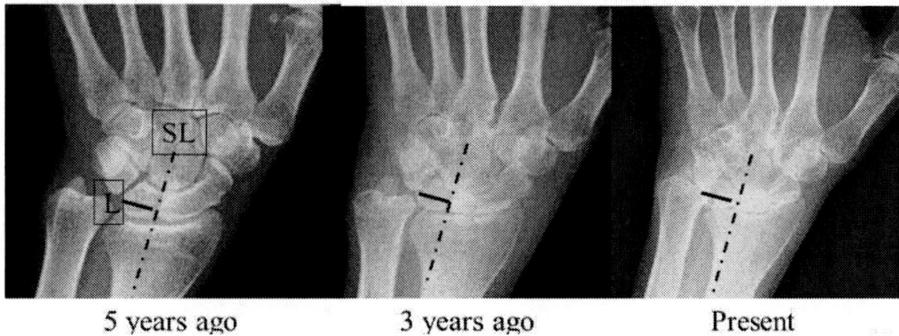

Figure 16. A 32-year-old female with RA shows that, gradually, the line (SL) between the scaphoid and the lunate has shifted to ulnar side (L). It resulted in radial deviation.

Scapholunate Dissociation

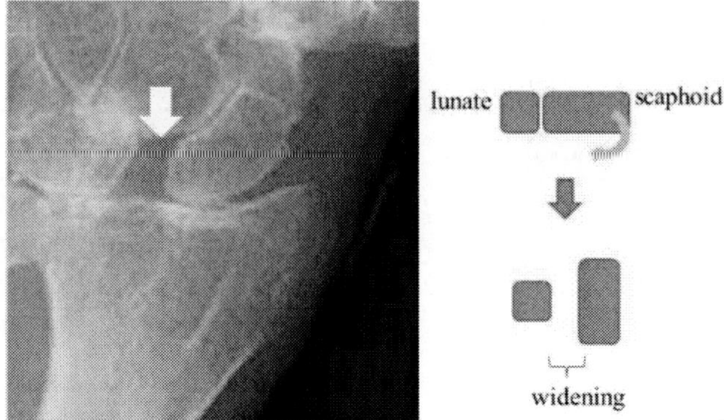

Figure 17. Widening between scaphoid and lunate suggests the rotatory subluxation of scaphoid in a patient with RA.

DEFORMITIES OF FINGER JOINTS

Swan-neck deformity

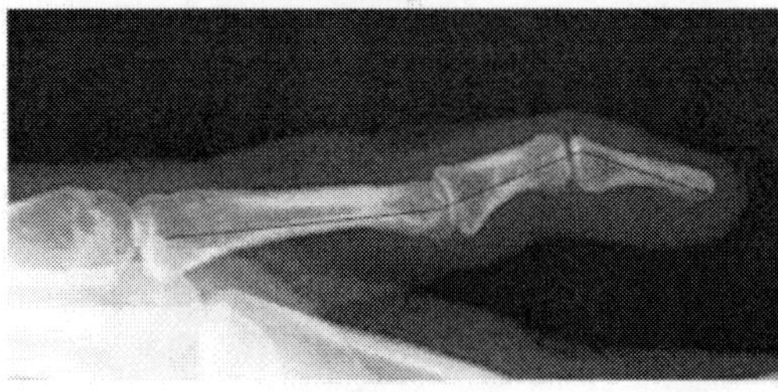

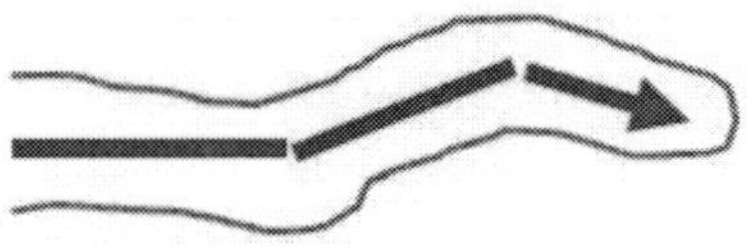

Button-hole deformity
(boutonnière deformity)

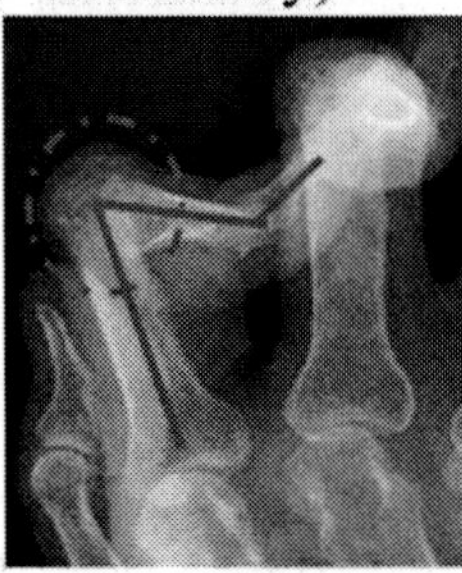

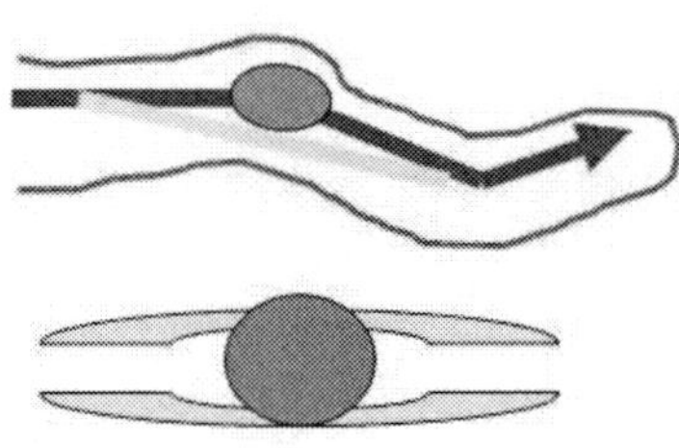

Figure 18. Swan-neck deformity: hyperextension in the PIP joint and flexion in the DIP joint. Button-hole deformity (boutonnière deformity): hyperextension in the DIP joint and flexion in the PIP joint.

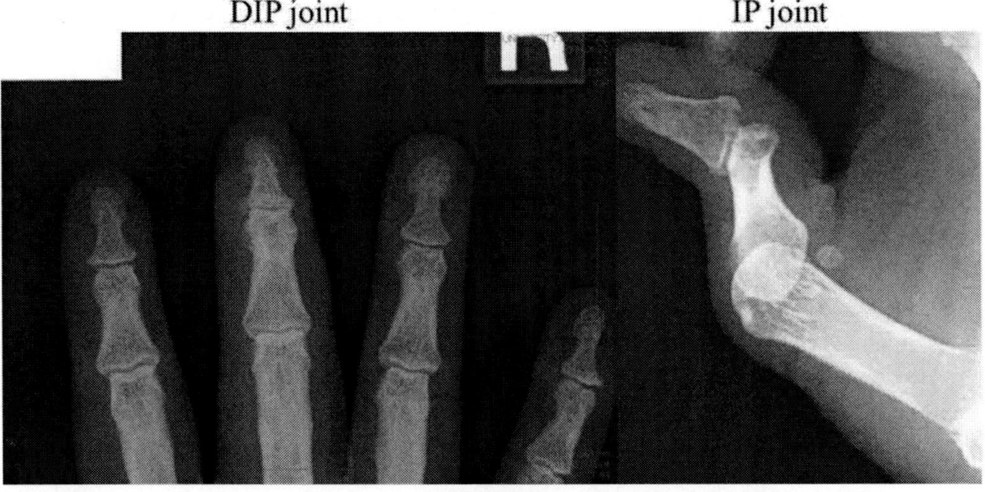

Figure 19. Deformity of dip joint and ip joint.

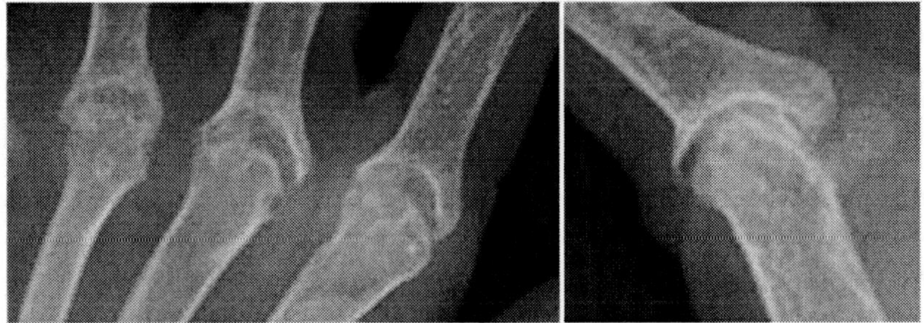

Figure 20. Cup-and-saucer deformity.

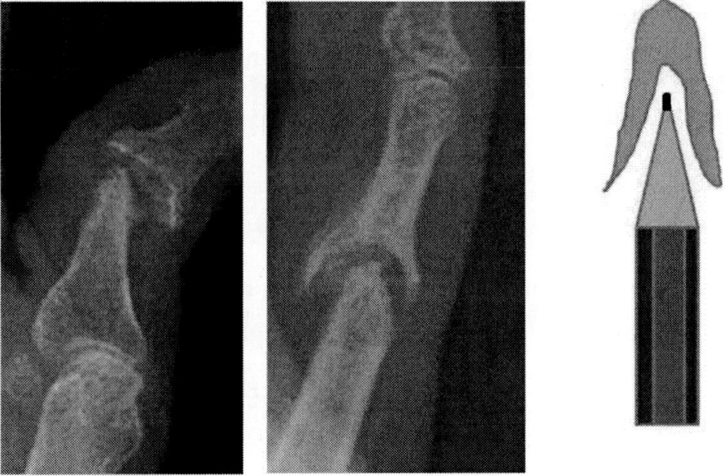

Figure 21. Pencil in cup deformity.

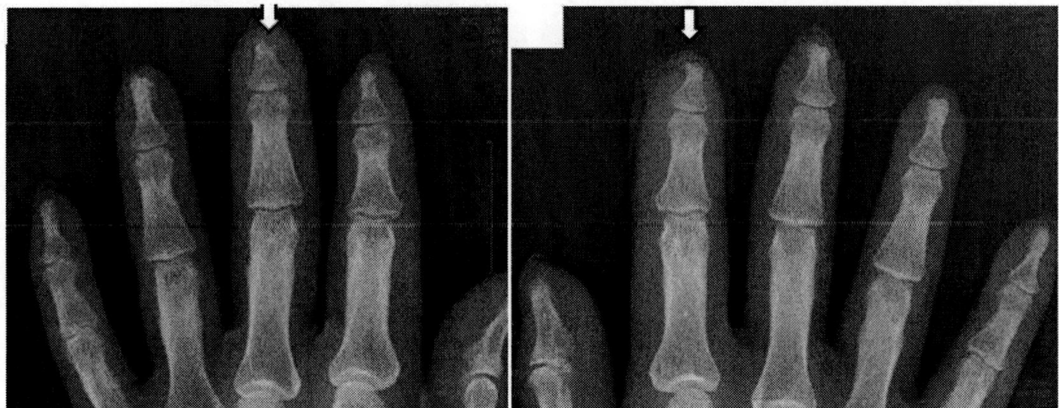

Figure 22. Acro-osteolysis is found at the distal phalanx in systemic sclerosis.

MAL-ALIGNMENT IN RA

"A=mal-alignment" in RA

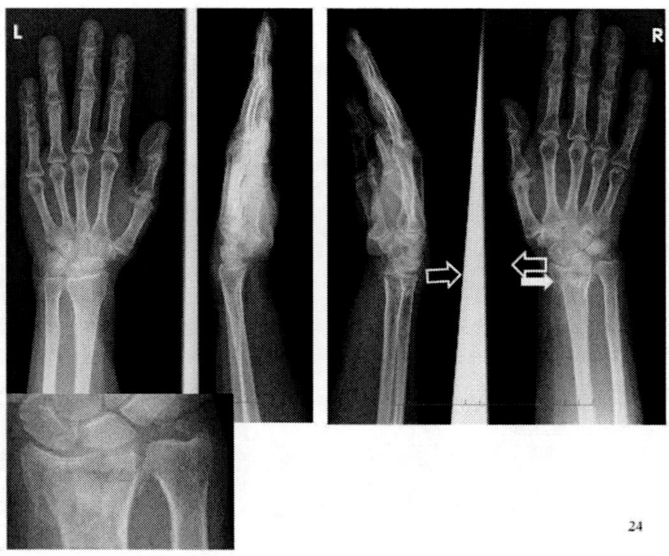

Figure 23. There are many mal-alignment in RA. The drawing shows some typical changes.

BONE FRACTURES

Colless' Fracture

Figure 24. A PA view of the hand showing the characteristic Colles' fracture (solid arrow) with displacement and radial deviation of the distal end of the radius (blank arrows) in a 62-year-old female with SLE

LUXATION

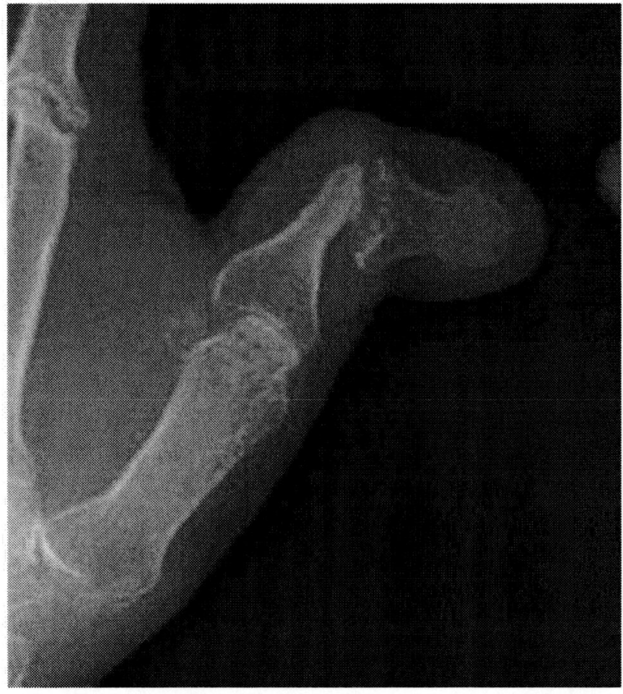

Figure 25. Luxation of 1st IP of advanced PsA

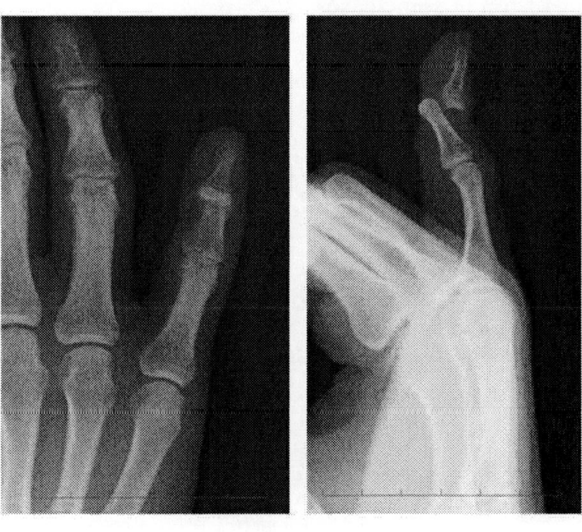

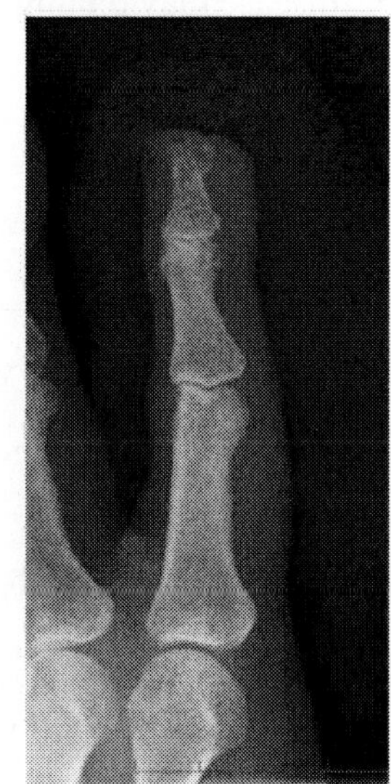

Figure 26. Luxation Due to Injury.

OTHER IMPORTANT ABNORMALITY OF ALIGNMENT IN RA

The alignment of the spine

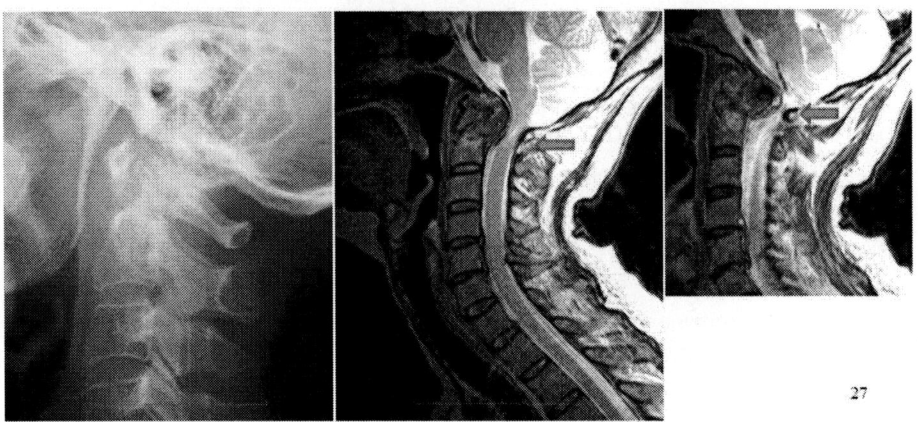

Figure 27. Lateral views of the C1-C2 in patient with rheumatoid arthritis.

Atlantoaxial disease is most commonly seen in the cervical spine. The laxity of the transverse ligament that holds the odontoid to the atlas is frequently found in RA patients. In this case, the dens is disappeared in plain radiograph.

Sagittal T2-weighted MR images confirms large nodule at C1/C2 and marked compression of the spinal cord between the dens and posterior arch of C1 (arrows).

This disease may require posterior fusion in some cases.

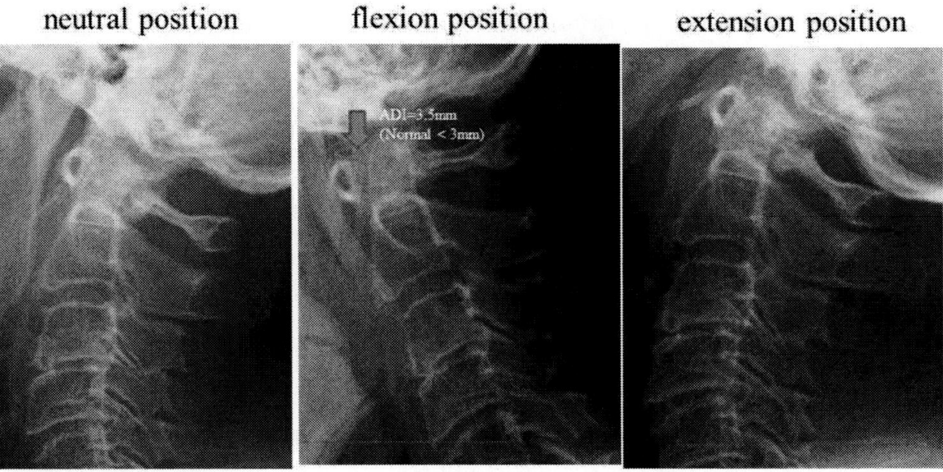

Figure 28. Mild Adi Abnormality in Patient with Rheumatoid Arthritis.

Lateral Views of the Cervical Spine in Patient with Rheumatoid Arthritis

Atlantodens interval (ADI): Lateral flexion radiograph is useful to detect widening of atlantodens interval because of increased distance between the atlas and odontoid (arrows). The flexion position excellently shows the laxity of the transverse ligament. However, when there is a definitive subluxation exists, this position may be dangerous. In the population of patients with rheumatoid arthritis, the radiography of cervical spine in the flexed position, more than 30 percent patients have ADI abnormality.

In this patient, the radiography in the neural position shows almost normal findings. However, the laxity of the transverse ligament becomes apparent in the flexion position of the cervical spine. In this patient, ADI is 3.1mm.

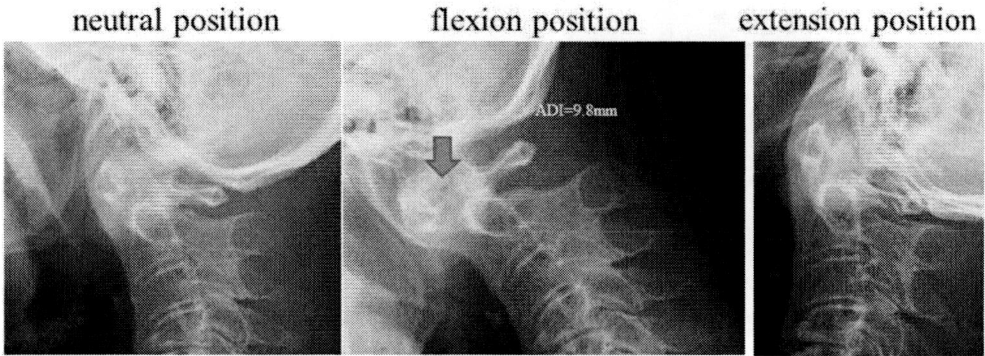

Figure 29. Severe ADI abnormality in patient with late rheumatoid arthritis.

Lateral Views of the Upper Cervical Spine in Patient with Late Rheumatoid Arthritis

A radiography of the neck in a flexed position shows increased distance between the atlas and odontoid (arrow). ADI is 9.8mm (>3.5mm) and severely damaged C1/C2. This findings suggest the laxity of the transverse ligament. The distance between the atlas and the odontoid is greater than 8 mm. Therefore, the narrowing of the spinal canal between the dens and posterior ring of C1 is evident (arrow). Usually, greater than 8 mm of ADI requires posterior fusion.

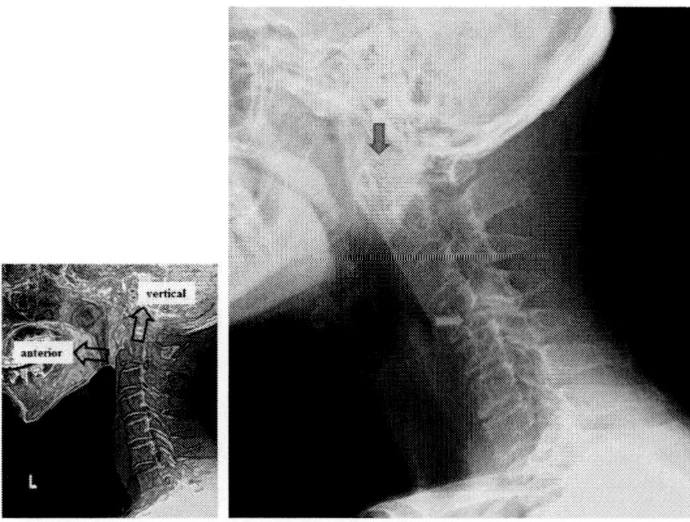

Figure 30. In a patient with rheumatoid arthritis, the dens is unclear and enlarged ADI in plain radiograph. Also, dis-alignment of C4/5.

In some cases, vertical subluxation of the dens is a severer manifestation of atlantoaxial change.

Lateral Views of the Cervical Spine in Patient with Adult Onset Still's Disease

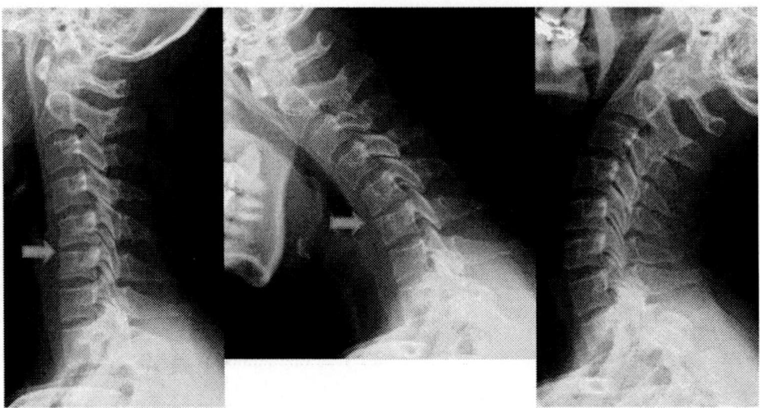

Figure 31. Lateral view of cervical spine shows anggulation of C5/6.

SUBLUXATION OF THE KNEES DUE TO SEVERE RA

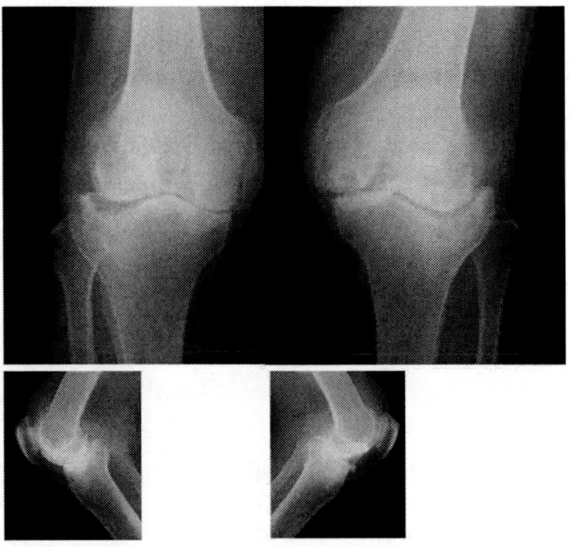

Figure 32. Subluxation of the knees due to severe RA.

Bipartite Patella

A bipartite patella, that develops differently and there are two separate parts to the bone, separated by a fibrousarea, is found in about 1% of the population.

Most patients with the bipartite patella show no pain or other symptoms. However, in some patients with a bipartite patella have joint pain of the knee(s).

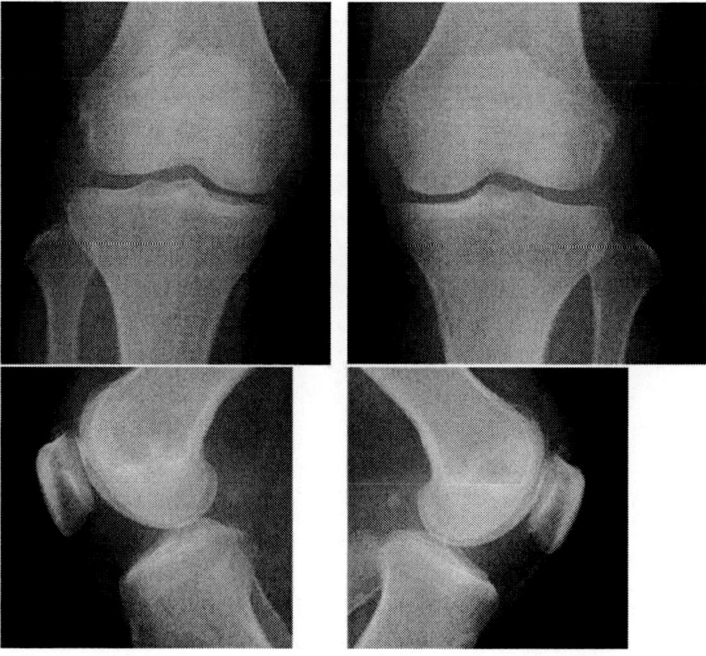

Figure 33. A 58-year-old Female with SLE complained pain of the knees. She was diagnosed as having bipartite patella.

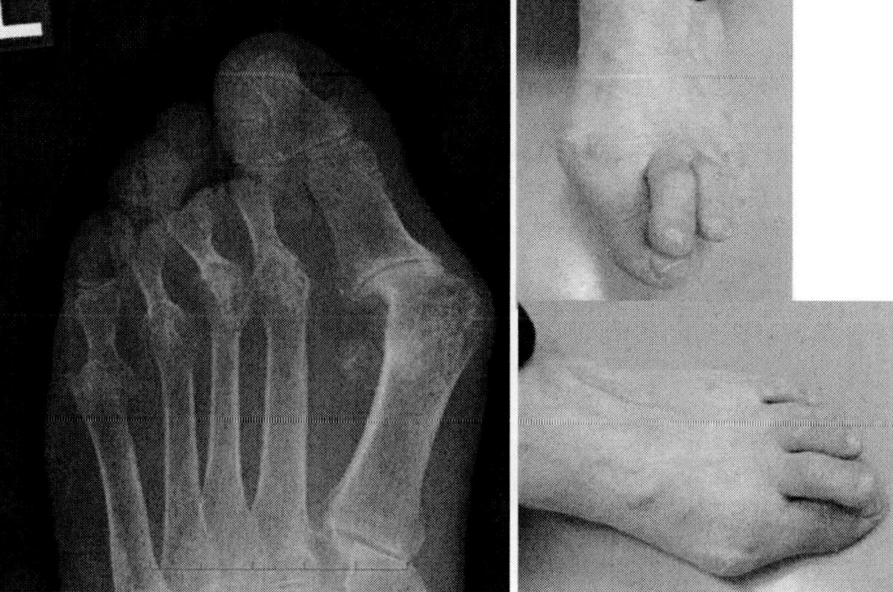

Figure 34. Cock-up Deformities of the Foot in RA Patients.

Chapter 3

BONE MINERALIZATION

BONE DENSITY

Bone Density is speculated by evaluation of the metacarpal shaft of the 2nd or the 3rd digit in PA view of the hands.

Evaluation of mineralization is performed by checking the cortices at the center of the metacarpal shaft of the 2nd or the 3rd digit. In normal persons, the sum of the lateral side of cortices of the shaft is more than 50% of the width of bone of the digit. The generalized osteoporosis can be estimated by the cortices of the shaft.

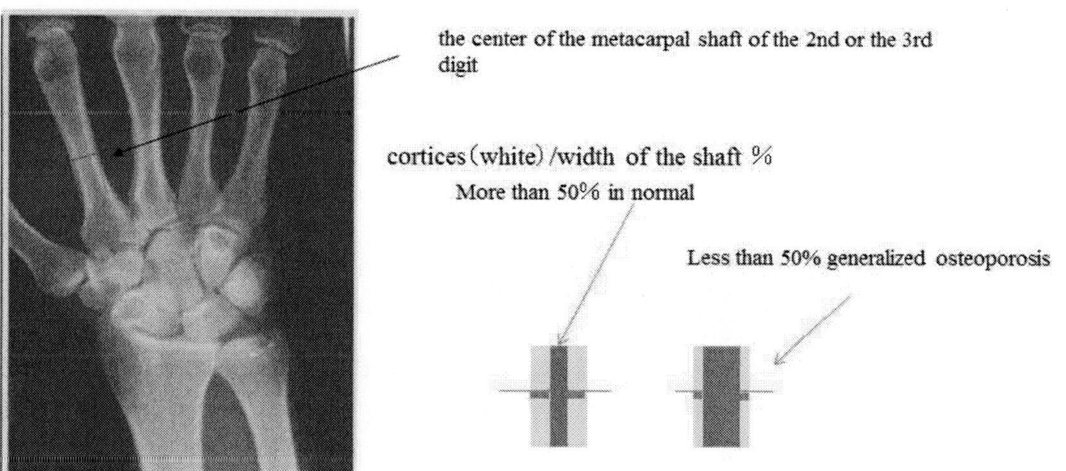

Figure 1. Evaluation of mineralization.

Normal Mineralization

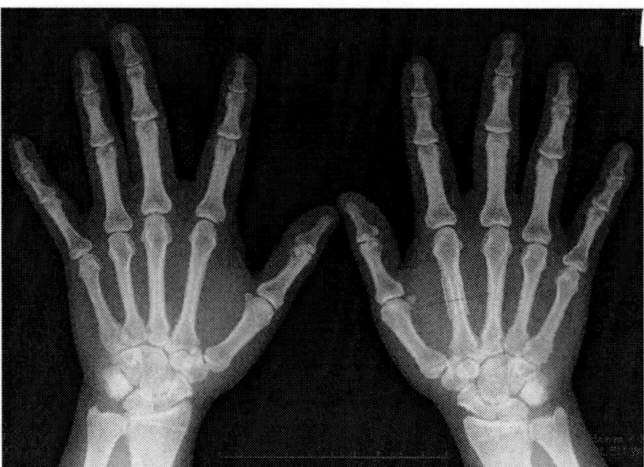

Figure 2. A 48-year-old healthy female shows that the cortices (white)/width of the shaft % is clearly more than 50%.

OSTEOPOROSIS

Decreased Mineralization

Diffused Osteoporosis (Primary Osteoporosis)

This condition may be found in primary osteoporosis, glucocorticoid-induced, hyperthyroidism, Cushing's disease and syndrome, advanced rheumatoid arthritis and so on. When diffuse osteoporosis exists, the evaluation of bone and general condition of the patient should be performed.

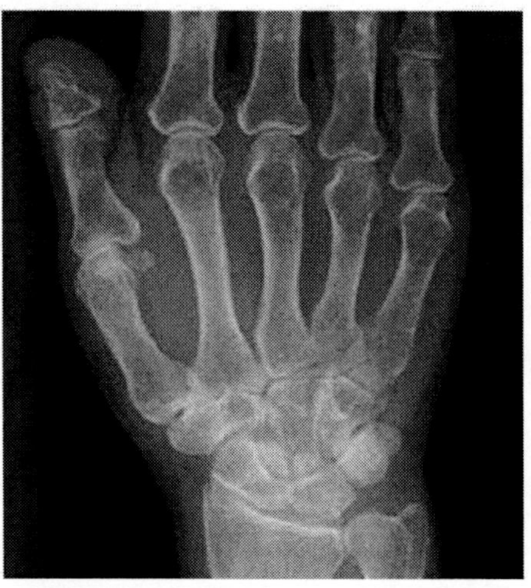
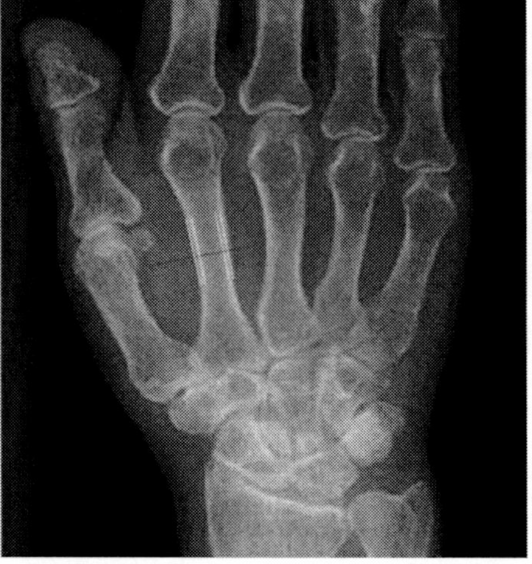

Figure 3. A 70-year-old female shows that white cortices is less than 50% of width of the shaft in the 2nd metacarpal bone.

Osteoporosis Induced by Cushing's Disease

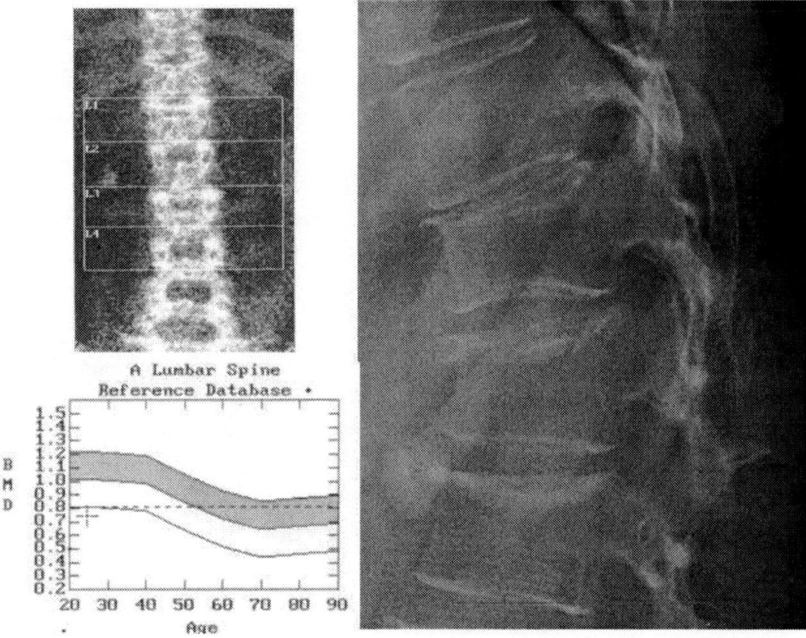

Figure 4. Bone densitometry (DEXA) evaluated osteoporosis showing low BMD in a 23-year-old female with Cushing's disease. Bone fractures at TH12 and L1 were also found.

Juxta-articular Osteoporosis

Even in normal persons, the metaphyseal-epiphyseal part of the digit is usually darker than the diaphysis because of the tinner cortical bone in the metaphysis and epiphysis. Although juxta-articular osteoporosis is a nonspecific finding, the blacked bones and dramatic differences may be found in inflammatory joints in RA patients. Inflammation of joints produces a lot of cytokines, and then the cytokines induce bone resorption. Juxta-articular osteopenia may be found in reactive arthritis, but its mineralization will recover.

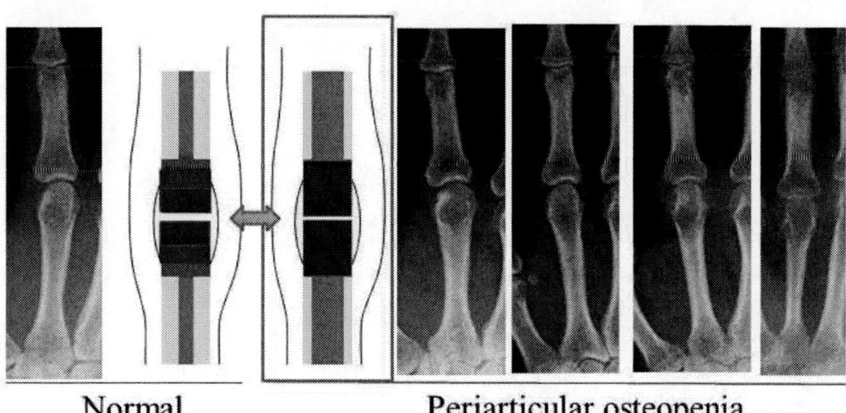

Figure 5. Mineralization of joint in normal persons may be slightly and gradual darkened in the plain films. On the other hand, osteoporosis at joint shows clearly and abruptly blackened.

Rheumatoid Arthritis

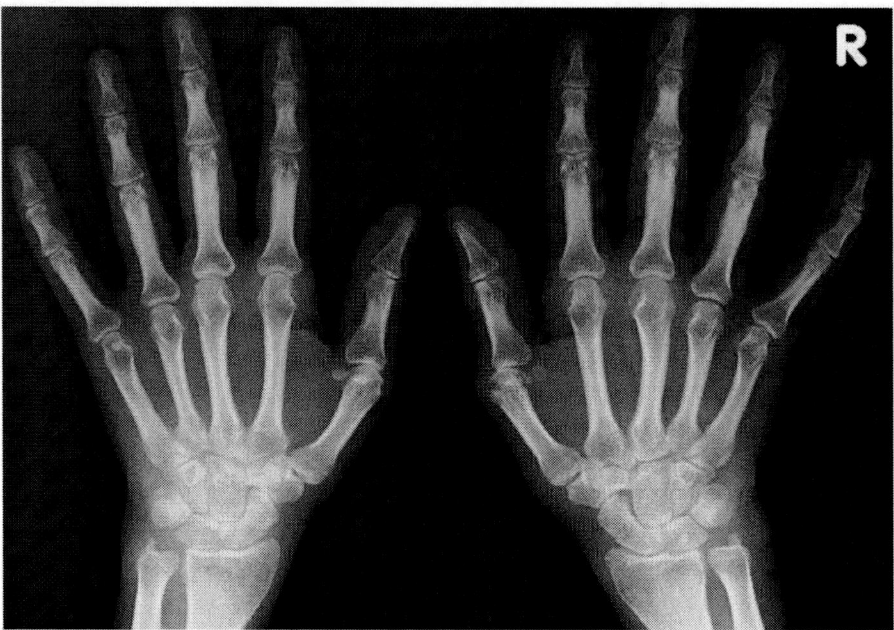

Figure 6. A 29-year-old female with RA shows juxta-articular osteoporosis of the MCP and PIP (IP) joints of the all digits.

Systemic Lupus Erythematosus (SLE)

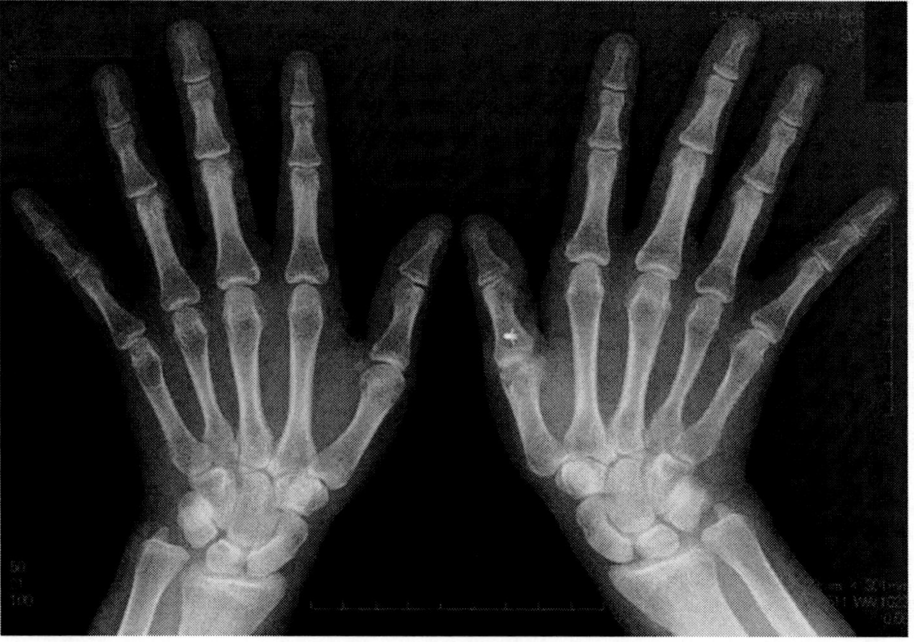

Figure 7. A 34-year-old female with SLE shows juxta-articular osteoporosis of the MCP and PIP joints of the all digits.

SLE+RA

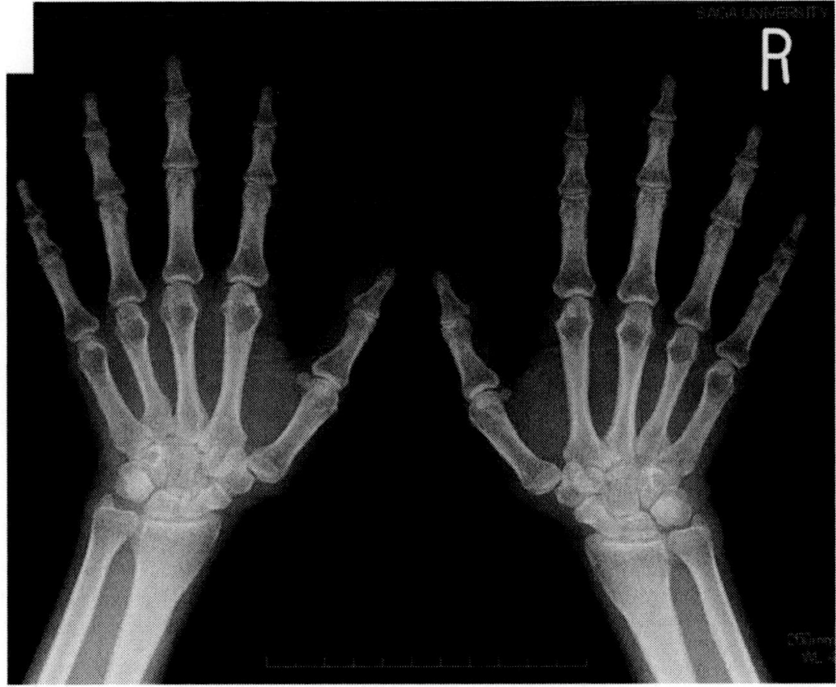

Figure 8. A 51-year-old female with SLE and RA shows juxta-articular osteoporosis.

Increased Mineralization

Osteosclerosis

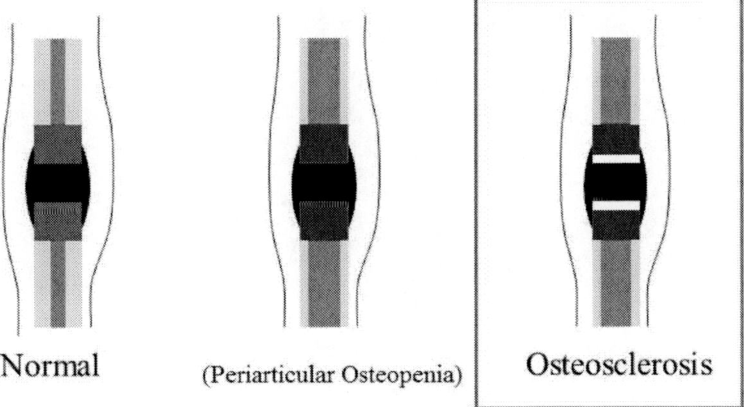

Figure 9. Growth factors, that are produced by chronic stress, repair subchondral bones. The subchondral bone has proliferative change and the color is strongly white.

Osteosclerosis in OA

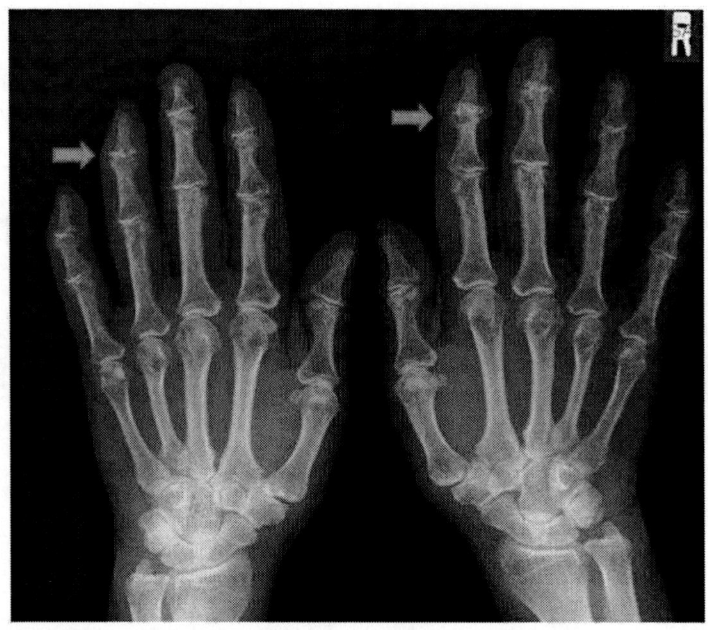

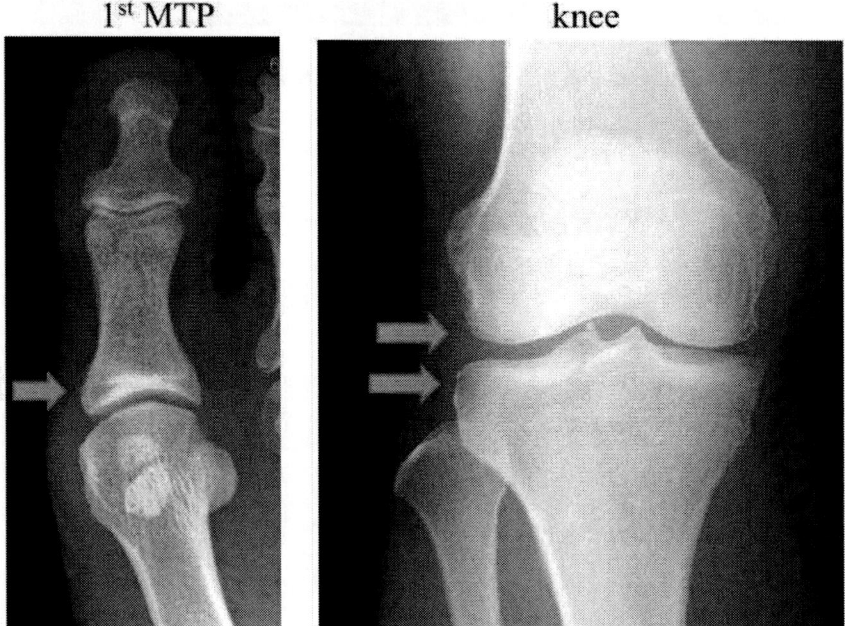

Figure 11. In OA patients, osteocslerosis at DIP joints are characteristic. However, osteosclerosis is found in other joints.

Kienbock's Disease

A 71-year old male with microscopic polyangiitis shows increased density of lunate suggesting avascular Necrosis of Lunate. The T1-weighted coronal MR image shows low intensity (black) of the lunate (arrow). The MRI is more sensitive than plain film to detect early change of avascular necrosis. The PA view of the hand shows sclerosis of the lunate caused by avascular necrosis that followed a glucocorticoid therapy.

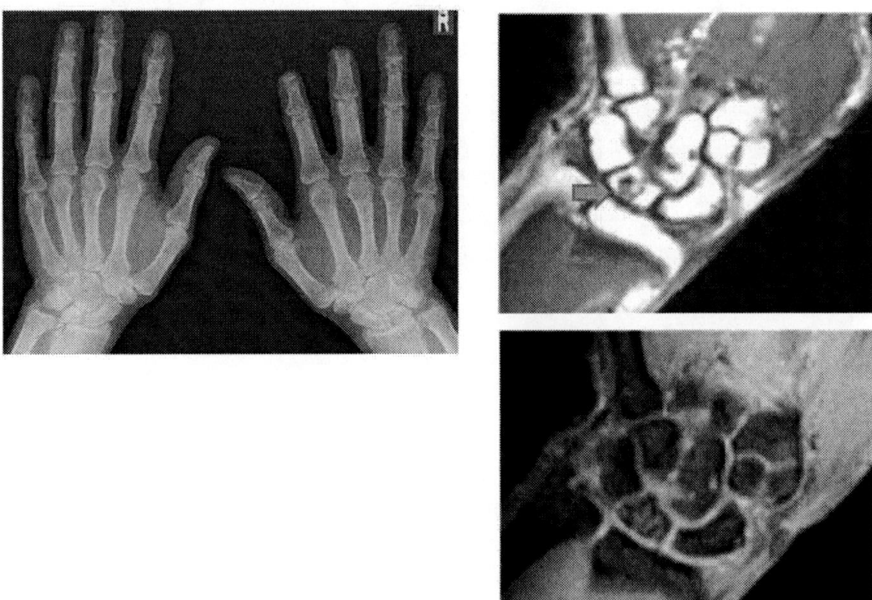

Figure 12. A 71-year old male with microscopic polyangiitis.

Osteonecrosis of Femoral Head

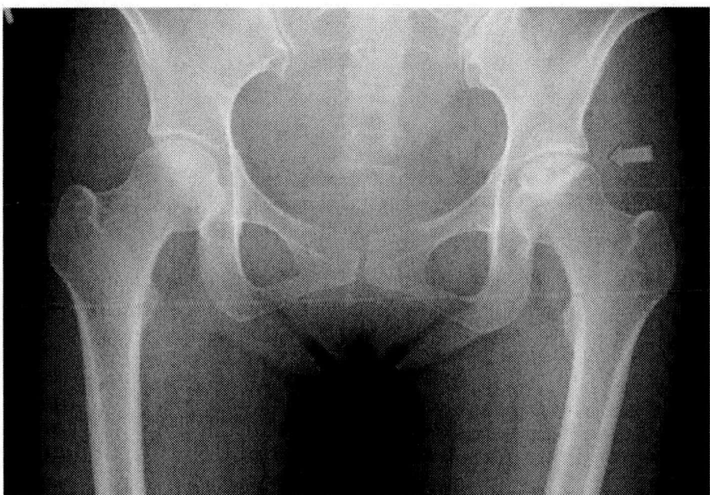

Figure 13. A 49-year-old female with mixed connective tissue disease (MCTD) shows increased density in the left femoral head. However, joint space is relatively maintained.

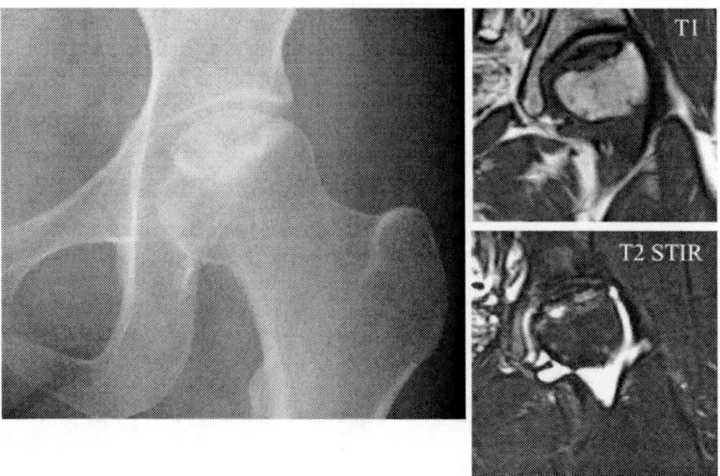

Figure 14. Severe Osteonecrosis of Femoral Head in SLE

AP View of Both Hips in a Patient with SLE

Severe osteonecrosis is found. AP view of both hips in a patient with SLE. Increased smudgy density is observed in the both femoral head. This is a severe radiographic change of osteonecrosis. Hip replacement arthroplasty was performed.

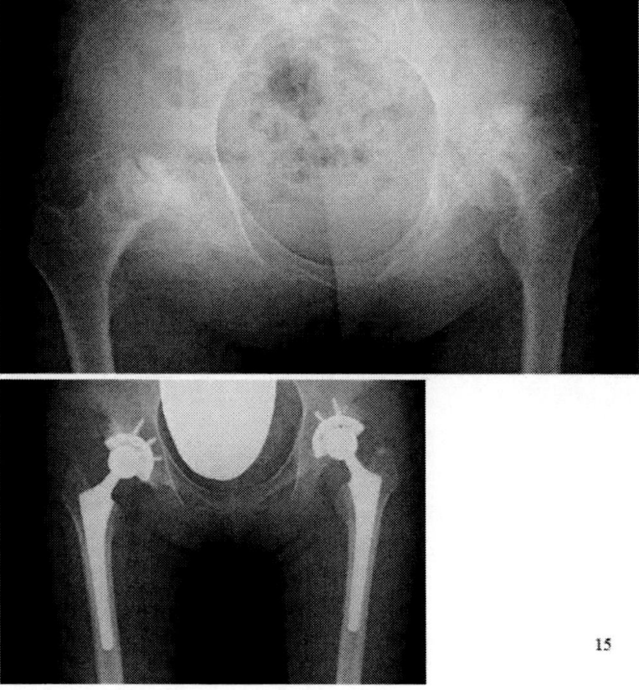

Figure 15. AP view of both hips in a patient with SLE.

Chapter 4

CARTILAGE

"C" cartilage is the main part of reading hand radiograph.

JOINT-SPACE NARROWING (JSN)

Joint space consists of the cartilage between two bones. If the cartilage is damaged, the joint space narrowing occurs.

Arthropathies except for osteoarthritis show joint-space narrowing uniformly. Uniform narrowing of joint space is found in inflammatory arthropathies including RA and various arthropathies due to deposition of extra substance including gout, CPPD, Wilson's disease, acromegaly and so on.

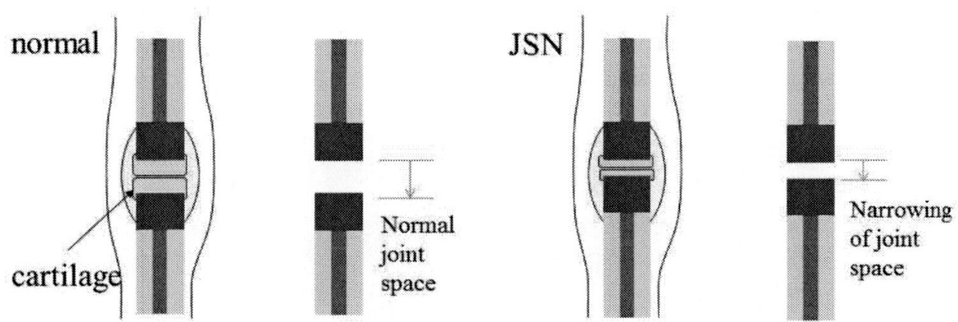

Figure 1.Joint Space Narrowing.

DIFFERENTIAL DIAGNOSIS OF JSN

- RA   uniform narrowing
- Gout   maintained in early stage and narrowing in advanced stage
- OA   non-uniform narrowing at stressed site
- Osteonecrosis   keeping joint space in the terminal stage

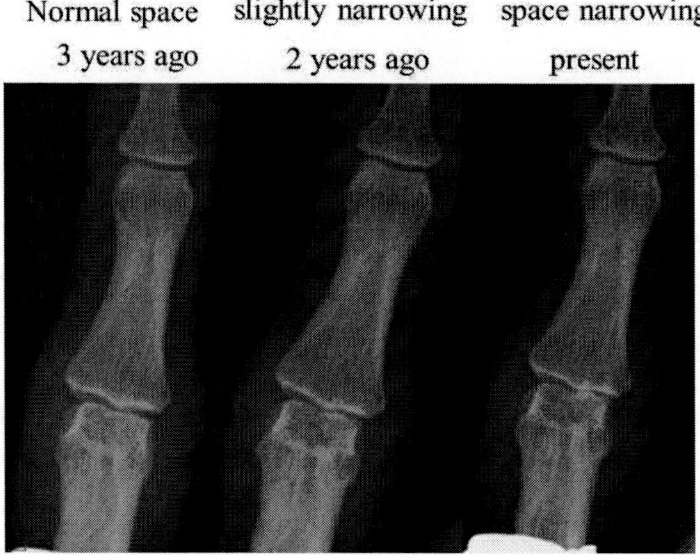

Figure 2. Time Course of Joint Space Narrowing in RA.

Uniform narrowing and soft tissue swelling of the MCP joints are progressive in RA during the disease course.

PITFALL OF READING JSN

In PA view, joint space narrowing can be simulated by palmar subluxation and by flexion deformity.

Oblique view can help to evaluate it.

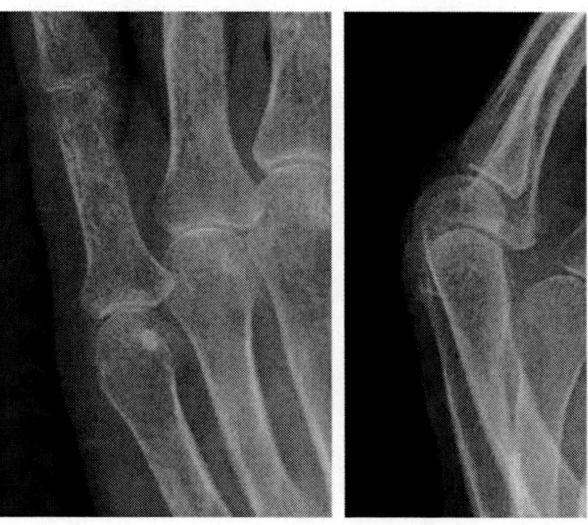

Figure 3. False jsn in pa view. Evidently keeping joint space in oblique view.

Joint Space Narrowing of other Joints

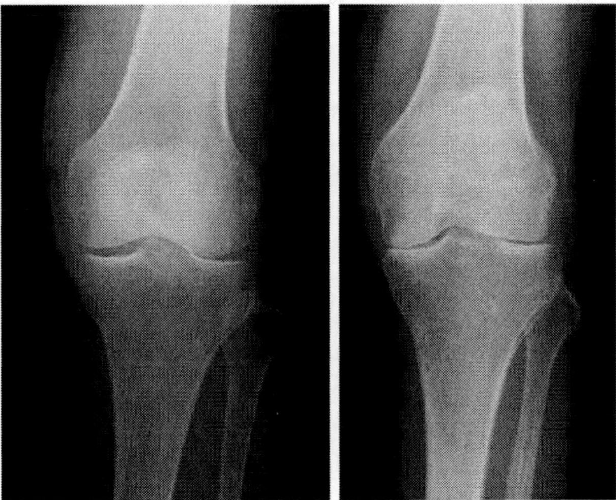

Figure 4. JSN of Knees in RA.

AP standing view of both knees in patients of rheumatoid arthritis showing uniform joint space narrowing of the medial and lateral compartments of knee and osteoporosis. However, erosions are very little.

In PA view, the uniform joint space narrowing is found and migration of humeral head proximally (inward) and superiorly (upward) in all compartments of the shoulder joint, the glenohumeral, the acromial humeral, and the acromioclavicular (AC) joint. Also, osteoporosis is found.

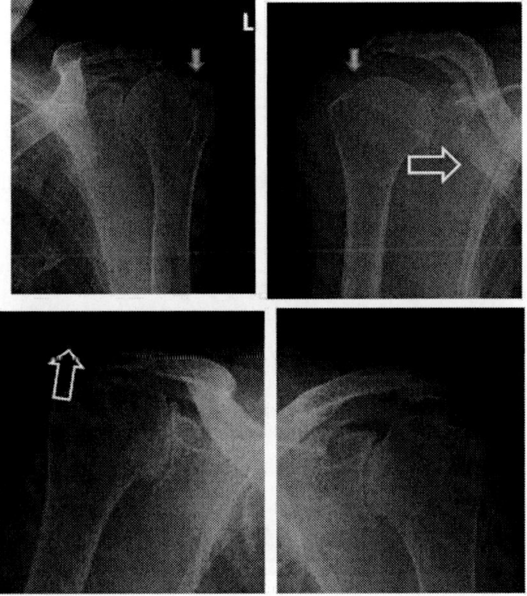

Figure 5. JSN of Shoulders in RA.

Erosions are seen at the rotator cuff attachment in shoulder joint.

Joint space narrowing induced proximal migration of the humeral head due to loss of cartilage in the glenohumeral join

The humeral head migrates superiorly usually associated with rotator cuff tear.

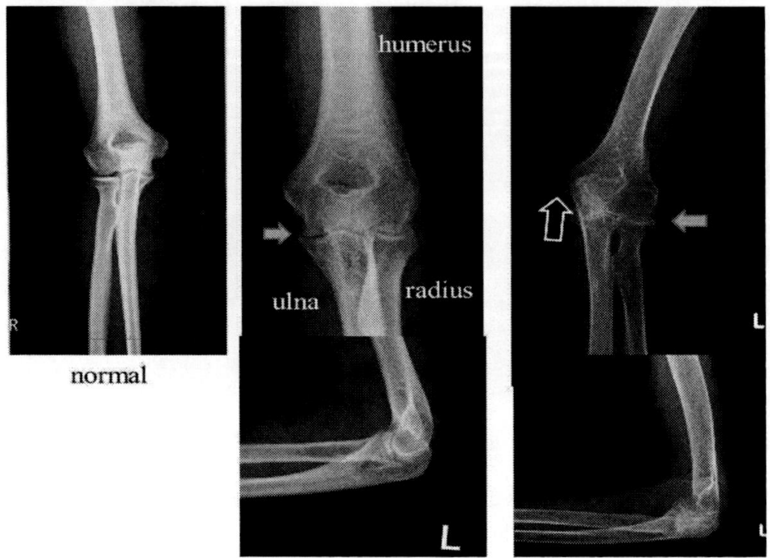

Figure 6. JSN of Elbows in RA.

In AP and lateral views of the elbow, uniform joint space narrowing or loss between the radius and the humerus as well as between the ulna and the humerus and generalized osteoporosis is found. However there is no reparative reaction and osteophytes.

EROSIONS

Basic information of anatomical aspects for understanding of erosions

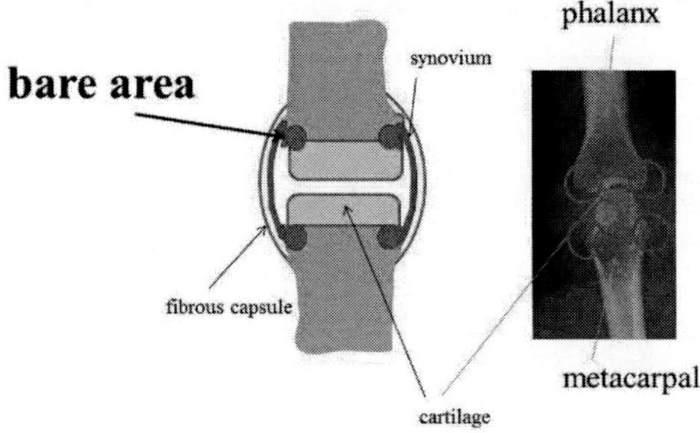

Figure 7. Structure of Joint.

Marginal erosions occur in the bare areas of the bone. In the joint fibrous capsule, cartilage does not cover the bone, or marginal areas, where synovium directly touches bones (designated with red circle).

Very Early Change of Erosion: Loss of the Continuity of White Cortical Line

Very early sign of erosions may be very subtle. Loss of the continuity of the white cortical line. PA view shows discontinuity of line at the margins (bare areas) of the PIP joints (2). The finding ends evident eriosions.

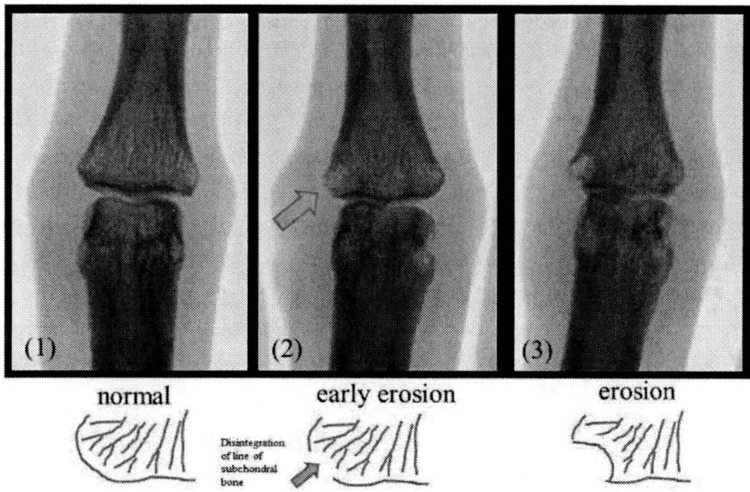

Figure 8. Dorsopalmar radiogarph of early change of erosion at the bare areas in the PIP joint.

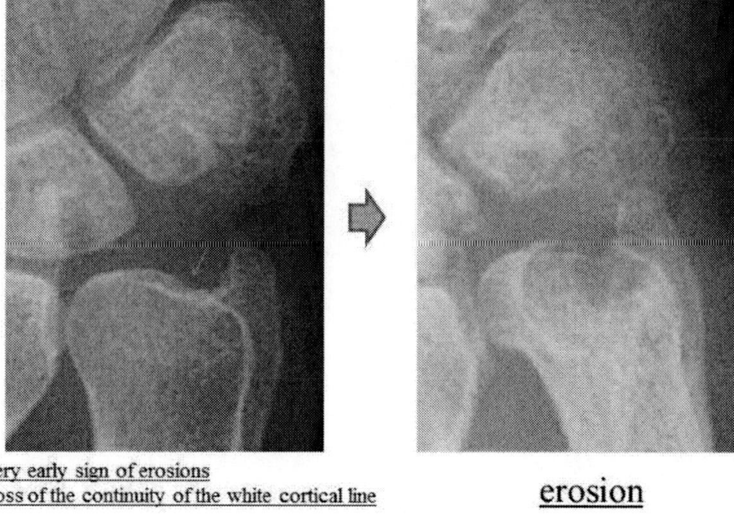

Figure 9. Loss of the Continuity of White Cortical Line.

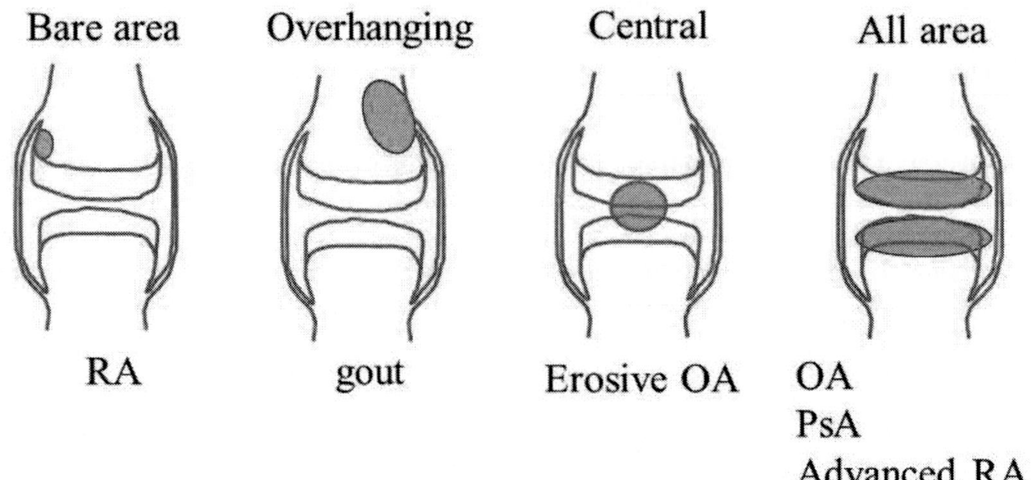

Figure 10. The patterns of erosion in the joint.

Marginal Erosions at Bare Areas

Various erosions found in RA.

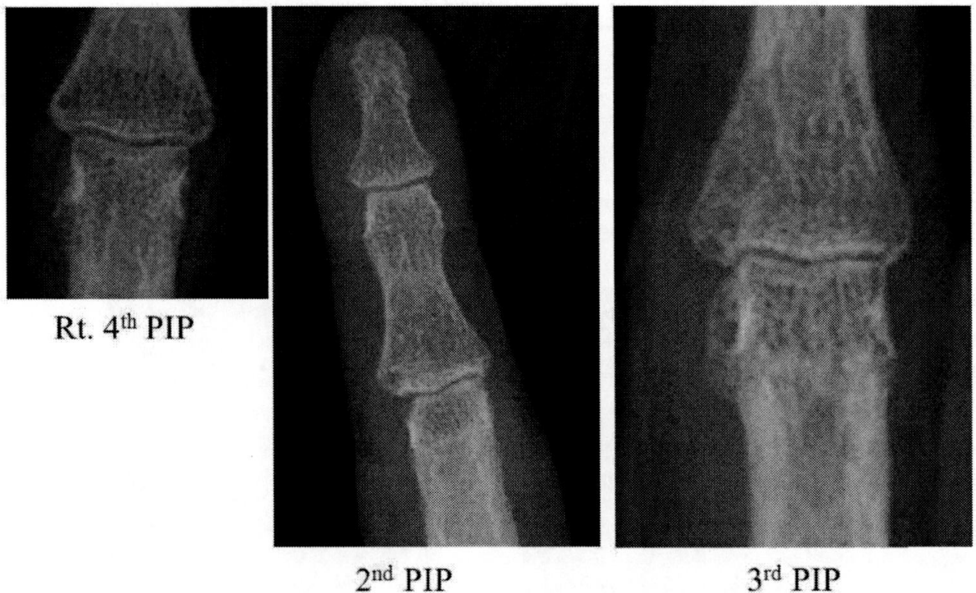

Figure 11. PIP Joints.

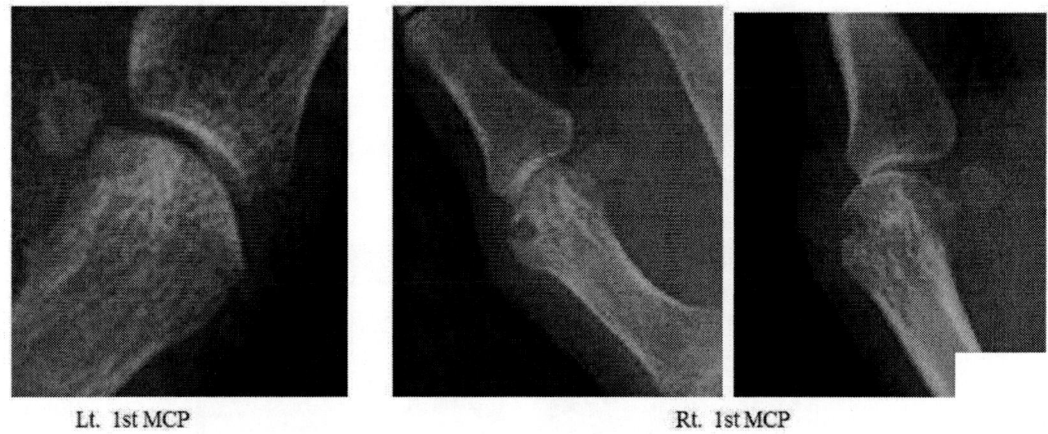

Lt. 1st MCP   Rt. 1st MCP

Figure 12. 1st MCP Joints.

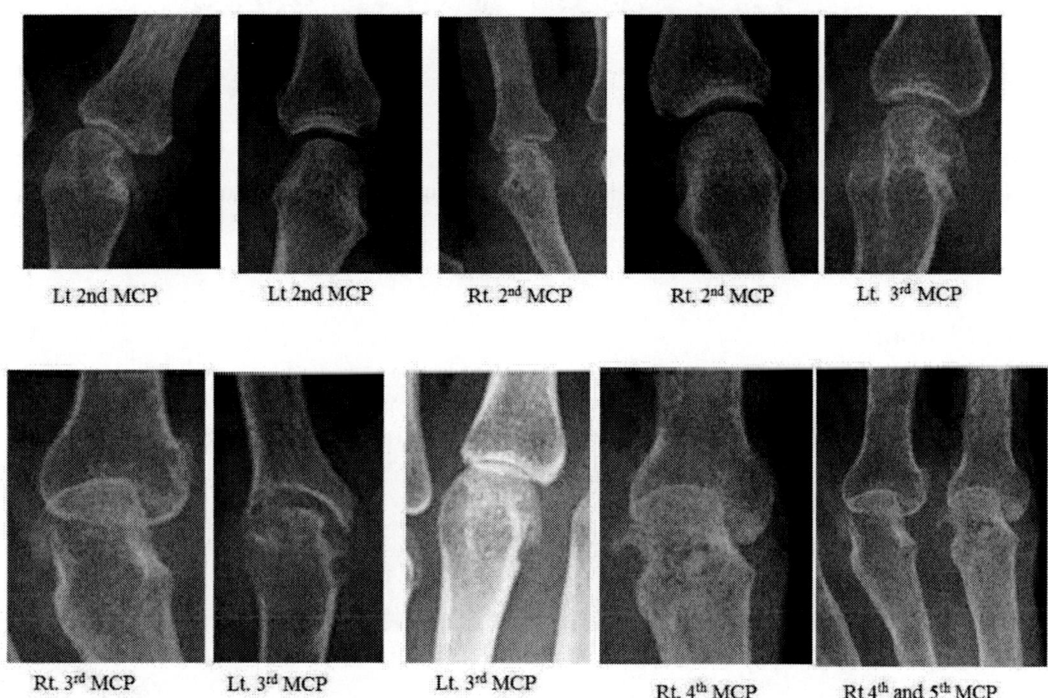

Lt 2nd MCP   Lt 2nd MCP   Rt. 2nd MCP   Rt. 2nd MCP   Lt. 3rd MCP

Rt. 3rd MCP   Lt. 3rd MCP   Lt. 3rd MCP   Rt. 4th MCP   Rt 4th and 5th MCP

Figure 13. MCP Joints.

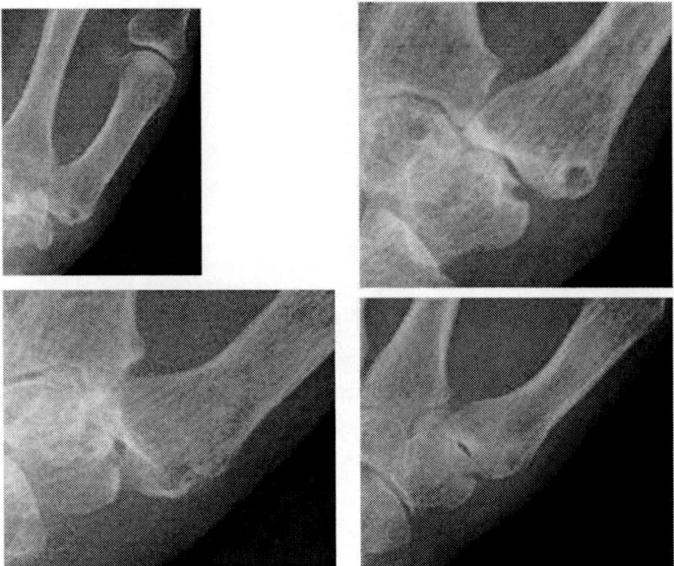

Figure 14. 1st CMC Joints.

Wrist

In the wrist, the locations of erosions are specific. However, to know the locations of normal notch is also important.

Normal Variant

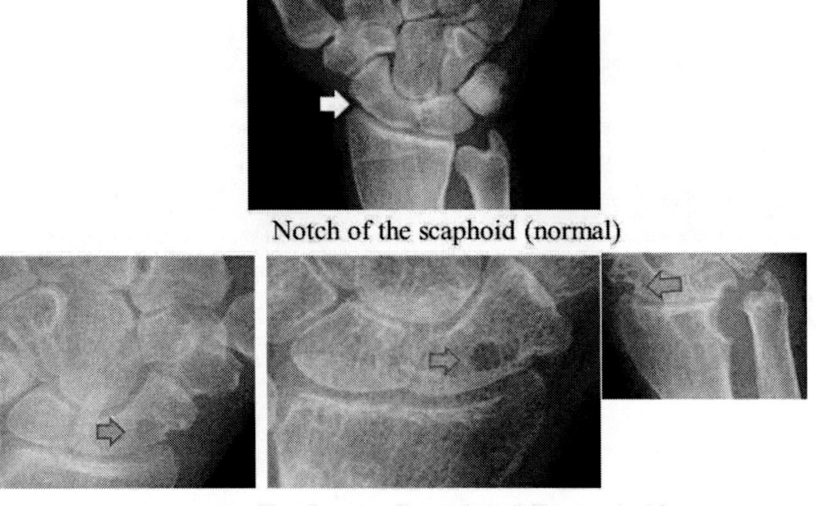

Figure 15. Notch of the scaphoid (normal) and Erosions at the waist of the scaphoid.

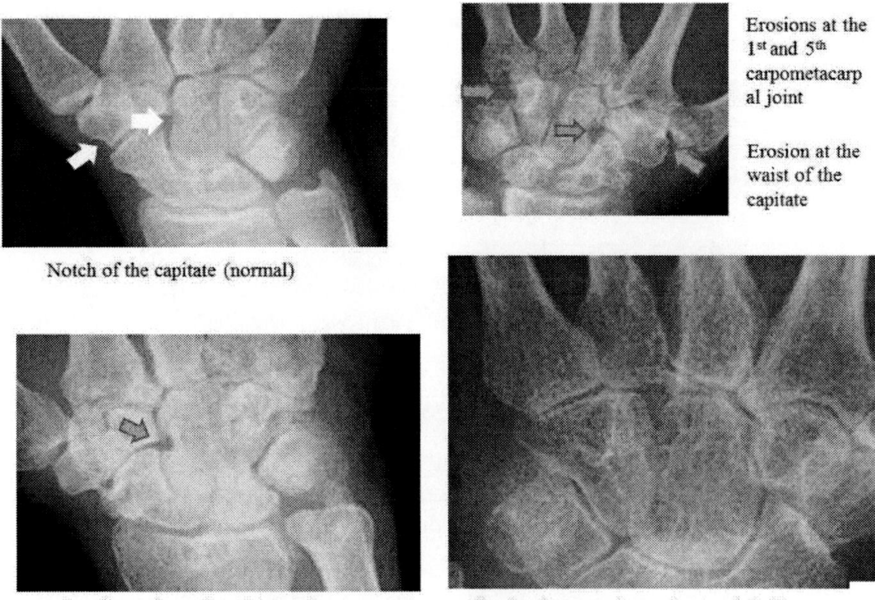

Figure 16. Notch of the capitate (normal) and Erosion at the waist of the capitate and wrist.

Ulnar styloid process

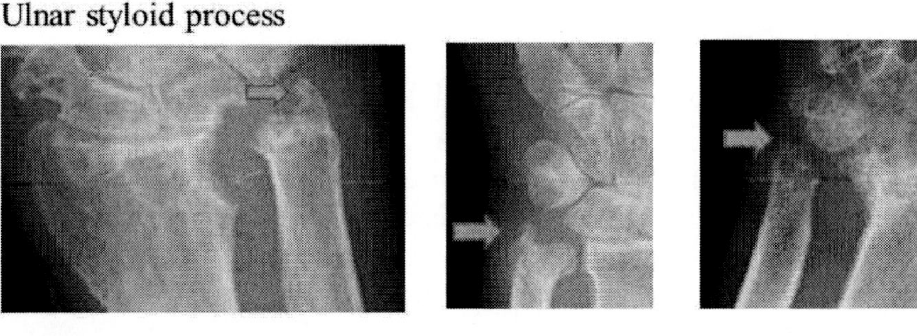

Radial styloid process

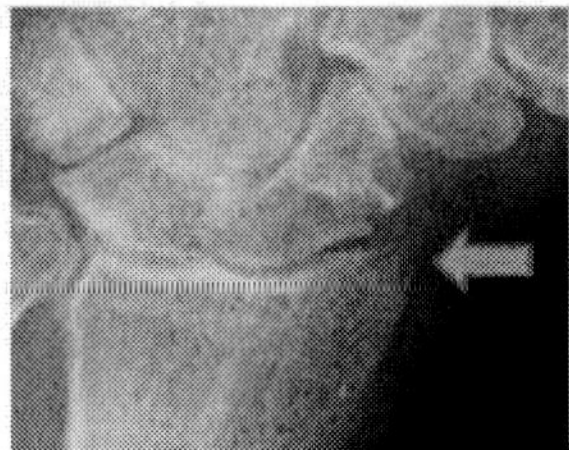

Figure 17. Erosions of Ulnar styloid Process and Radial styloid Process.

Clinical Course of Erosions in Rheumatoid Arthritis Over Five Years

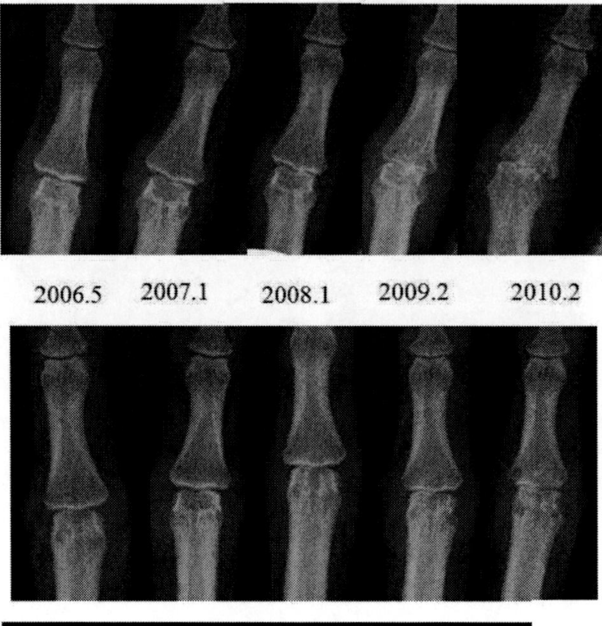

Figure 18. Time Course of Erosions in Rheumatoid Arthritis over Five Years.

The initial radiograph (2006) shows only soft tissue swelling around PIP joint and normal bone structure.

The second view (2007) suggests mild periarticular osteopenia of PIP joints.

In the third pictures (2008), beginning disintegration of the subchondral bone plate is found.

The forth picture shows (2009) marginal erosions of PIP joints and newly appearing "dot-dash appearance."

In advanced stage, shown in the last radiograph (2010), these marginal erosions enlarged and expand toward the center of joint, resulted in marginal destructions on PIP joints.

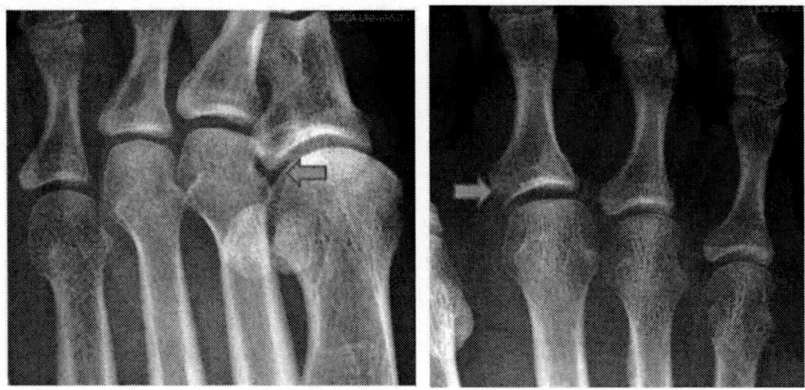

Figure 19. Erosion of Foot.

Marginal Erosions in other Joints of RA Patients

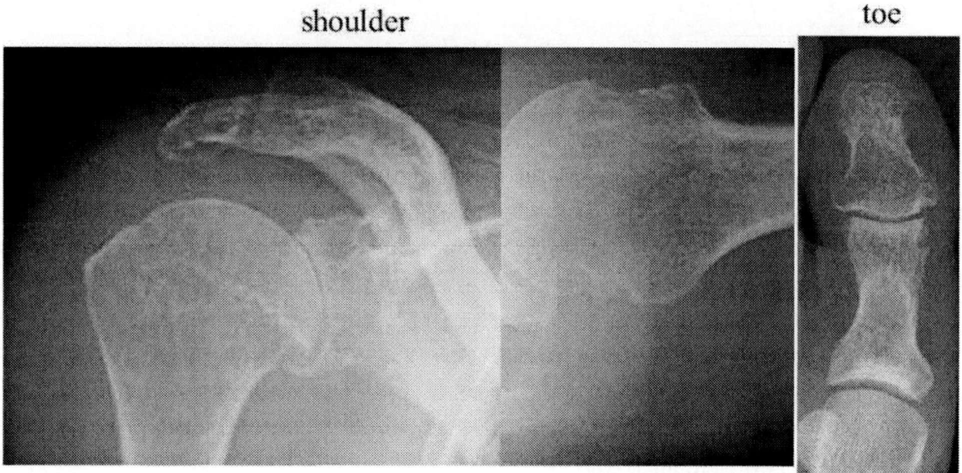

Figure 20. Shoulder and Toe.

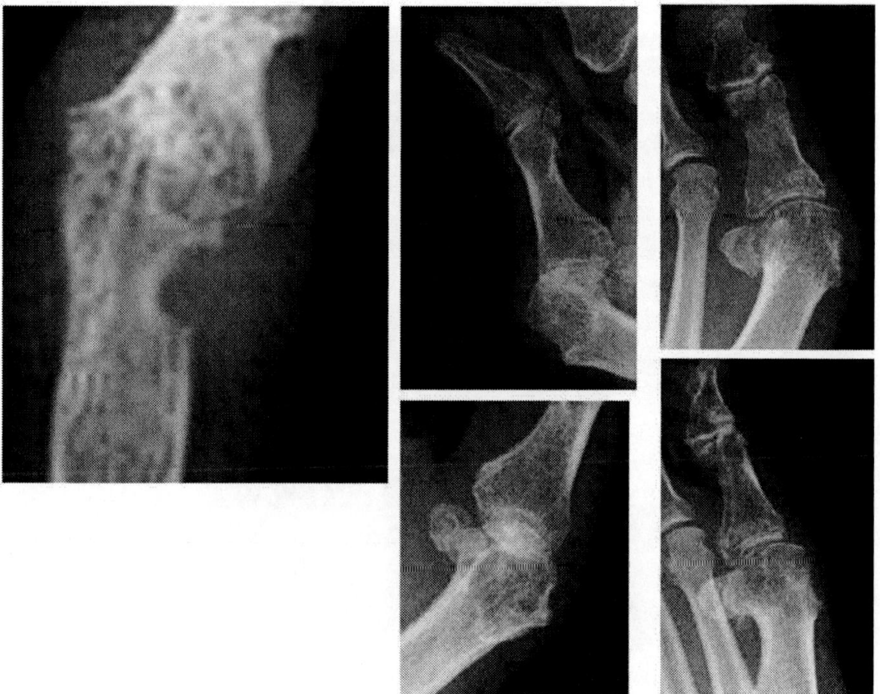

Figure 21. Overhanging Erosions in Gout.

Central Erosions

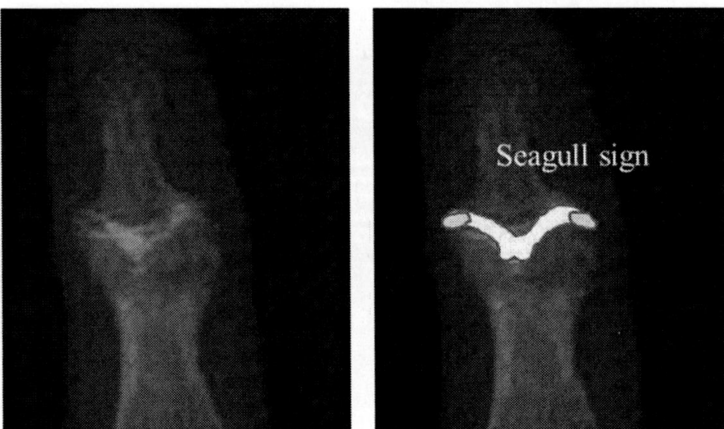

Figure 22. Erosions of OA: Combined with Osteophytes to Produce "Seagull" Sign.

OA

Seagull sing is found at DIP joints.

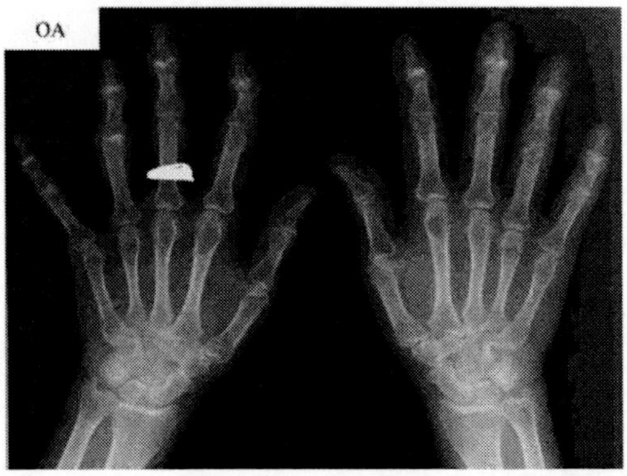

Figure 23.

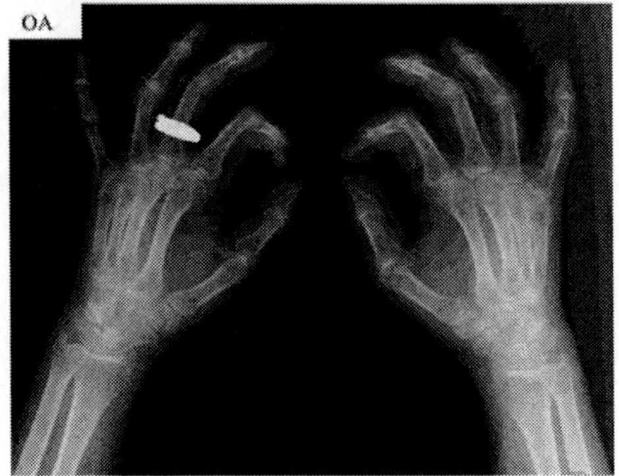

Figure 24.

GENERALIZED EROSIONS

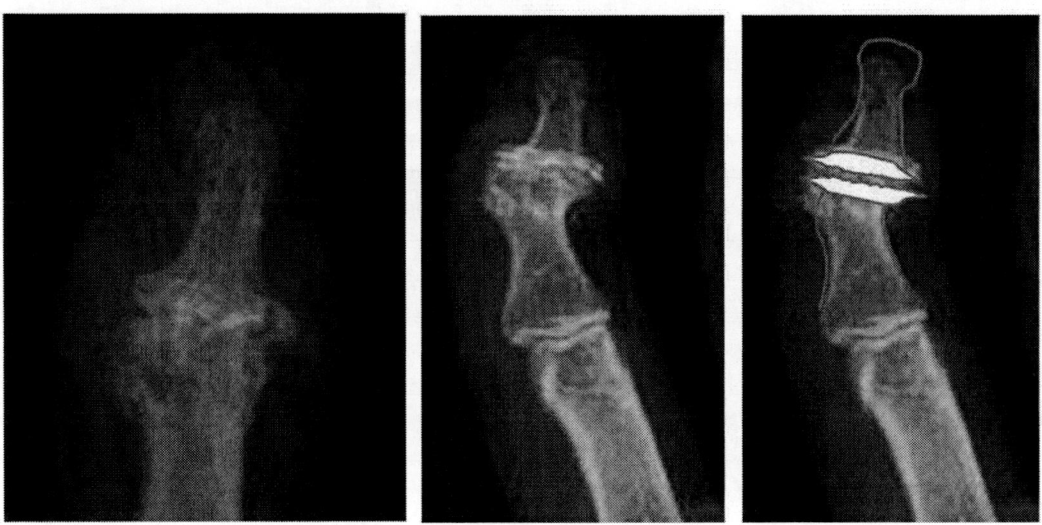

Figure 25. OA: Joint space narrowing with osteophyte formation

Psoriatic Arthritis (PsA)

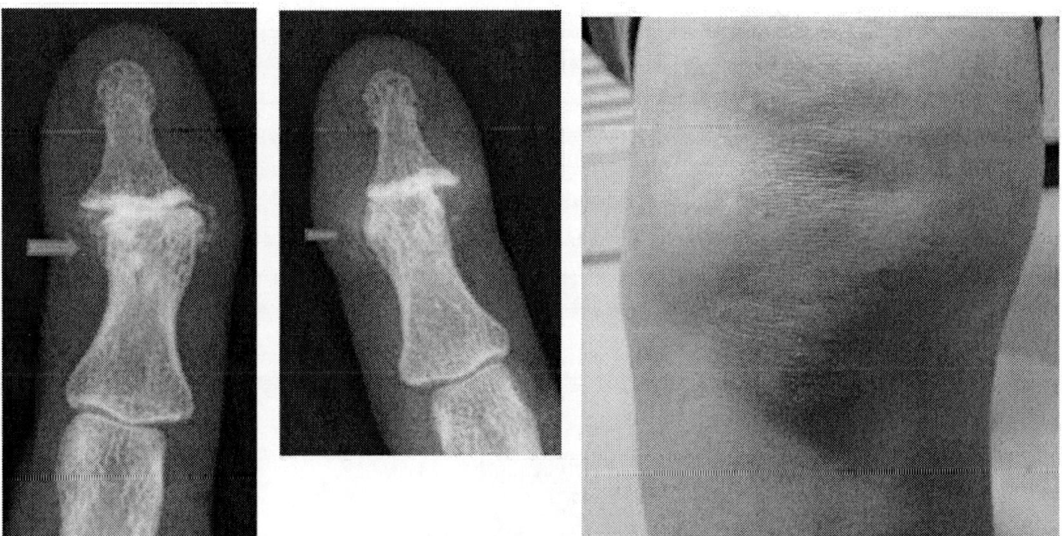

Figure 26. The PA view of finger shows joint space narrowing and irregular bone erosions at distal interphalangeal joint. Also, bone proliferation and periostitis throughout phalanges (arrows). Skin lesion is psoriasis at the right knee.

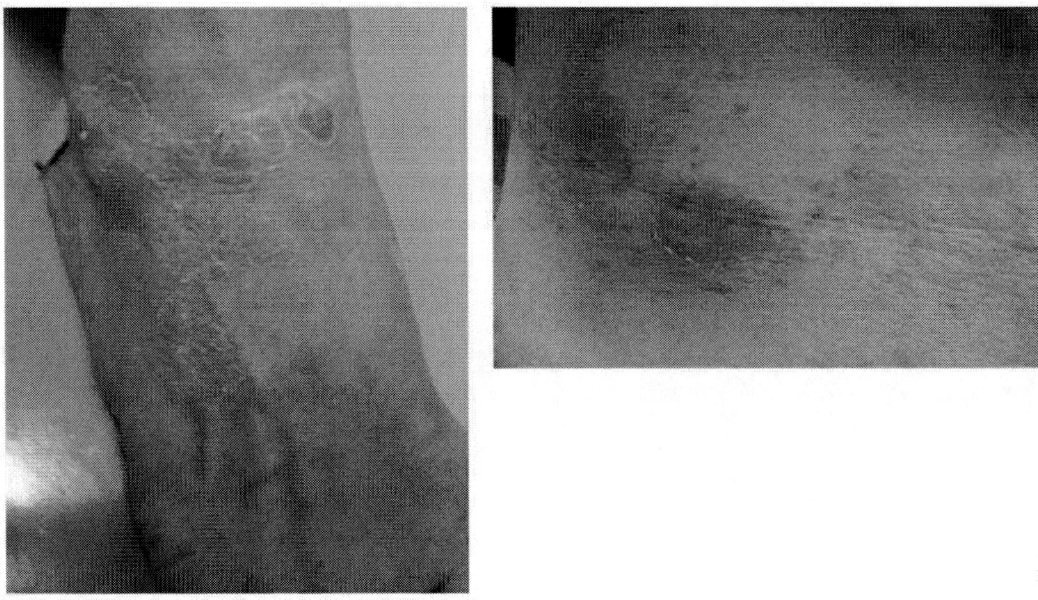

Figure 27. Skin eruptions of psoriatic arthritis are found at the right foot and the abdomen.

PsA

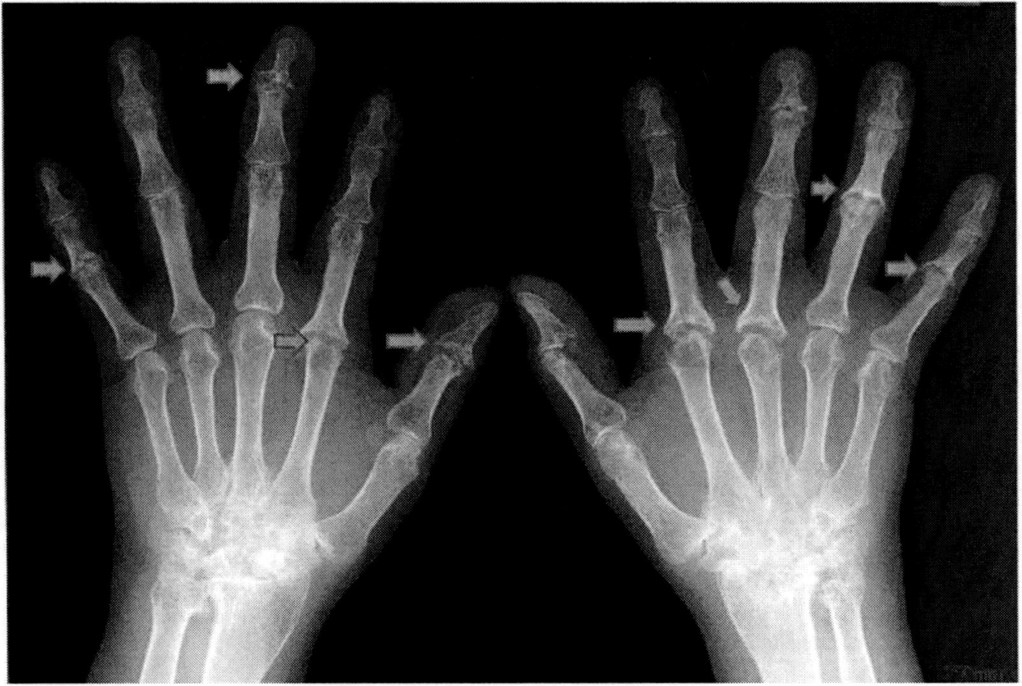

Figure 28. No periarticular osteopenia even at the erosive joints. Changes of bone formation, osteosclerosis and osteophytes are found.

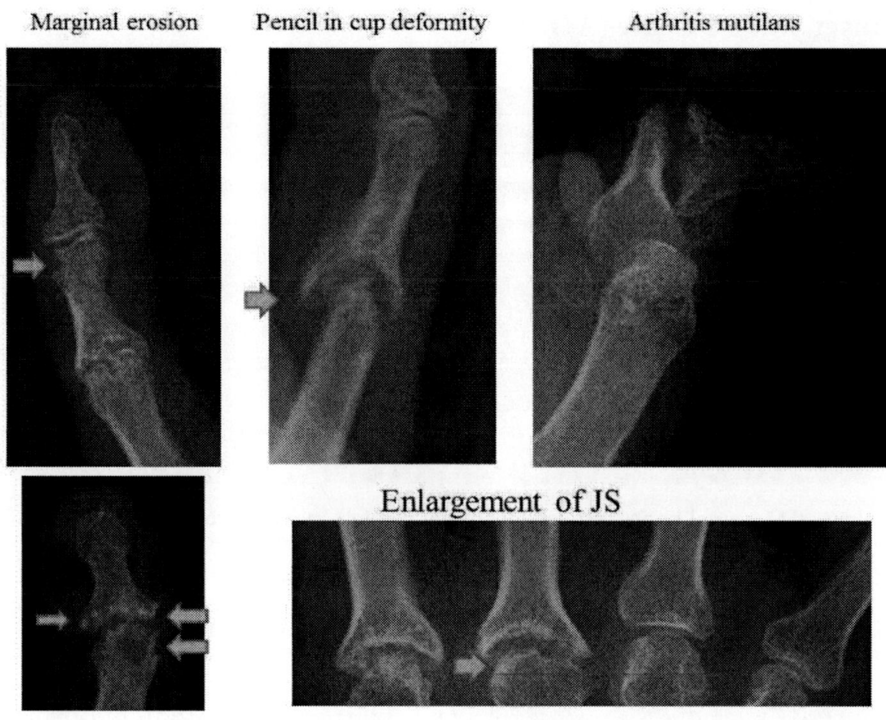

Figure 29. Various Findings of Arthritis in PsA.

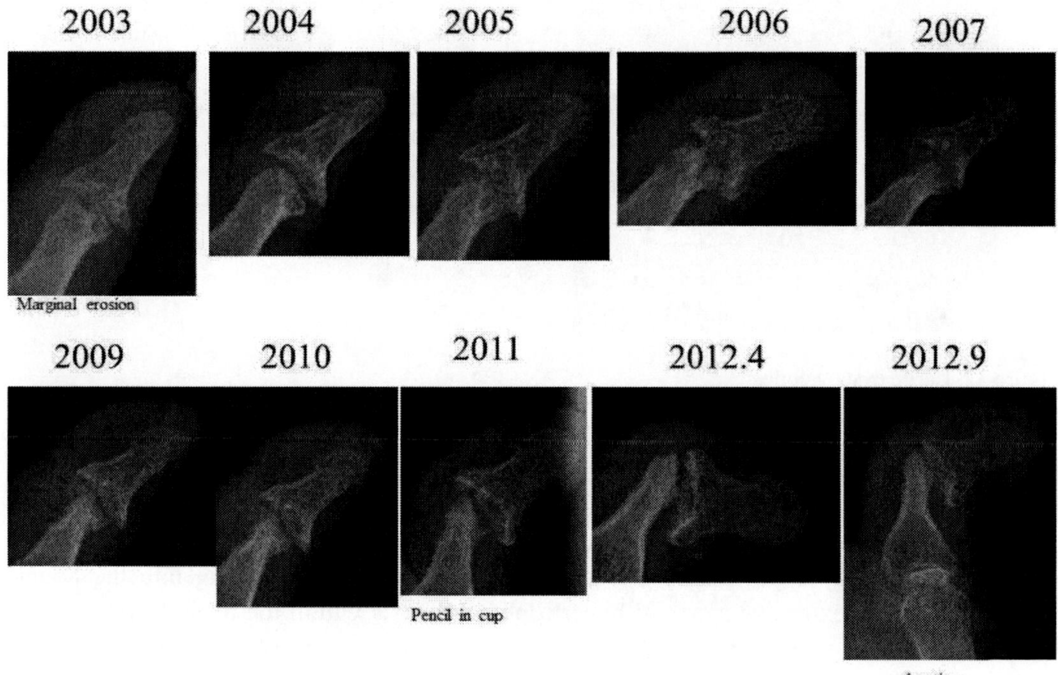

Figure 30. Time Course of PsA - From Marginal Erosion to Luxation through Pencil in Cup.

Adult Onset Still's Disease (AOSD)

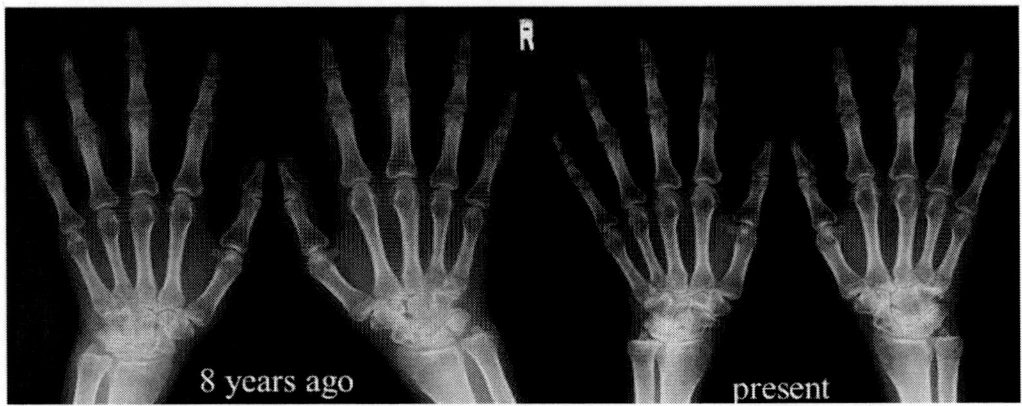

Figure 31. In AOSD, carpal bones, especially around capitate, are preferentially affected and result in ankylosis.

INTRAOSSEOUS SYNOVIAL CYSTS

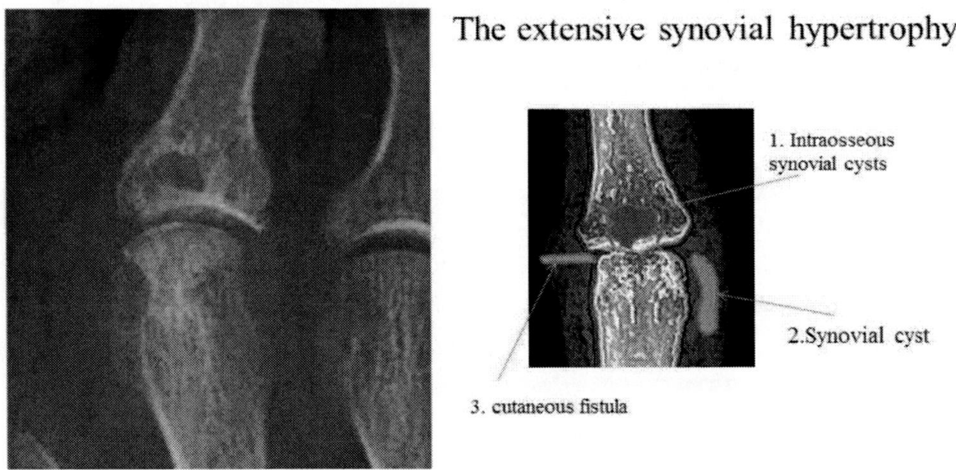

Figure 32. Large cysts"geodes"

AP view of the digit of patient with rheumatoid arthritis shows lucent lesion in base of proximal phalanx with thin sclerotic margination.

1. Intraosseous large synovial cysts, called "geodes," are found in the joint, that is produced by synovium breaking through the cartilage infiltrating into the bone of joint. The extensive synovial hypertrophy and cysts within the bone. Geodes may be caused by invagination of synovium through the cortical surface leading to large cyst-like lesions below the cortex of bone. Geodes may be mistaken for a bone tumor.
2. Synovial cyst extends into the soft tissues
3. Cutaneous fistula is a extension to the skin.

OSTEOPHYTE FORMATION

Proliferation of Bones at the Joint

osteophytes→OA
DIPs
PIPs
Knees, hips and other joints

Osteophyte Formation at DIPs

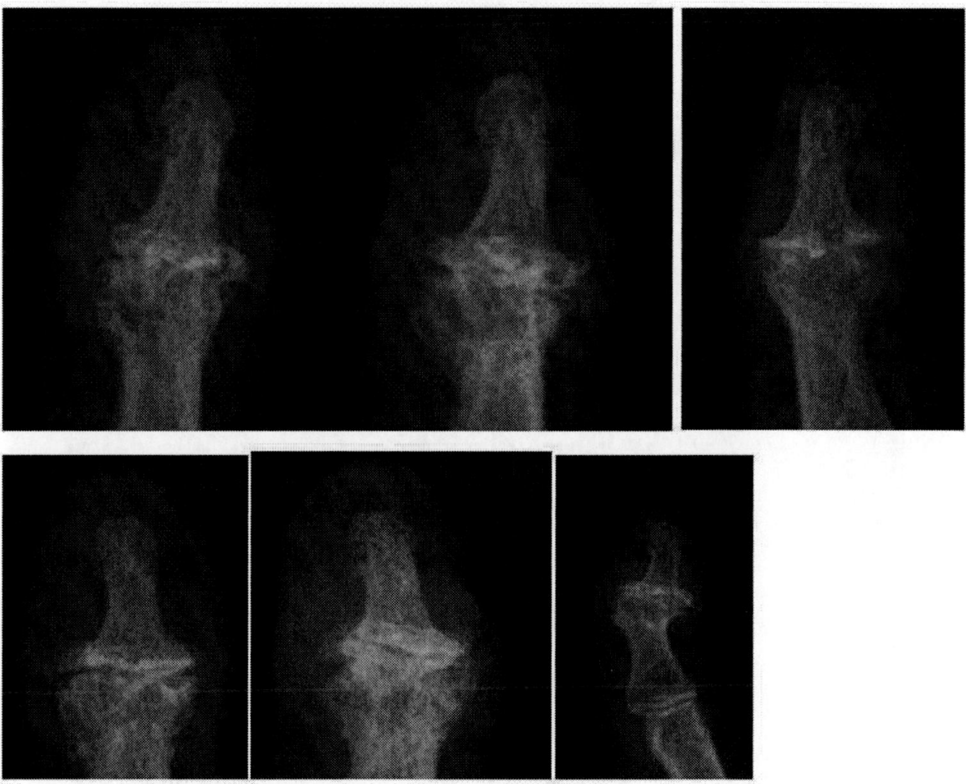

Figure 33. DIP: Heberden's nodes.

The swelling of soft tissue due to osteophyte formation at DIP joint is called Heberden's node.

Osteophyte Formation at PIPs

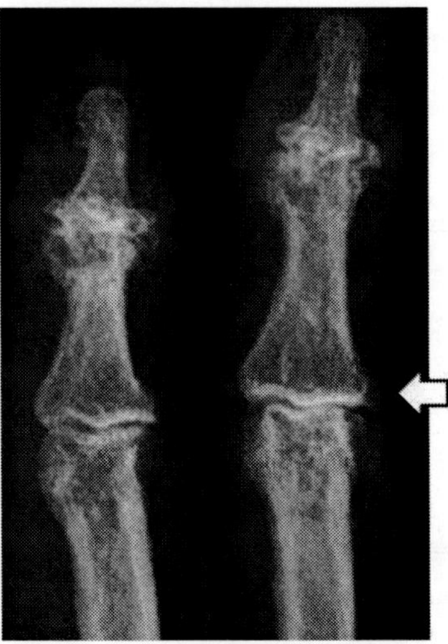

Figure 34. PIP: Bouchard's nodes. PA view of two digits in patient with osteoarthritis.

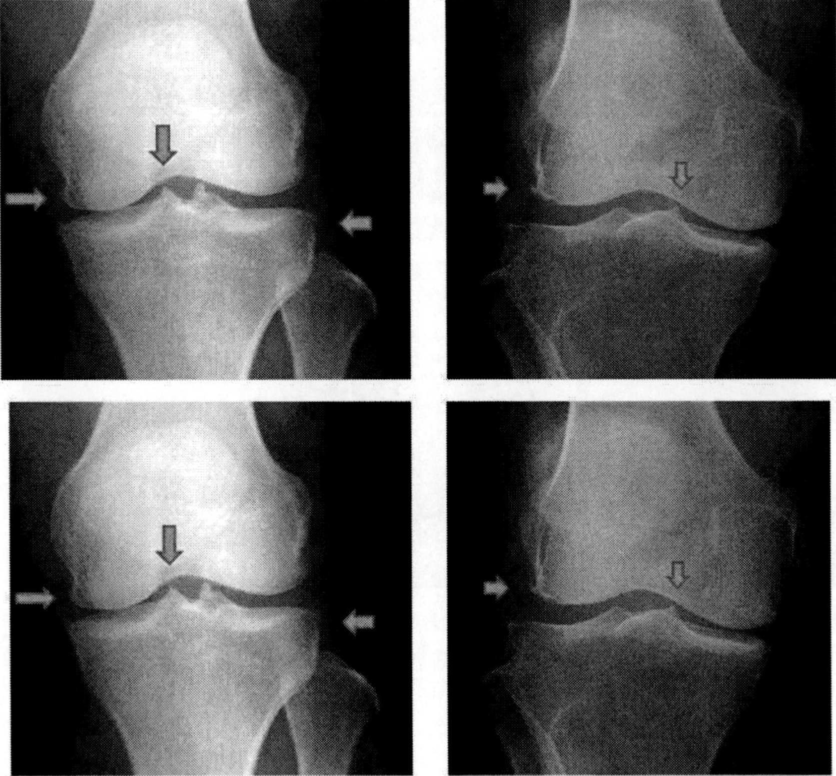

Figure 35. Osteophyte Formation at Other Joints, at the Knees.

The nodules due to osteophytes are found in PIP joints.

The swelling of soft tissue due to osteophyte formation at PIP joint is called Bouchard's node.

CARTILAGE CALCIFICATION (CHONDROCALCINOSIS)

Calcium pyrophosphate dihydrate (CPPD) deposition disease

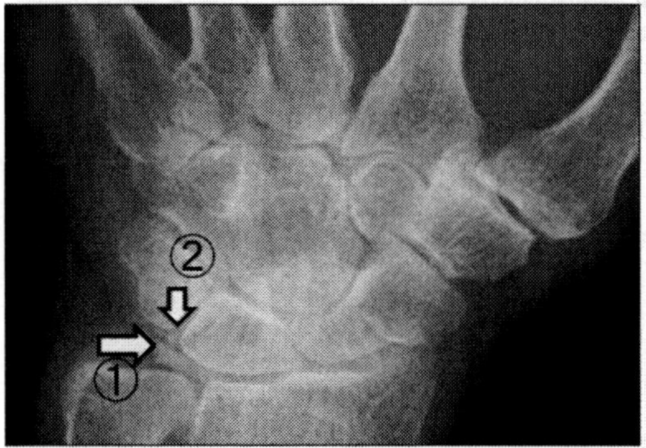
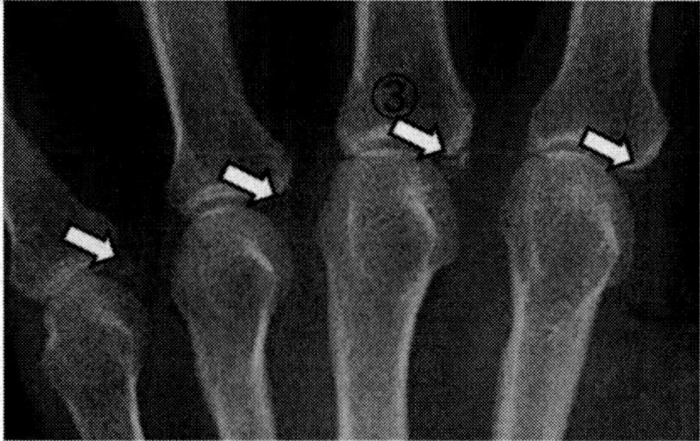

Figure 36. Calcification in the triangular fibrocartilage of the wrist (arrow).

Cartilage calcification in the triangular cartilage and hyaline cartilage of the left wrist (CPPD).

Calcification is presented in the capsules of MCP joints of patient with CPPD.

Calcification
1.   triangular cartilage (fibrous cartilage)
2.   between lunate and triquetrum (hyaline cartilage)
3.   MCP joints

Idiopathic CPPD ctystal deposition disease
1.   Gout with CPPD
2.   Hyperparathyroidism
3.   Hemochromatosis

Calcification, calcium pyrophosphate dihydrate crystals deposit in triangular cartilage (fibrous cartilage) (1), hyaline cartilage between lunate and triquetrum (2) and the MCP joints (3), is found in a PA view of the hands.

Calcium pyrophosphate dihydrate (CPPD) deposition disease is diagnosed when more than two joints are affected.

This condition is found in idiopathic CPPD ctystal deposition disease, Gout with CPPD, Hyperparathyroidism, and Hemochromatosis.

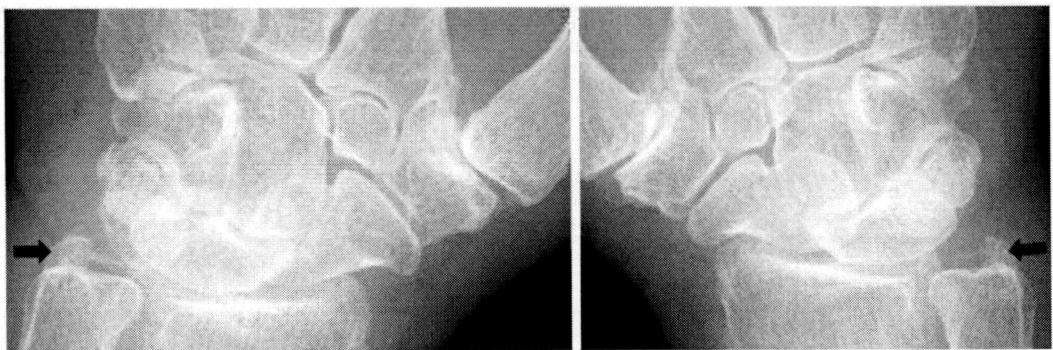

Figure 37. Triangular Cartilage (Fibrous Cartilage).

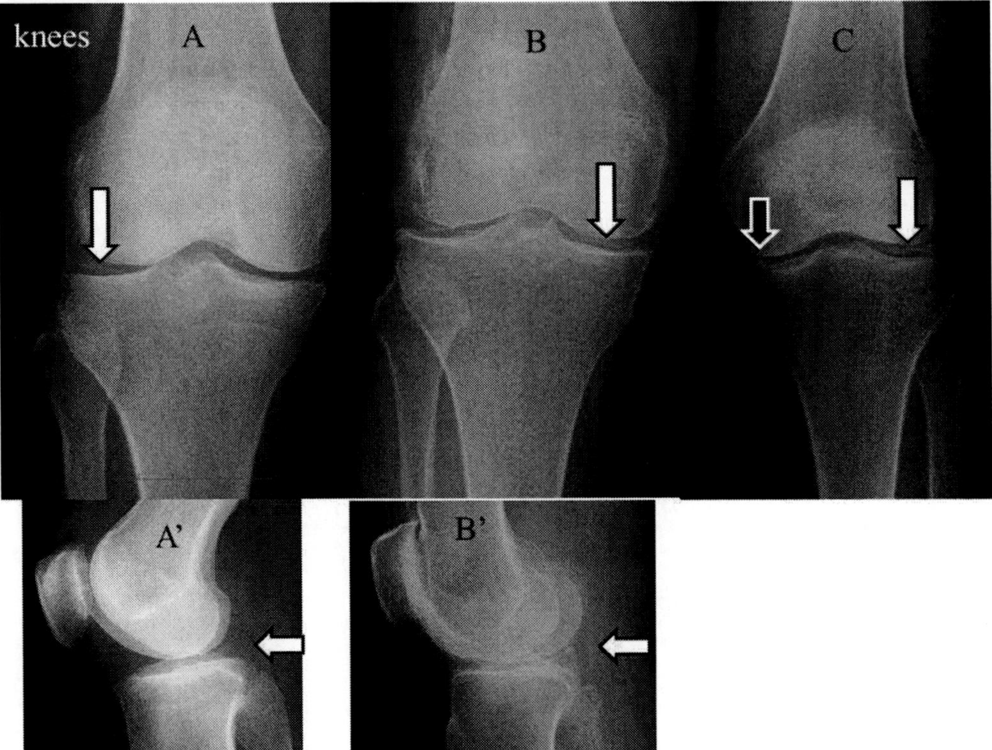

Figure 38. CPPD at the Knee.

Chondrocalcinosis (arrows) in the knee. Anteroposterior (AP) view and lateral view of the knees in the patients of CPPD. Thin-line (A), bold-line (B) and wedge-shaped (C) calcification are seen in the fibrocartilaginous meniscus (black arrows). However, the joint space narrowing is not seen.

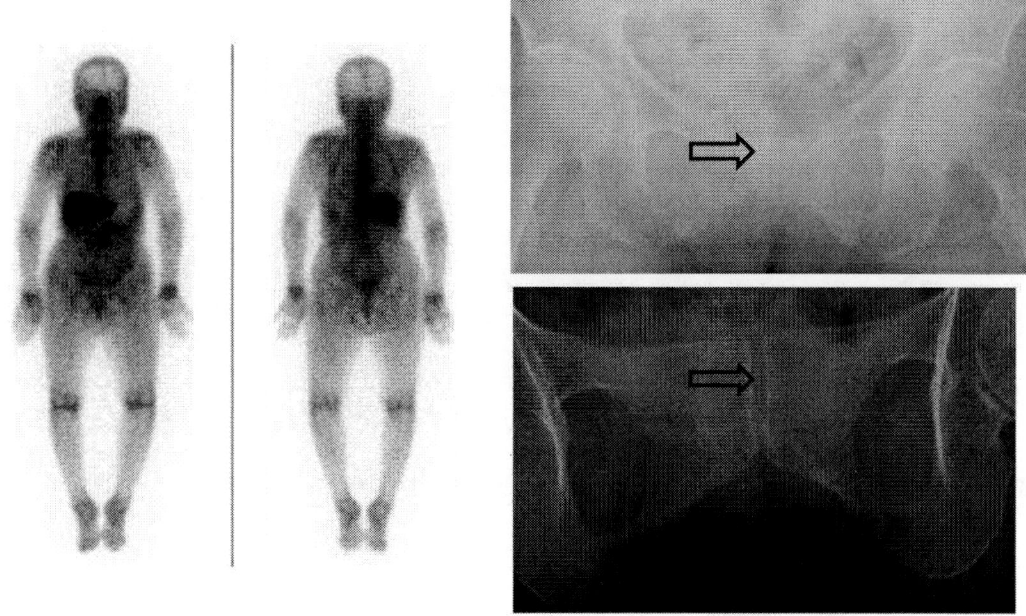

Figure 39. 67Gallium scintigram suggests arthritis in a patient with CPPD.

CPPD crystal deposition disease are characterized chondrocalcinosis and osteoarthritic changes in a specific distribution. Cartilage calcification is present in wrists, the knees, pubic symphysis, shoulders, ankles and so on.

In the hip joints, calcification in joints parallels the femoral head and the center of pubic symphysis.Chondrocalcinosis present in the fibrous cartilage of the pubic symphysis (arrows). Linear cartilage calcification in the public symphysis of the patient with CPPD.

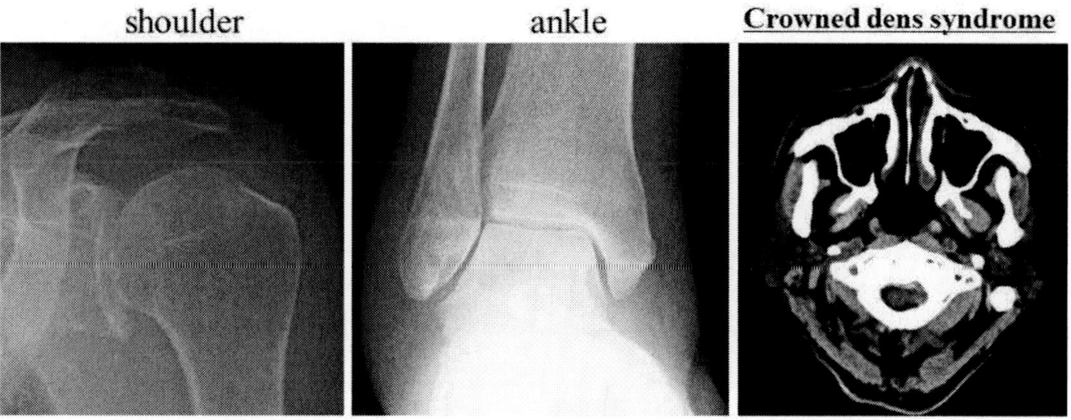

Figure 40. CPPD at the Shoulder, Ankle, and Spine.

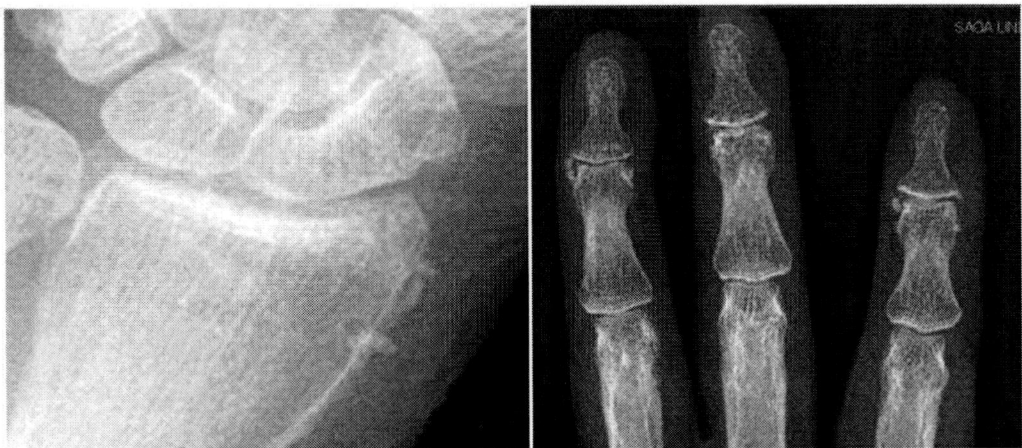

Figure 41. Hydroxyapatite Deposition. Hydroxyapatite deposition into soft tissues surrounding joints.

Chapter 5

DISTRIBUTION

"D"; DISTRIBUTION

4 points of "D"

1.   Distribution in the hand
2.   Distribution in the other joint
3.   Distribution in the body
4.   Distribution in the time

The pattern of joint involvement provides important diagnostic evidence.

1. Distribution in the Hand

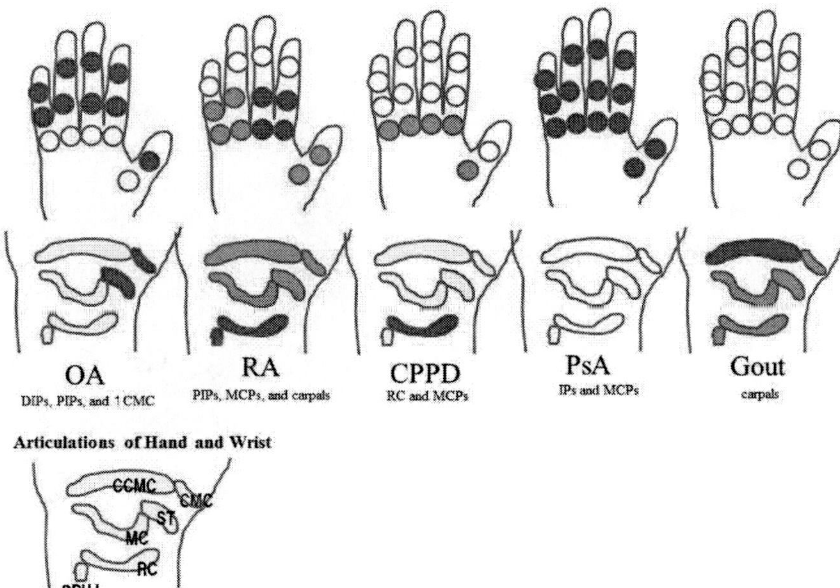

Figure 1. The distribution of the radiologic changes within the hands makes an approved diagnosis.

Osteoarthritis (OA) of the hands involves the DIP and PIP joints, but not the MCP joints. However, the patient with rheumatoid arthritis (RA) shows the PIP, MCP and carpal joints, but not the DIP joints. Psoriatic arthritis may affect all or some of DIP, PIP and MCP joints. Crystal-induced arthritis, CPPD and gout may affect the MCP and RC joints and carpal joints, respectively. (Figure 1)

Sarcoidosis may involve all of these joints. Chronic Lyme disease does not show synovitis of hand. (Figure 2)

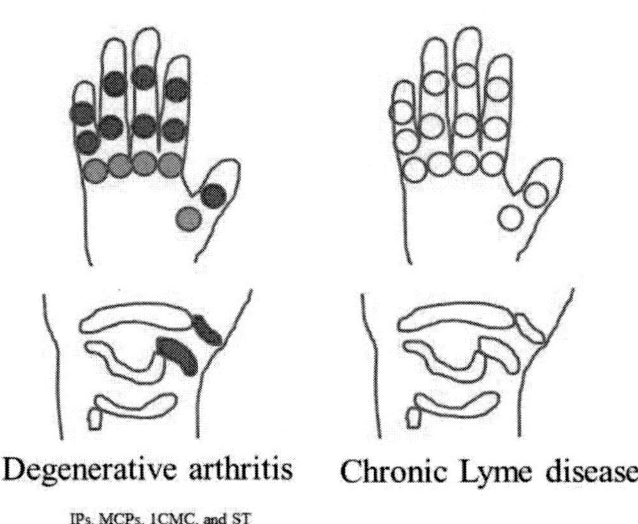

Figure 2.

Distribution in the hands of RA

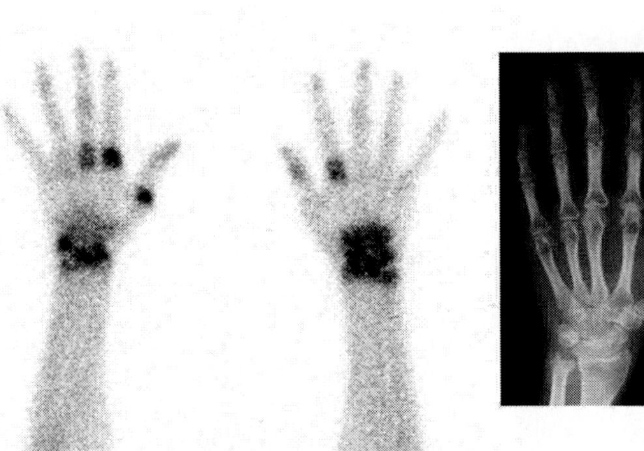

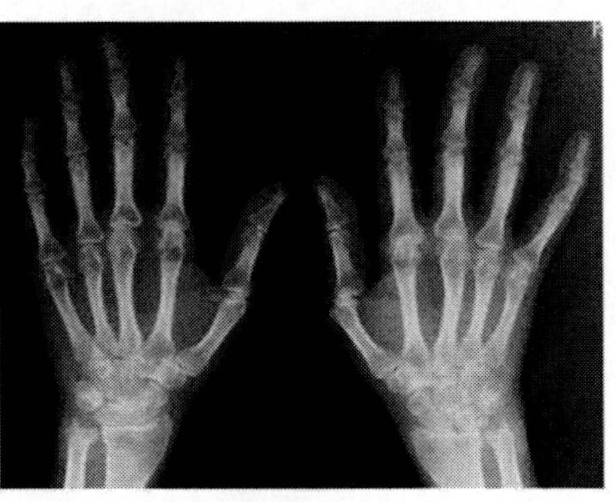

Figure 3. Bone scintigraphy can confirm disease presence. In this RA patient, arthritis in the hand distributes carpal and MCP joints.

It may help to evaluate distribution of arthritis in the hand and the body.

2. Distribution in other Joint

Bare	RA
Overhanging	gout
Central	erosive OA
All area	OA, PsA, advanced RA
OA	non-uniformly, the portion of stress
RA	uniformly

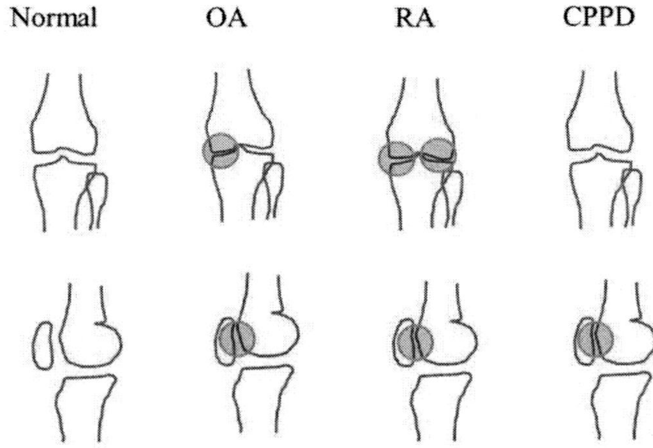

Figure 4. Distribution in the knee joint.

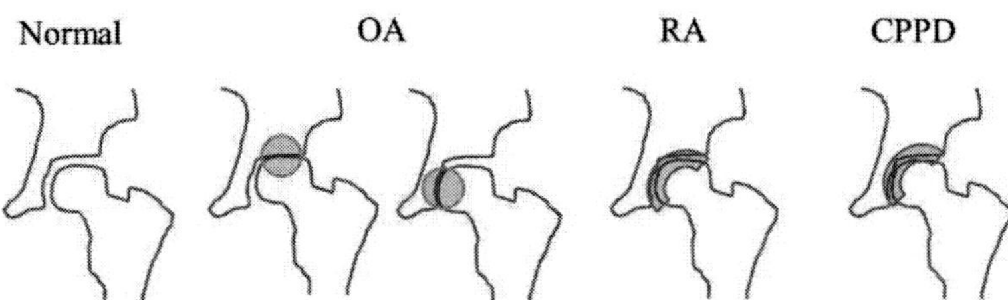

Figure 5. Distribution in the Hip join.t

3. Distribution in the Body

The distribution of arthritis in the whole body may be a helpful indicator in the evaluation of peripheral joint pain.

Poly-:	more than 4 joints
	RA and many other diseases
oligo-:	2-3 joints

Chronic Lyme disease: knee
Mono-: 1 joint
     Septic arthritis
     Gout
     CPPD
     Early stage of polyarthritis

The arthritis is initially seen involving one joint only, even in disease with polyarthritis. The distribution as the monoarthritis could lead to a misdiagnosis of septic arthritis.

Differential Diagnosis of Polyartritis

Systemic rheumatic disease
- Rheumatoid arthritis
- Systemic lupus erythematosus
- Polymyositis/dermatomyositis
- Adult onset Still's disease (AOSD)
- Juvenile rheumatoid arthritis
- Scleroderma
- Sjögren's syndrome
- Polymyalgia rheumatica

Systemic vasculitis disease
- Schönlein-Henoch purpura
- Hypersensitivity vasculitis
- Polyarteritis nodosa
- Microscopic polyangiitis
- Eosinophilic granulomatosis with polyangitis; EGPA Churg-Strauss syndrome; CSS
- Wegener's granulomatosis (Granulomatosis with polyangiits; GPA)
- Behçet's syndrome
- Giant cell arteritis
- Takayasu aortiris

Spondyloarthropathies
- Ankylosing spondylitis
- Psoriatic arthritis
- Inflammatory bowel disease
- Reactive arthritis (Reiter's syndrome)

Endocrine disorders
- Hyperparathyroidism
- Hyperthyroidism
- Hypothyroidism

Malignancy
- Metastatic cancer
- Multiple myeloma

Viral infection
        Human parvovirus (especially B19)
        Enterovirus, adenovirus
        Epstein-Barr
        Coxsackievirus (A9, B2, B3, B4, B6)
        Cytomegalovirus
        Rubella
        Mumps
        Hepatitis B
        Varicella-zoster virus (human herpes virus 3)
        Human immunodeficiency virus
Indirect bacterial infection (reactive arthritis)
        Neisseria gonorrhoeae (gonorrhea)
        Bacterial endocarditis
        Campylobacter species
        Chlamydia species
        Salmonella species
        Shigella species
        Yersinia species
        Tropheryma whippelii (Whipple's disease)
        Group A streptococci (rheumatic fever)
Direct bacterial infection
        N. Gonorrhoeae
        Staphylococcus aureus
        Gram-negative bacilli
        Bacterial endocarditis
Other infections
        Borrelia burgdorferi (Lyme disease)
        Mycobacterium tuberculosis (tuberculosis)
        Fungi
Crystal-induced synovitis:
        Gout
        Pseudogout (calcium pyrophosphate deposition disease)
        Hydroxyapatite
Others
        Osteoarthritis
        Hypermobility syndromes
        Sarcoidosis
        Fibromyalgia
        Osteomalacia
        Sweet's syndrome
        Serum sickness

(Richie AM and Francis ML. Diagnostic Approach to Polyarticular Joint Pain. Am Fam Physician. 2003 Sep 15;68(6):1151-1160.)

Bilateral

Symmetrical distribution — RA (rheumatoid arthritis)
Some of OA
SLE (systemic lupus erythematosus)
PMR (polymyalgia rheumatica)
Viral arthritides
Human parvovirus B19 infection
Serum sickness reactions
Fibromyalgia
Ankyosing spondilitis

Asymmetric — reactive arthritis
Psoriatic arthritis
Gout
Some of OA

Axial involvement
Positive — OA cervical
Lumbar
Fibromyalgia
Ankylosing spondilitis
PSA

Negative — RA (however, cervical +)
Human parvovirus B19 infection
SLE
PSA

Small or large joints
Small — human parvovirus B19 infection
SLE

Small and large — RA
OA
Fibromyalgia
PSA

Large — ankylosing spondylitis

RA

In rheumatoid arthritis (RA), peripheral arthritis with large joint arthritis. However, lower back pain due to the arthritis for itself is very rare.

OA

Primary osteoarthritis (OA) spares the wrists, elbows, and ankles. In addition to these peripheral joints, osteoarthritis (OA) may involve the lower back, the neck, or both.

Table 1. Distribution in the body

	RA ranking	RA	CPPD	OA	PsA		reactive
hands	1			frequent	1	Most frequent	less frequent
wrists	1		Most frequent				
elbows	7	34%	frequent	rare			
shoulders	5	60%	frequent	rare			
pubic symphysis			Most frequent				
hips	6	50%					less frequent
knees	3	80%	The most frequent	frequent			frequent
ankles	4			rare			frequent
feet	2	80-90%			2	frequent	most frequent
sacroiliac (SI)					3	frequent	frequent
spine cervical	6	atlantoaxial 50%		frequent			less frequent
thoracic and lumbar areas		Very rare		frequent	4	frequent	frequent 6

Spondyloarthropathies

(Ankylosing spondylitis, psoriatic arthritis, inflammatory bowel disease-associated arthropathy, and reactive arthritis)

Typically, involving the larger joints of the lower extremities

Involve peripheral arthritis accompanied by the larger joints

Low back pain

Prolonged morning stiffness

These symptoms improve with exercise

Enthesitis (inflammation of the muscular or tendinous insertions)

    Achilles tendonitis

    Plantar fasciitis

    Dactylitis: inflammation of the finger or toe

4. Distribution in the Time: Disease Chronology

The pattern of arthritis may change over time depending the original disease.

```
Acute monoarthritis
      gout and septic arthritis:   an acute onset
                                   reaching a peak within days
                                   Early gout usually affects only one joint

Acute polyarthritis (< 6 weeks)
      Viruses
            human parvovirus B19
             hepatitis viruses)
      Crystals (gout, CPPD)
      serum sickness reactions
      The acute stage of Lyme disease
      (bacterial infections in joints seldom cause polyarthritis)
      early stage of rheumatic diseases (RA, SLE and so on)

chronic oligo-arthritis
            the chronic phase of Lyme disease

Chronic (slower onset) polyarthritis
      RA               usually over weeks to months
      SLE
      OA
       PsA
      ankylosing spondylitis
      fibromyalgia

insidious onset, but sometime abruptly
       RA
```

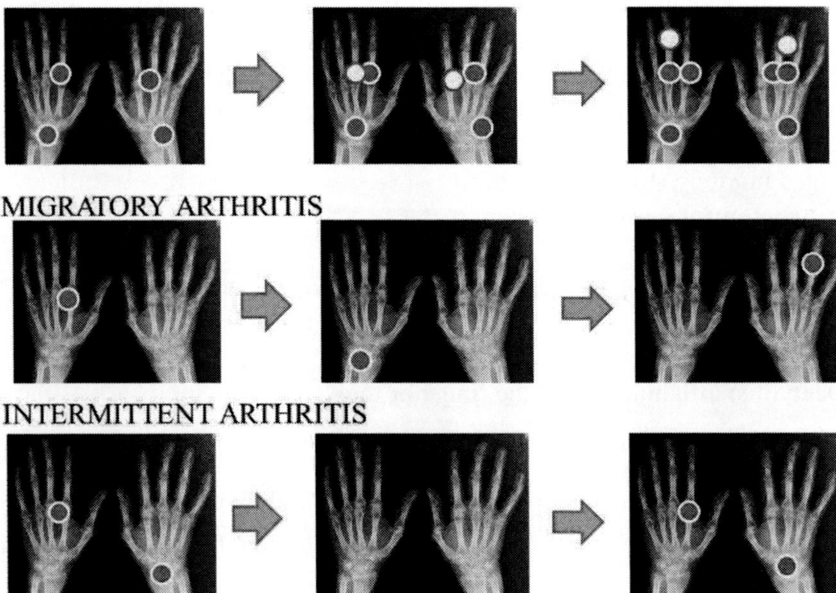

Figure 7. Aditive, migratory and intermittent arthritis.

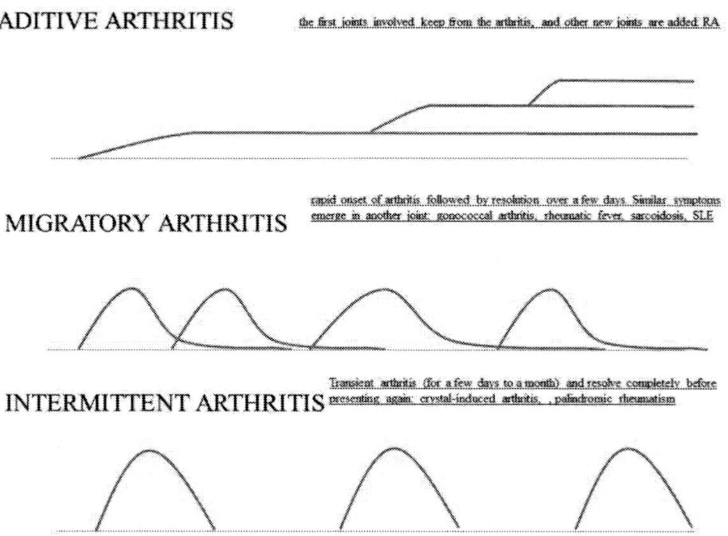

Figure 8. Aditive, migratory and intermittent arthritis.

ACUTE MONOARTHRITIS

Gout and septic arthritis: an acute onset
reaching a peak within days
early gout usually affects only one joint

Acute polyarthritis (< 6 weeks)
    Viruses
        human parvovirus B19
        hepatitis viruses
    Crystals (gout, CPPD)
    serum sickness reactions
    The acute stage of Lyme disease
    (bacterial infections in joints seldom cause polyarthritis)
    early stage of rheumatic diseases (RA, SLE and so on)
    chronic oligo-arthritis
    the chronic phase of Lyme disease
Chronic (slower onset) polyarthritis
        RA   usually over weeks to months
        SLE
        OA
        PsA
    ankylosing spondylitis
    fibromyalgia
Insidious onset, but sometime abruptly
        RA
Acute polyarthritis (for less than six weeks)

Human parvovirus B19, hepatitis viruses, and other virus infection induce acute polyarthritis. However, the etiology of virus-induced arthritis is not always found. Therefore, in actual, the prevalence of virus-induced arthritis may be more often and more common.

In addition, crystal-induced arthritis, CPPD and gout may be the causes of acute polyarthritis.

The elderly female patients with acute polyarthritis taking diuretics and having OA in the fingers may have gout (Agudelo CA, Curr Opin Rheumatol. 2001).

Because many conditions with acute polyarthritis are self-limited arthritis, the physicians should avoid treating the arthritis with disease-modifying anti-rheumatic agents. Differential diagnosis of rheumatoid arthritis is important in this condition (Arnett FC, Arthritis Rheum. 1988).

Neisseria gonorrhoeae can cause acute polyarthritis. However, usually, other bacterial infections do not cause acute polyarthritis.

Classic reactive arthritis associated with enteric infections (Salmonella, Shigella, Campylobacter, or Yersinia species) and urogenital infections (Chlamydia trachomatis) may cause acute polyarthrits.

Some of drugs, including anticancer drugs, interferon, and so on, may induce arthritis. Sometimes, interferons may acceralate RA.

Chapter 6

EXTERNAL BONE

"E"; EXTERNAL BONE

Extra-articular Manifestations

- Extra-articular manifestations may provide important clues to the rheumatologic diseases, however, they are not always diagnostic for itself.
- Soft tissue swelling should be distinguished from hypertrophy of the bone, osteophytes, such as Heberden's and Bouchard's nodes in osteoarthritis
- Soft tissue swelling

PA view of the hands is excellent for imaging soft tissue swelling.

The Soft Tissues

Distance (b) of normal soft tissue distal to the distal tuft is more than 20 percent of the width of the distal phalanx (a).

b/a>0.2 in normal

a: the soft tissues distal to the distal tuft
b: the transverse dimension of the base of the distal phalanx

SSc

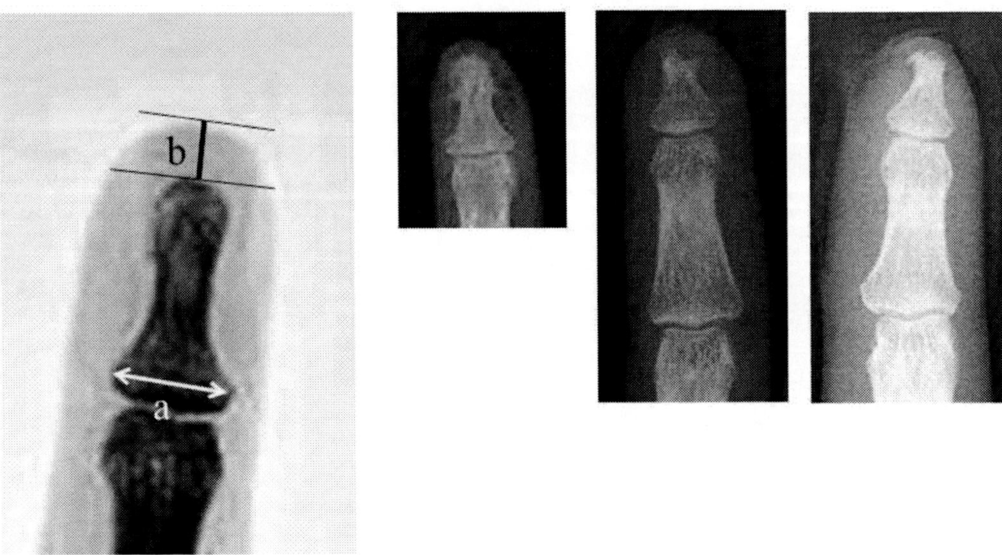

Figure 1. Index finger in patient with scleroderma shows marked atrophy of distal soft tissues due to the resorption of the soft tissue of the fingertip.

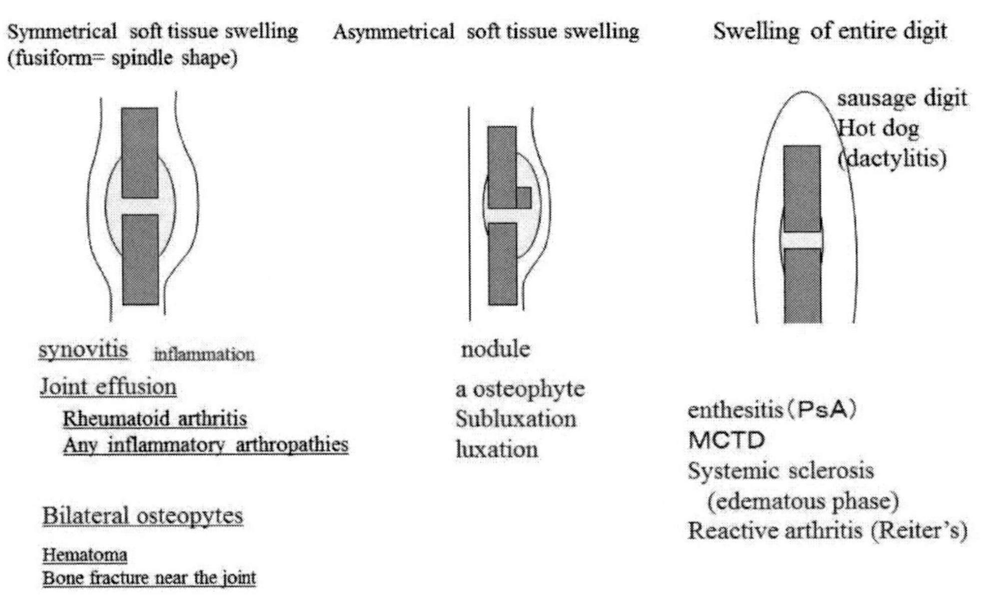

Figure 2. Soft Tissue Swelling at the Joints.

Symmetrical soft tissue swelling (fusiform= spindle shape)
Asymmetrical soft tissue swelling
Swelling of entire digit
Normal

Symmetrical Soft Tissue Swelling

Shape of Spindlehape

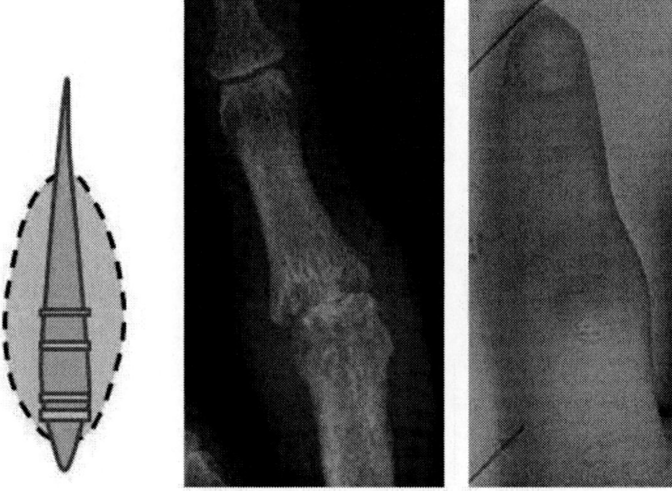

Figure 3. Shape of spindle (left), PA view (middle) and photograph (right) of symmetrical soft tissue swelling like as a spindle at the PIP joint in a RA patient.

Symmetrical soft tissue swelling, synovitis, joint effusion, shaping of spindle, at a joint is found in any inflammatory arthropathies, especially in RA.

Various other conditions, such as bilateral osteophytes, hematoma, and bone fracture near the joint may also form symmetrical soft tissue swelling.

The evaluation of soft tissue swelling at PIP, MCP and wrist joints are performed in PA view of the hands.

Recently, swelling due to synovitis and joint effusion have been screened by ultrasound with color doppler.

    Inflammatory arthritis
        infectious arthritis
        gout
        rheumatoid arthritis
        systemic lupus erythematosus
        reactive arthritis

Inflammatory signs are erythema, warmth, pain, and swelling.

Patients with severe inflammatory arthritis or systemic disease may have generalized symptoms, fatigue, weight loss, or fever (El-Gabalawy HS, JAMA. 2000).

Reumathoid Arthritis (RA)

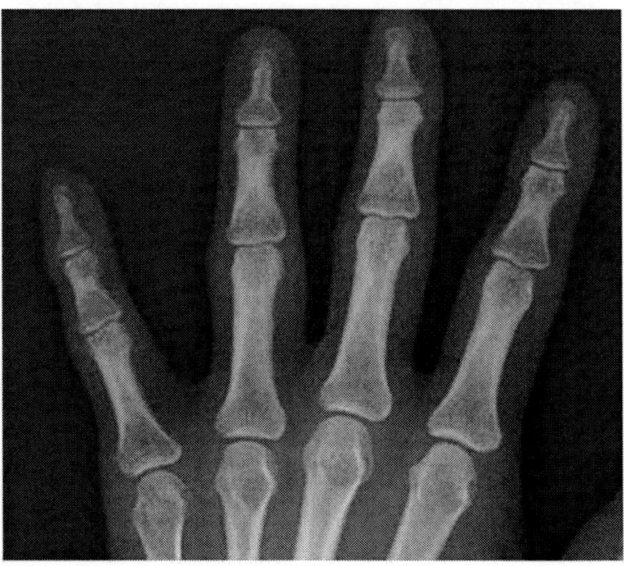

Figure 4. PA view of four digits in patient with rheumatoid arthritis.

Symmetrical soft tissue swelling like as spindles around the 2nd, 3rd 4th and 5th PIP joints in rheumatoid arthritis.

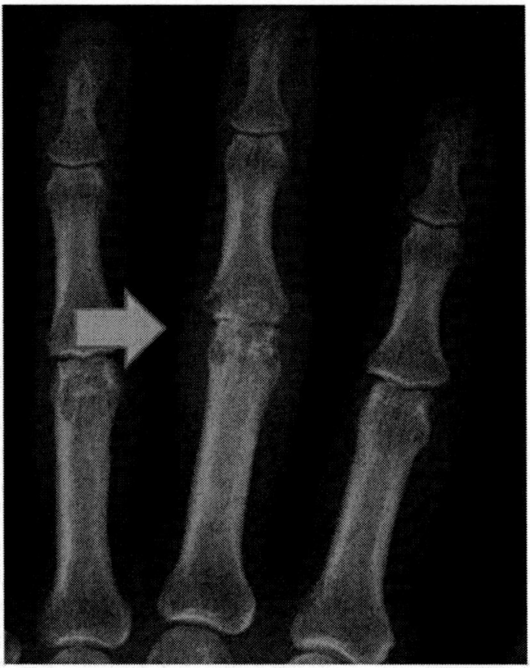

Figure 5. Symmetrical soft tissue swelling at the joints.

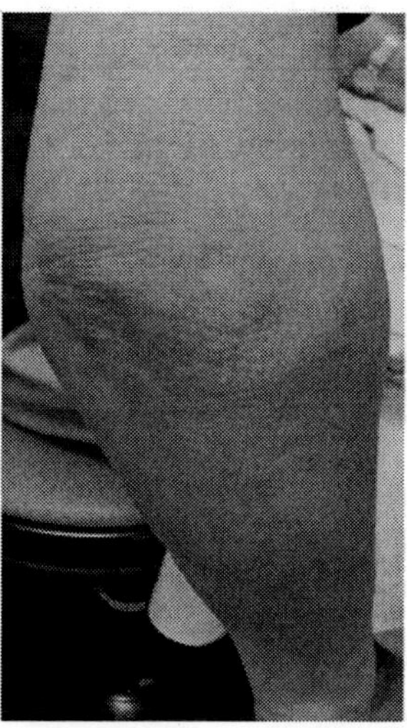

Figure 6. Joint swelling at elbow of a RA patient.

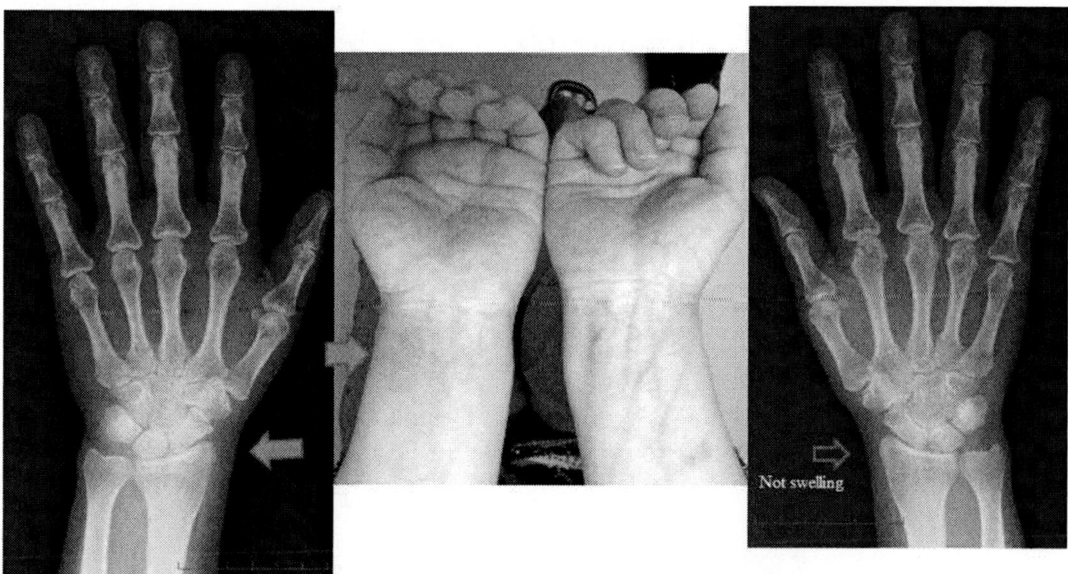

Figure 7. Swelling of Left Wrist in Relapsing Chondoritis. Redness of wrist and soft tissue swelling.

Power Doppler US of the joint in a RA patient shows vascularization of synovial proliferation.

Syuichi Koarada and Yoshifumi Tada

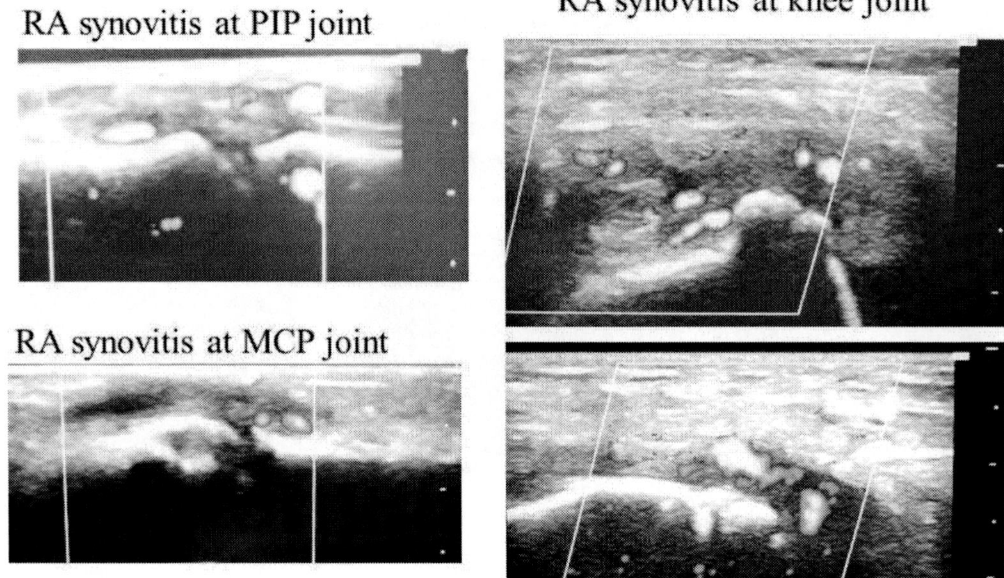

Figure 8. RA synovitis at joints is detected ultrasound.

OA

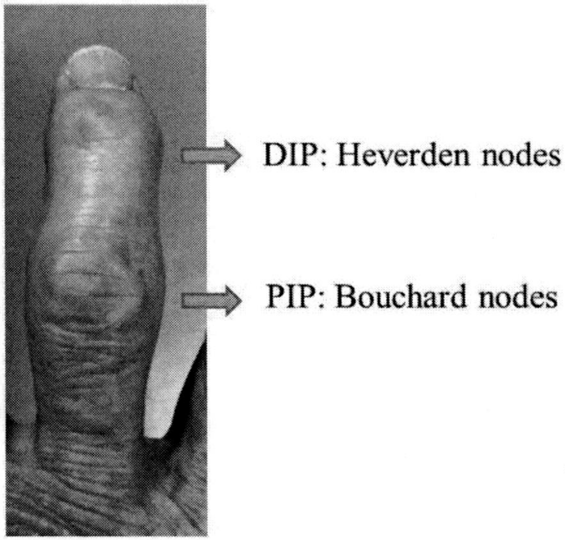

Figure 9. Soft tissue swelling due to osteophyte(s) is seen in the patient with OA.The swelling at DIP joints is called Heberden nodes. PIP joints' swelling is also called Bouchard nodes.

OA Changes in US

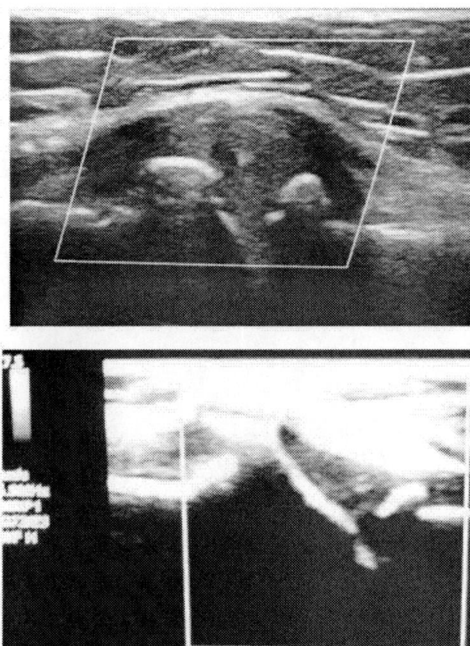

Figure 10. Power Doppler US of the knee in an OA patients shows osteophytes and synovial proliferation with few vascular spots.

Sjögren's Syndrome

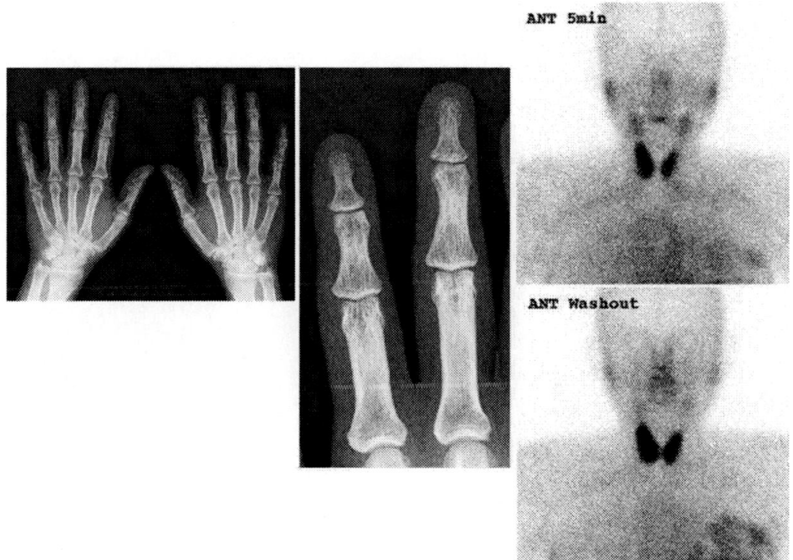

Figure 11. A 58-year-old female shows symmetrical soft tissue swelling due to Sjögren's syndrome.

Laboratory finding is ANA 160X, RF 66, ESR 55/h, CRP 0.03, MMP-3 <10, Anti-SS-A 500, and anti-SS-B 22.9.

Symmetrical and Non-symmetrical Soft Tissue Swelling

Microgeode Disease

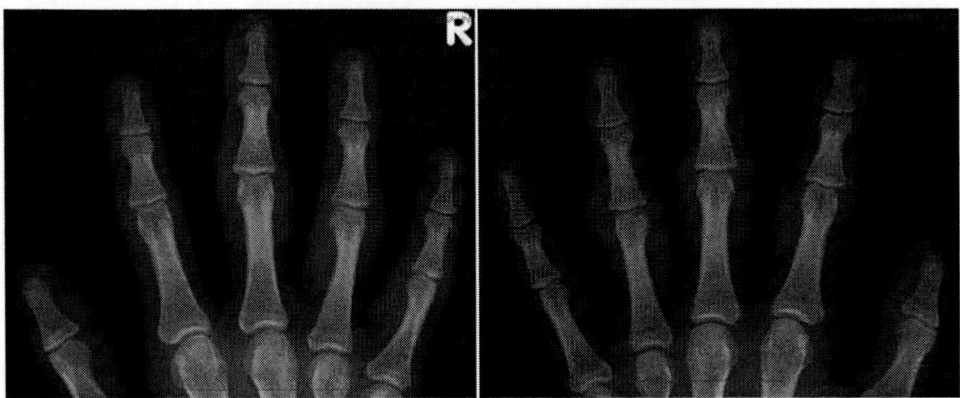

Figure 12. A 15-year-old male. PA view shows swelling of four digits in patient with microgeode disease. Symmetrical and non-symmetrical soft tissue swelling around the 2nd, 3rd 4th and 5th PIP joints.

Asymmetrical soft tissue swelling

Nodule

A nodule, an osteophyte or subluxation around joint may form asymmetrical soft tissue swelling.

In OA and erosive OA, non-opaque cartilage cap of the osteophyte distorts the soft tissue around the joint.

Distortion of the soft tissue due to subluxation or luxation is also found.

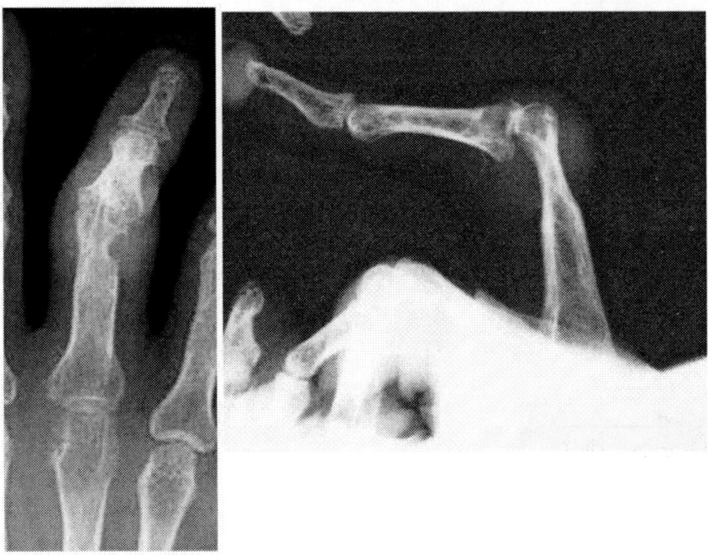

Figure 13. Gout.

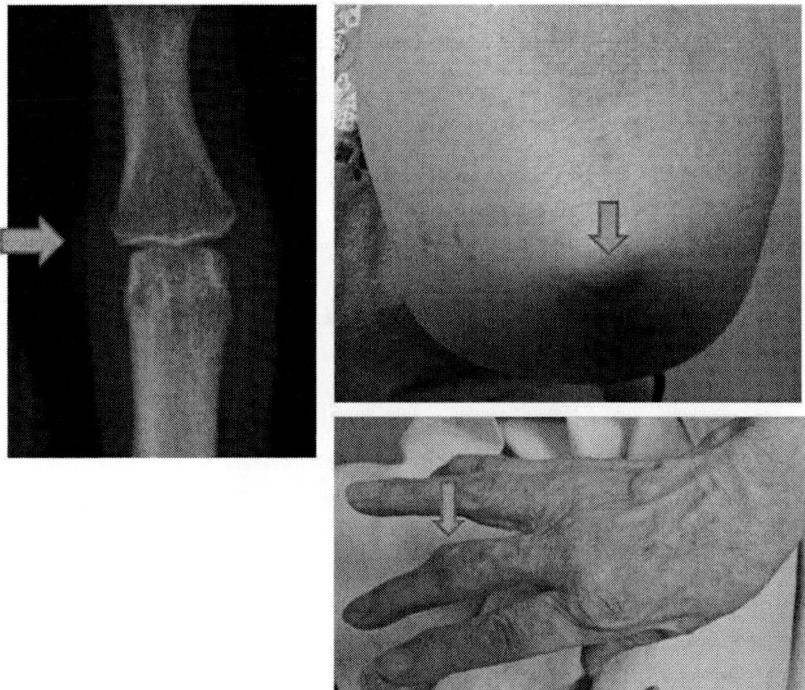

Figure 14. Asymmetrical soft tissue swelling due to a nodule distributed around the PIP joints of the 3rd digit in a patient with gout.

Rheumatoid Nodule

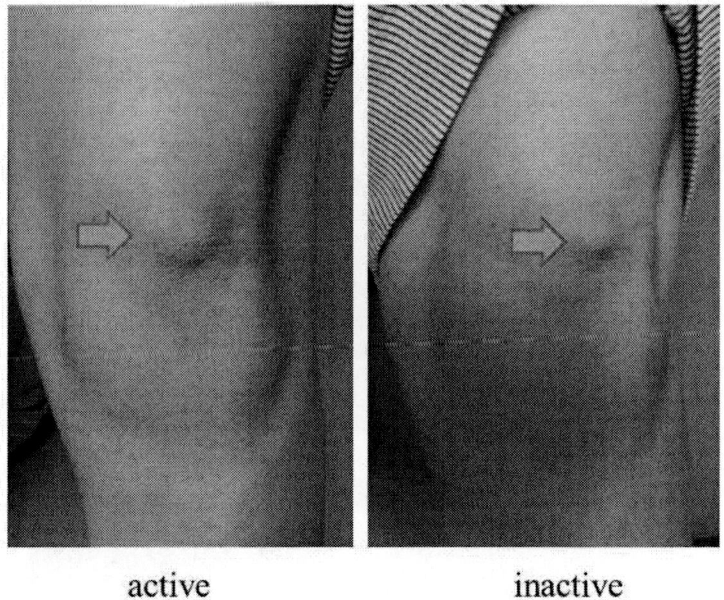

Figure 15. Fluctuating size of a rheumatoid node during the treatment of RA.

The size of rheumatoid nodule enlarge in active disease. In the same patient, the size can be changeable on the next visit due to inactive disease by the treatment.

Bursitis

Olecranon Bursitis
Caused by inflammation of the elbow's bursa.

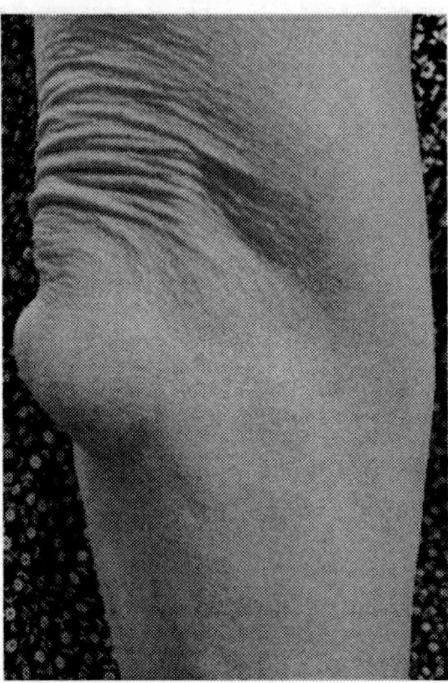

Figure 16. Olecranon Bursitis.

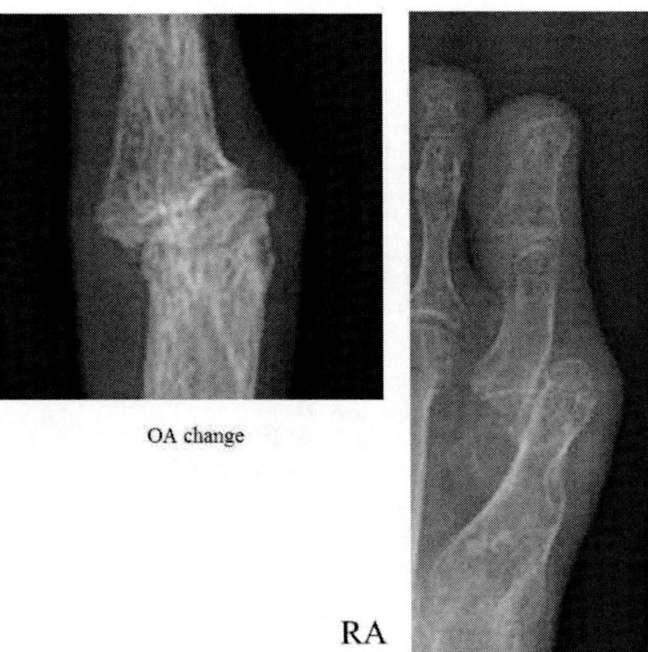

Figure 17. Luxation.

Osteophyte with subluxation: OA change

Distortion of the soft tissue due to osteophytes and subluxation in the PIP joint of a patient with OA.

Luxation of metatarsophalangeal of big toe in RA patient makes soft tissue swelling.

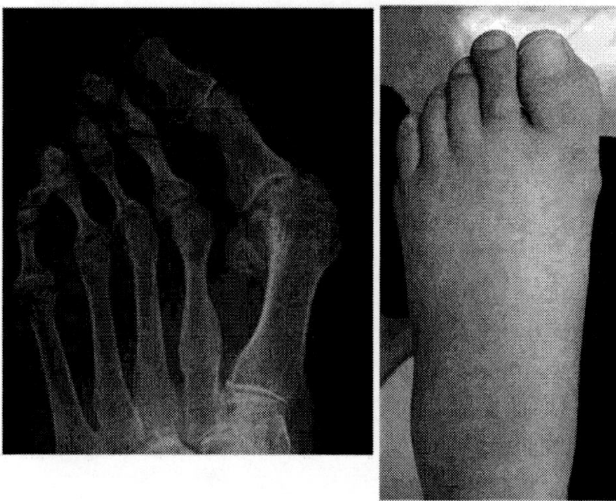

Figure 18. Hallux valgus.

Swelling of the entire digit

"sausage digits"
Dactylitis (inflammation of the finger or toc)
Classic sign of spondyloarthropathies
Caused by a combination of synovitis and enthesitis

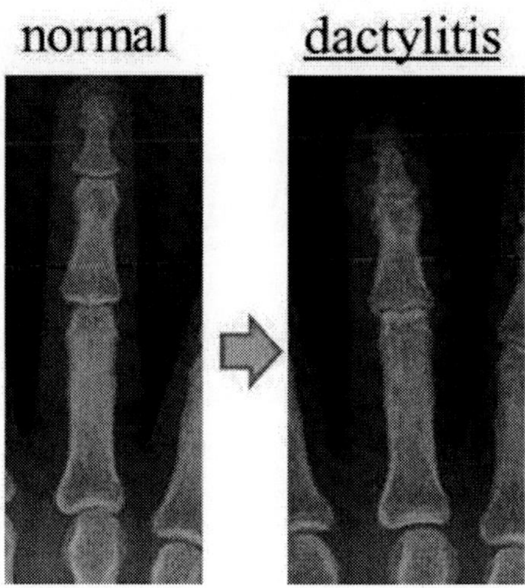

Figure 19. Psoriasis.

Swollen digit (dactylitis)

There is soft-tissue swelling of entire digit resembling a sausage or hot dog in psoriatic arthritis.

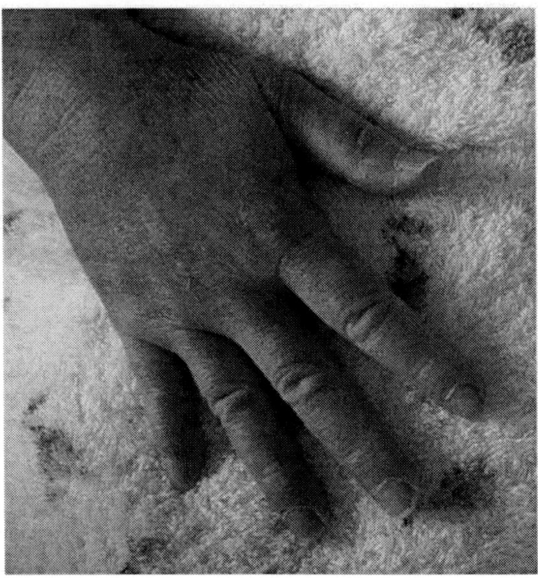

Figure 20. MCTD.

Swollen Hands

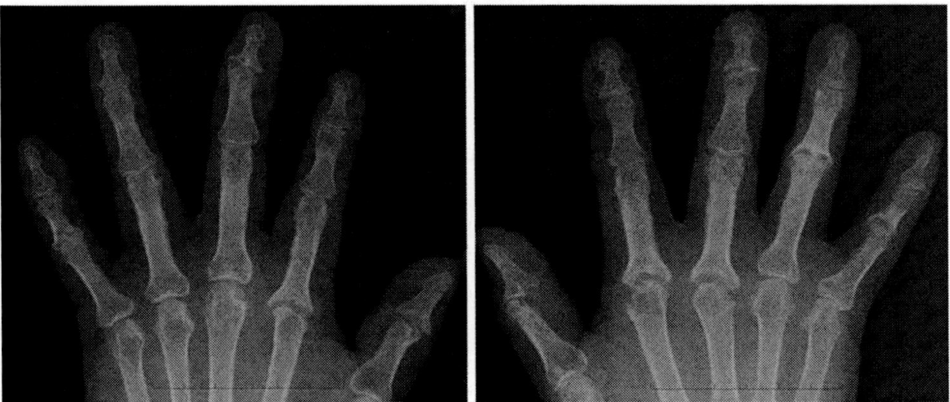

Figure 21. Sausage-like Appearance in Psoriasis.

RS3PE syndrome

Swelling of fingers, hands and feet

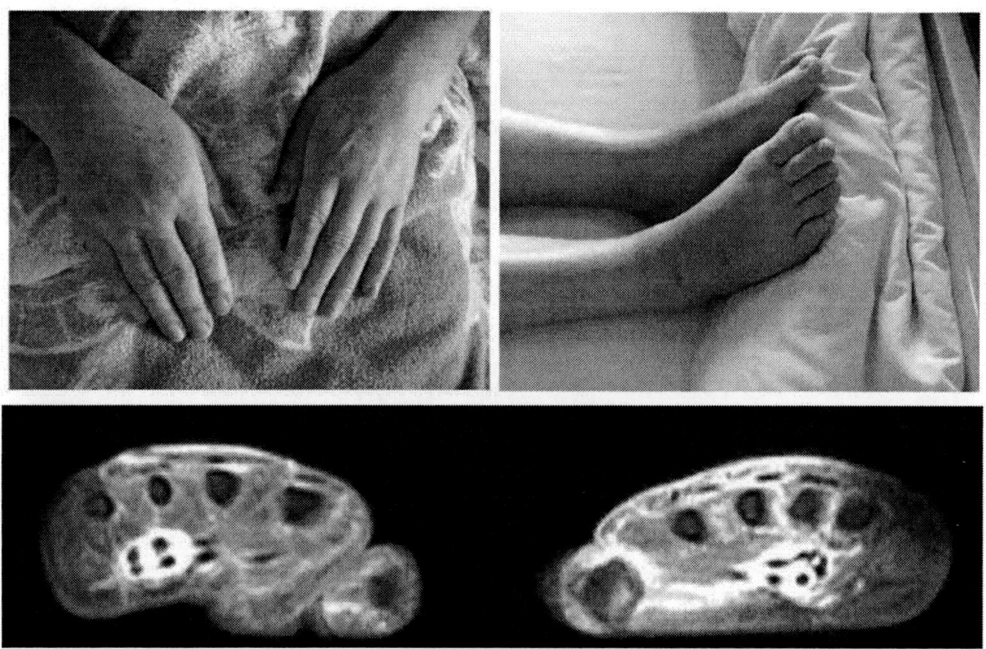

Figure 22. Primary RS3PE Syndrome.

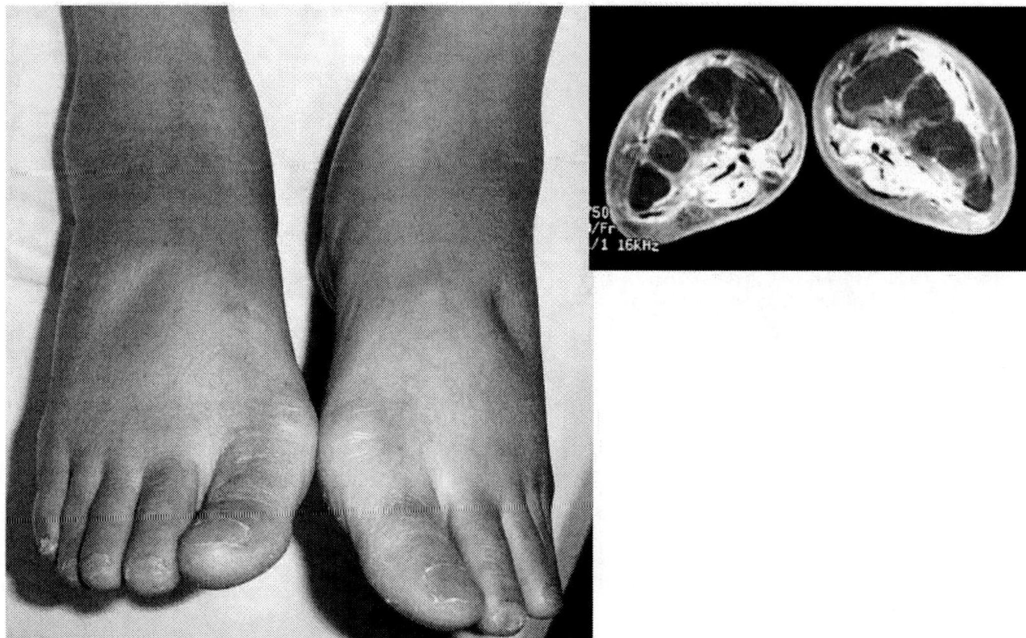

Figure 23. Secondary RS3PE (autoimmune, RA, associated).

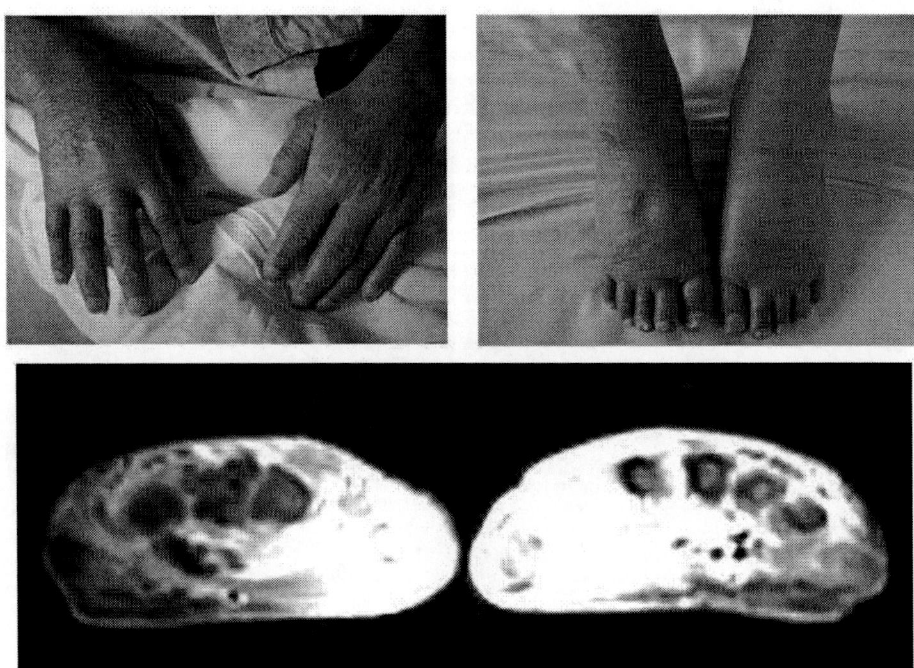

Figure 24. Secondary RS3PE [Malignant-associated (lung cancer).]

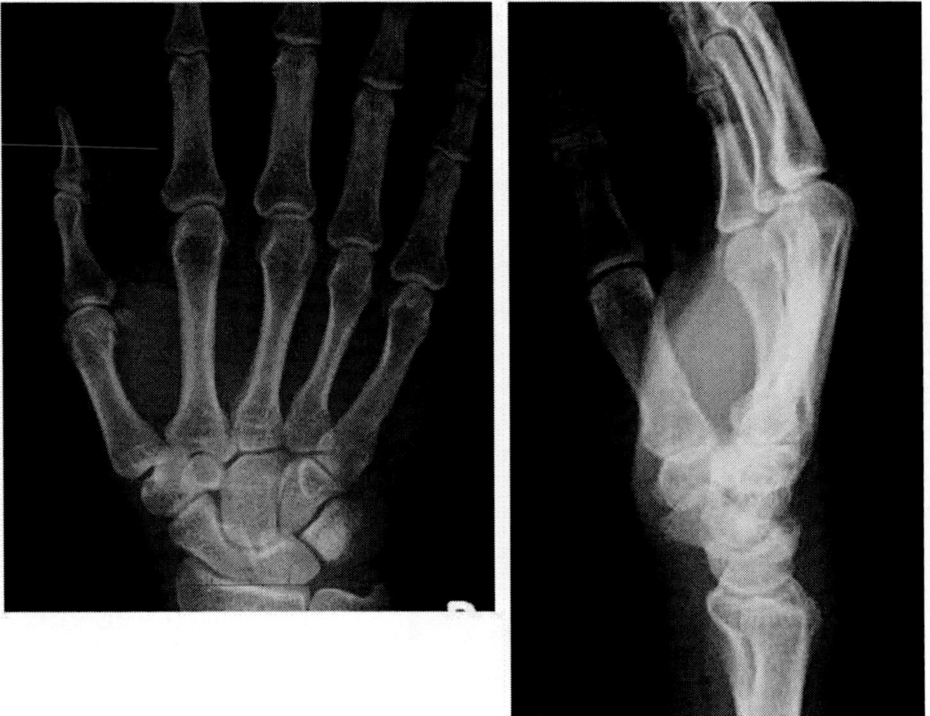

Figure 25. Subcutaneous Hematoma in Hemophilia.

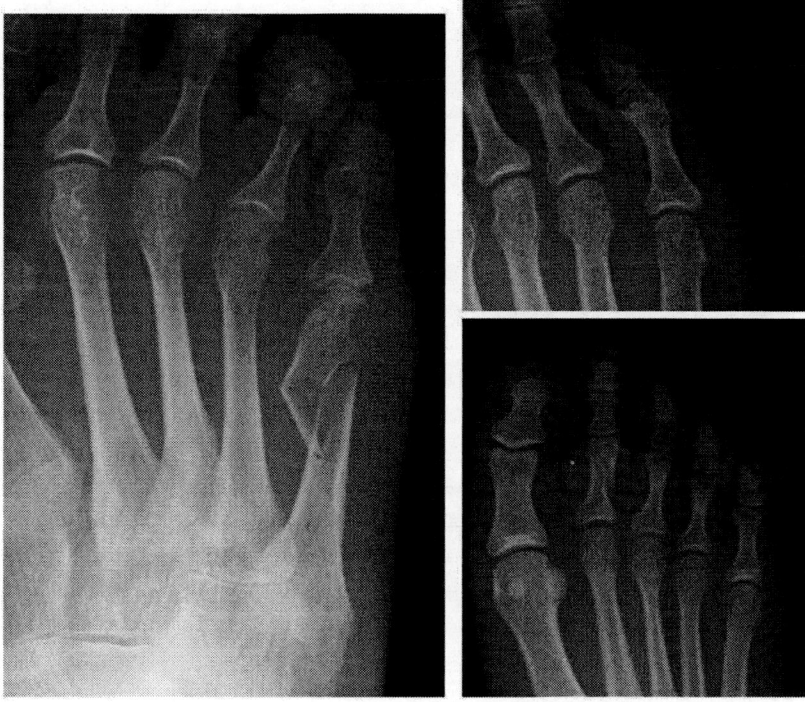

Figure 26. Bone Fracture.

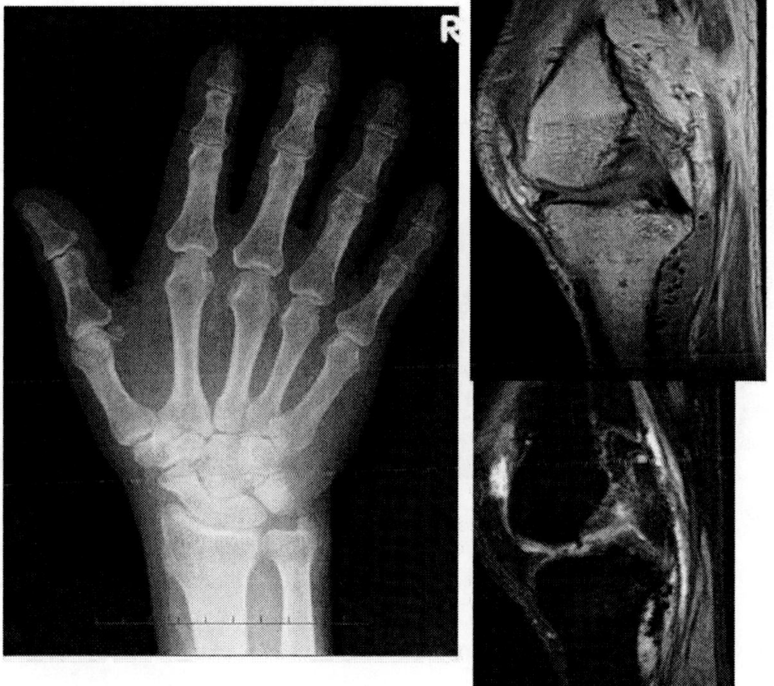

Figure 27. Amyloidosis. Swelling of the hands and the knees.

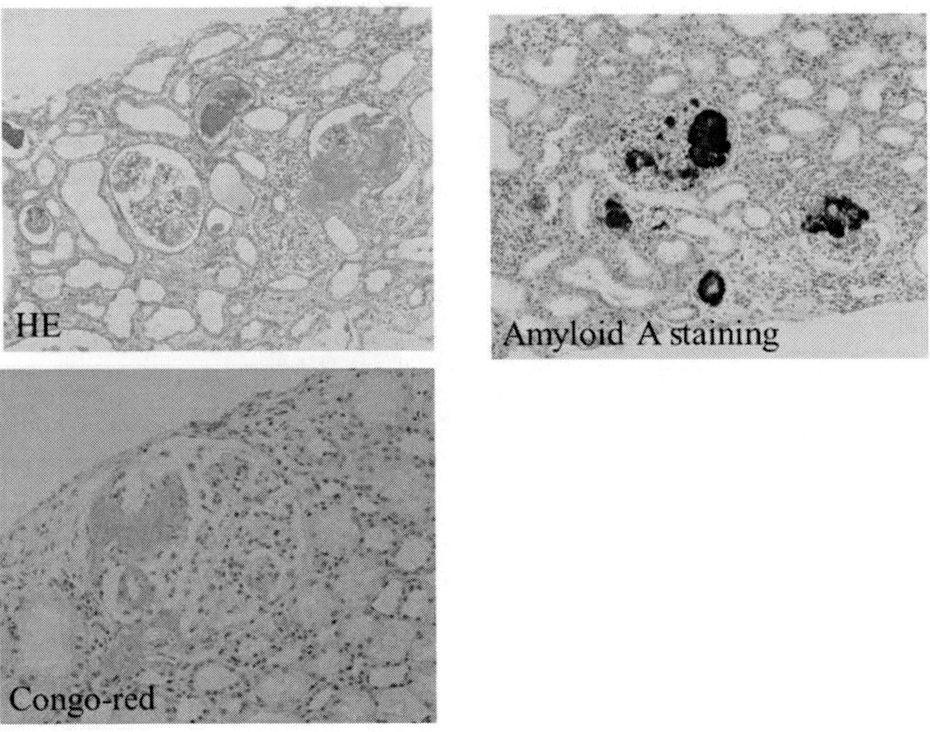

Figure 28. Biopsy of the kidney shows amyloidosis.

Plantar Fasciitis in MRI

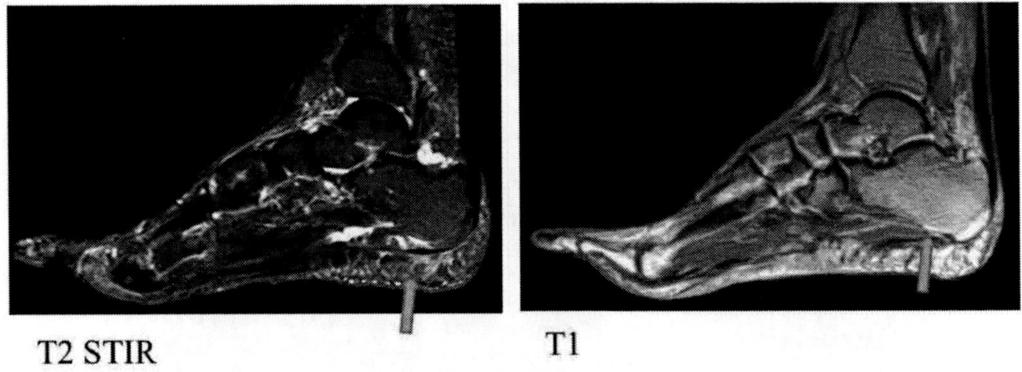

Figure 29.Mild thickness of the plantar aponeurosis. High intensity at subcutaneous lesion (arrow).

CALCIFICATION

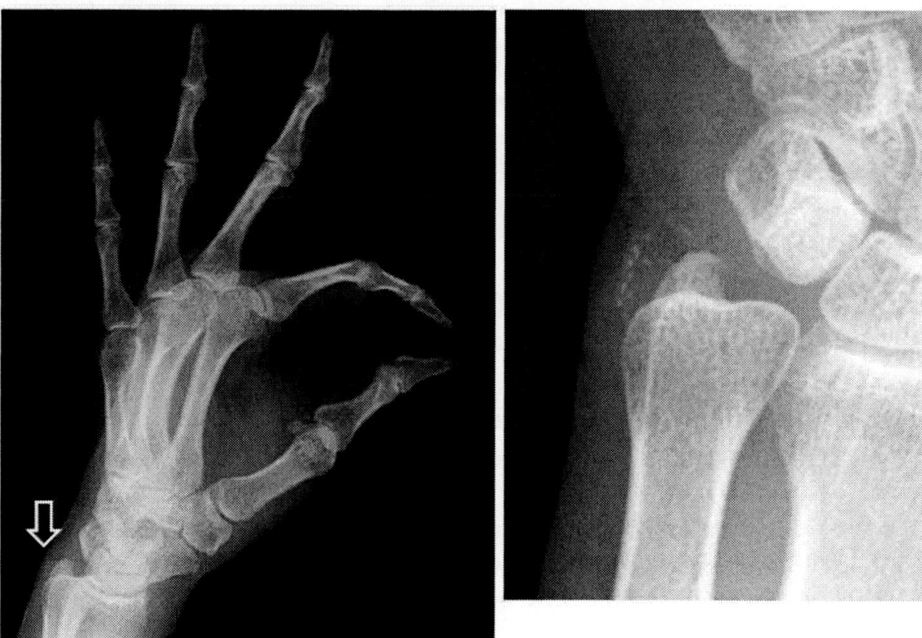

Figure 30. Palpable as a nodule: Scleroderma.

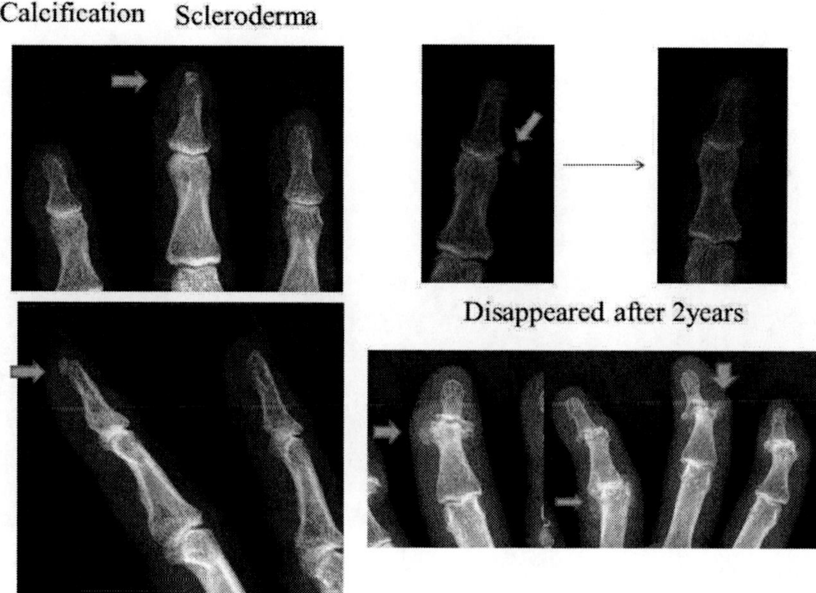

Figure 31. Calcification in SSc.

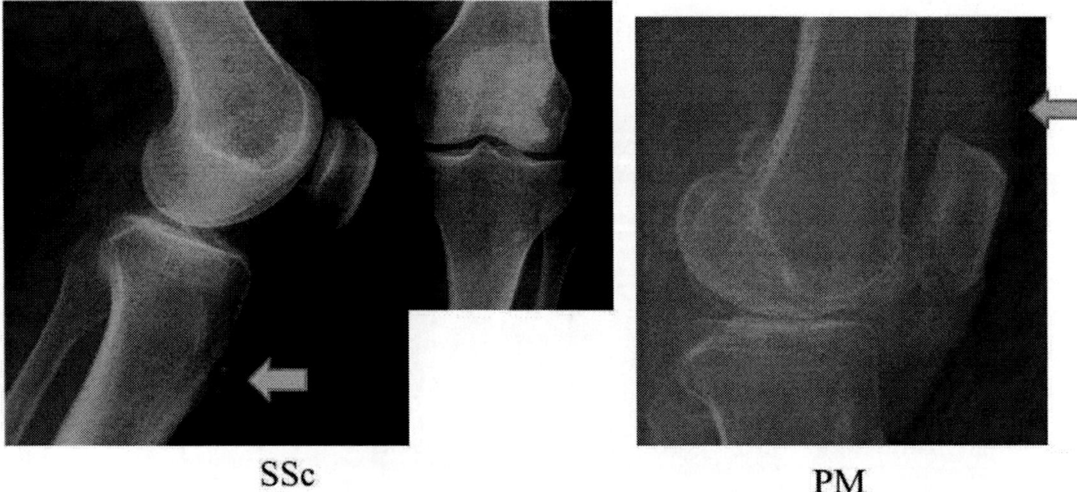

Figure 32. Calcification at the Knee in SSc and Polymyositis (PM).

Baker's Cyst

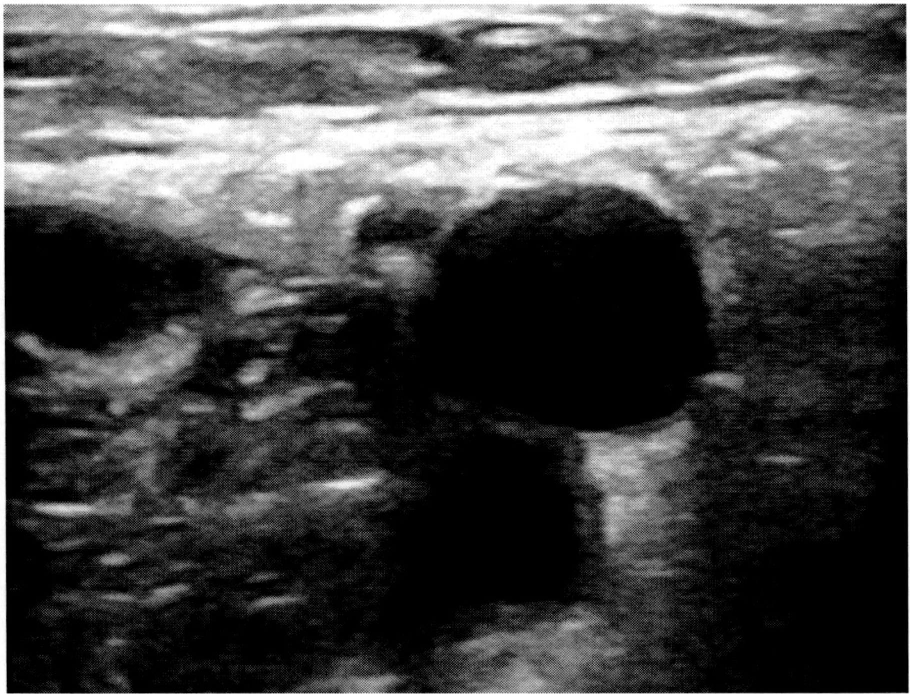

Figure 33. Baker's Cyst.

A Baker cyst is a synovial cyst that extends into the soft tissues. Baker cyst is a common manifestation in rheumatoid arthritis. The cyst in the back of knee extends posteriorly, inferiorly or superiorly into the soft tissues. Ultrasound is commonly used to detect the cyst.

Rupture of Baker Cyst

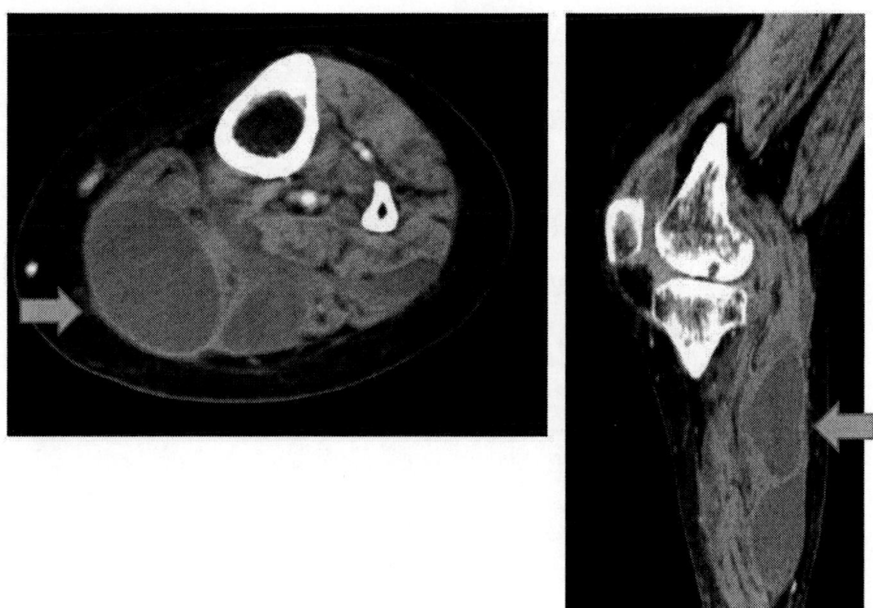

Figure 34. Rupture of Baker Cyst.

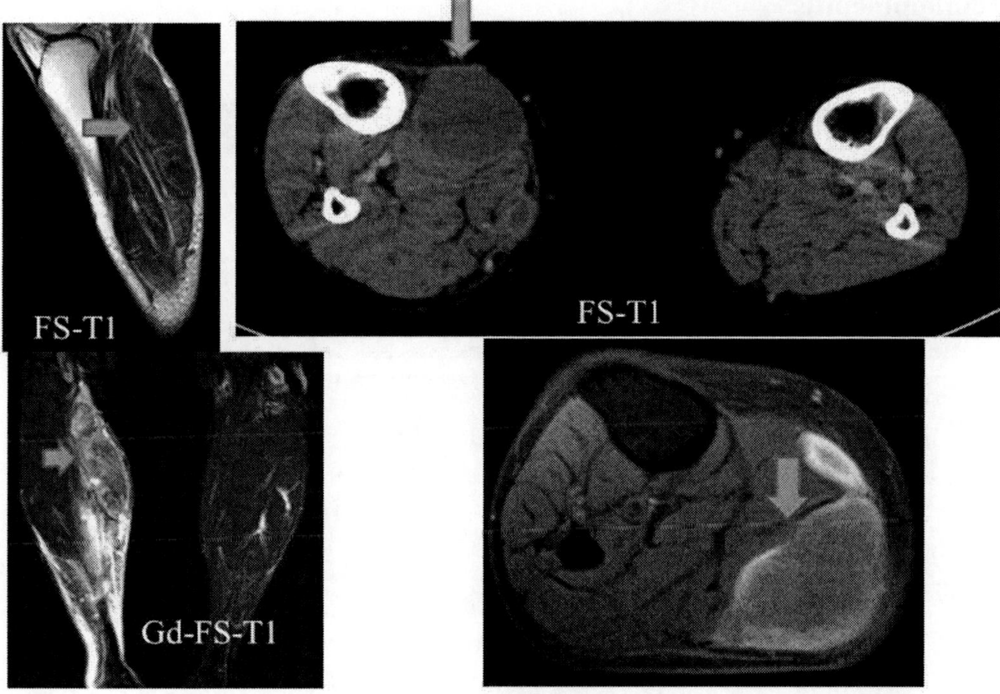

Figure 35. Rupture of Baker Cyst.

MRI finding shows that Baker cyst may rupture into the surrounding muscle.

Gd-enhanced coronal fat-suppressed T1-weighted image shows enhancement of soft tissue around the cysts.

Ganglion Cyst

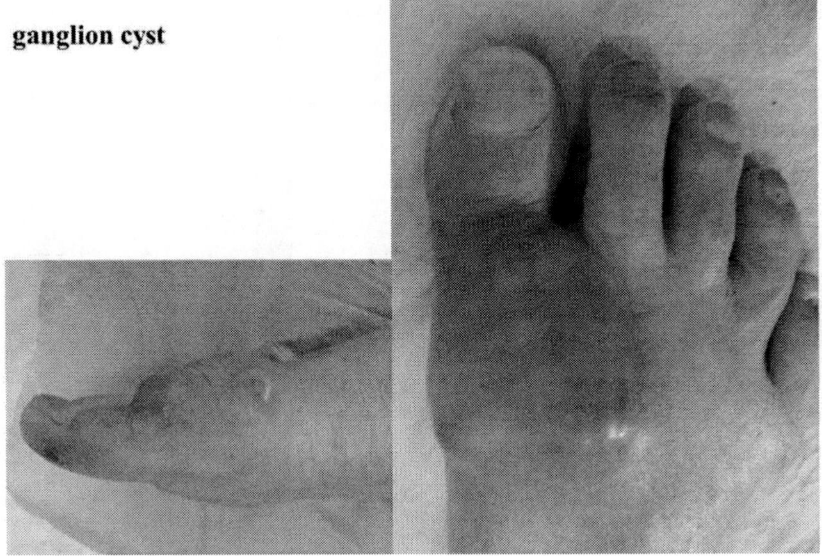

Figure 36. Ganglion cyst.

Thrombophlebitis

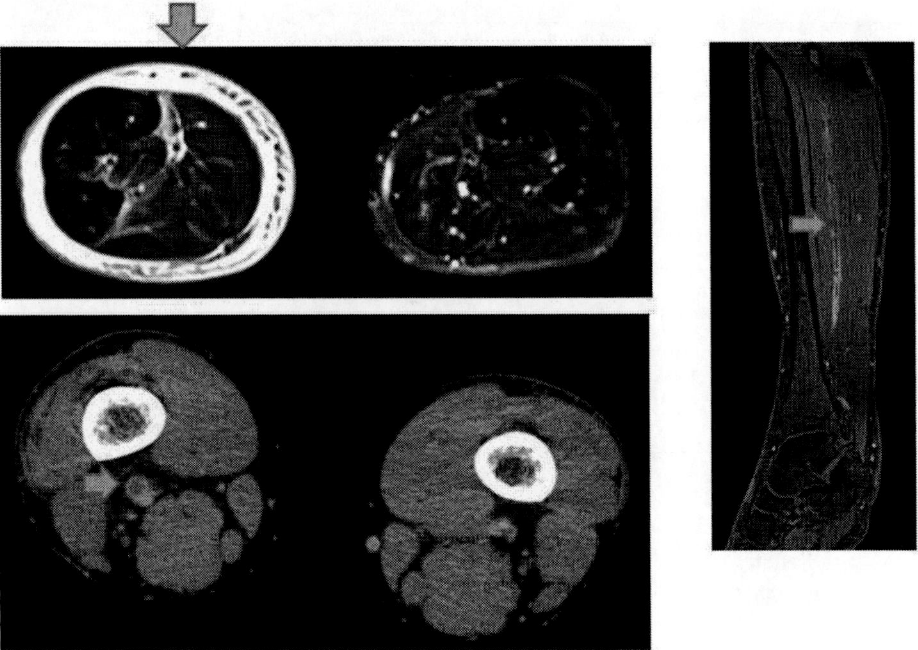

Figure 37.

The symptoms of thrombophlebitis in RA may be similar that of rupture of Baker cyst. Presence of ruptured Baker cyst increases the risk of thrombophlebitis due to high pressure on the deep venous system.

HADD (hydroxyapatite deposition disease)

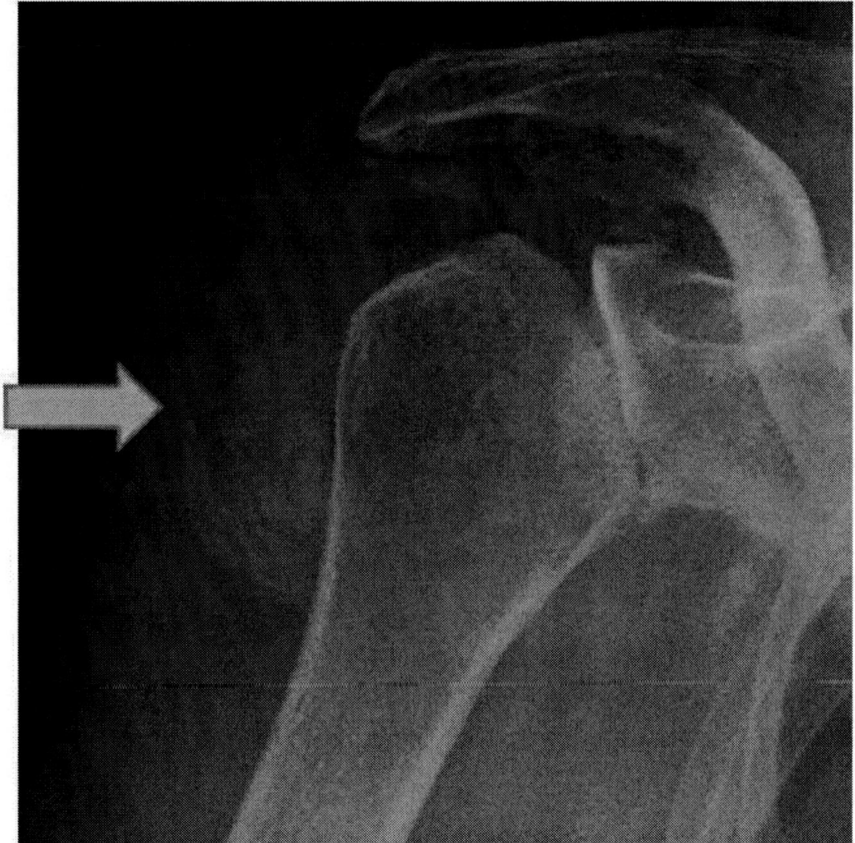

Figure 38. Soft tissue swelling due to HADD.

Fibromyalgia

No soft tissue swelling

Chapter 7

FURTHER INFORMATION

"F"; FURTHER INFORMATION

In the absence of definitive finding through radiological examination, further information including the history, physical examination, rheumatologic testing are important to make the early diagnosis and treatment. For physicians (not radiologists), this part is the most important and their work for itself.

Age
Sex
History
Family history
Occupation
Life style
Race
Geographical
Physical examination
Other radiographies
Laboratory findings
Immunological findings

Basic information
Age

	Age of Onset	arthrpathies
Juvenile	< 20 years	Juvenile Idiopathic Arthritis
		Hemophilia
		Septic arthritis
Young (> 20 years)	15 - 35 years	Ankylosing spondylitis
		Reiter's disease
		SLE
		Behçet's disease
		Takayasu
	Young adults	Enteropathic arthropathies

	25 - 55 years	Rheumatoid arthritis
		Psoriatic arthritis
		Sjögren's syndrome
		inflammatory bowel disease–associated arthropathy
		reactive arthritis
Elder	> 55 years	Osteoarthritis
		DISH
		CPPD
		RS3PE
		PMR

Female or Male Predominance

Female Predominance

	F:M ratio
Sjögren's syndrome	20:1
SLE	9:1 to 10:1
Fibromyalgia	9:1
Human parvovirus B19 infection	4:1 to 3:1
Rheumatoid Arthritis	4:1 to 2:1
OA >45 years	2:1 to 1:1

CPPD 1:1
Crohn's disease 1:1

Male Predominance

	M:F ratio
Ankylosing spondylitis	10:1 to 4:1 (to 1:1)
Psoriatic	2:1 to 3:1 (to 1:1)
Reiter's	5:1 to 50:1
Gout	20:1
DISH	3:2
Enteropathic arthropathy	
Ulcerative colitis	4:1
OA <45 years	

Morning stiffness
Typical

      Rheumatoid arthritis
      PMR
      AOSD
      Viral infection

Prolonged but improves with exercise

      Spondyloarthropathies
      Ankylosing spondylitis
      Psoriatic arthritis
      Inflammatory bowel disease-associated arthropathy
      Reactive arthritis

SECTION 1. PHYSICAL EXAMINATION

Skin

Rash

Malar rash	SLE*, Sjögren's syndome*, dermatomyositis*, human parvovirus B19 infection
	Lyme disease, rosacea, seborrhea
Heliotrope	Dermatomyositis*
Plaques (scalp, navel, gluteal cleft)	Psoriasis*
Erythema nodosum	Behçet's disease*, Sarcoidosis, Crohn's disease, Weber-Christian disease*
Pyoderma gangrenosum	IBD, RA, SLE, anklyosing spondylitis, sarcoidosis, Wegener's granulomatosis (Granulomatosis with polyangiits; GPA)
Palpable purpura	Hypersensitivity vasculitis, Schönlein- Henoch purpura, PAN
Purpura	vasculitis (mPA*), rheumatoid vasculitis and so on
Livedo reticularis	Antiphospholipid-antibody syndrome, vasculitis, cholesterol emboli
Salmon pink rash	AOSD

Lesions

Lupus chilblain	SLE*
Gottron's papules or plaques	Dermatomyositis*
sclerodactylia and skin ulcer	systemic sclerosis*
Finger tip ulcers	systemic sclerosis*
Necrosis of fingertip	systemic sclerosis*, vasculitis, SLE and so on
Discoid skin lesions	Discoid lupus erythematosus, SLE, sarcoidosis
Nodules	RA: rheumatoid node
	Gout, Whipple's disease, rheumatic fever, amyloidosis, sarcoidosis
Tophi	Gout

Oral ulcer	Behçet's disease*, SLE, Oral ulcers, reactive arthritis, GPA

Nails

Perionychia	Dermatomyositis, scleroderma, SLE* and so on
Onycholysis	Psoriatic arthritis, hyperthyroidism
Pitting	Psoriatic arthritis
Clubbing	IBD, Whipple's disease, hyperthyroidism
Glossitis	Sjögren's syndrome*
Skin ulcers	vasculitis, rheumatoid vasculitis*, and so on

Scalp tenderness	Giant cell arteritis
Swollen of hands	rheumatic diseases, RS3PE
Raynaud's	rheumatic diseases, especially, MCTD, SLE, scleroderma, etc.
striate cutis induced by glucocorticoid*	
Telangiectasia	Scleroderma (CREST syndrome)
Thickened skin (sclerema)	Scleroderma, amyloidosis, eosinophilic fasciitis
Hair thinning	Hypothyroidism, SLE
Lymphadenopathy	viral infection, Tumor-associated arthritis, SLE

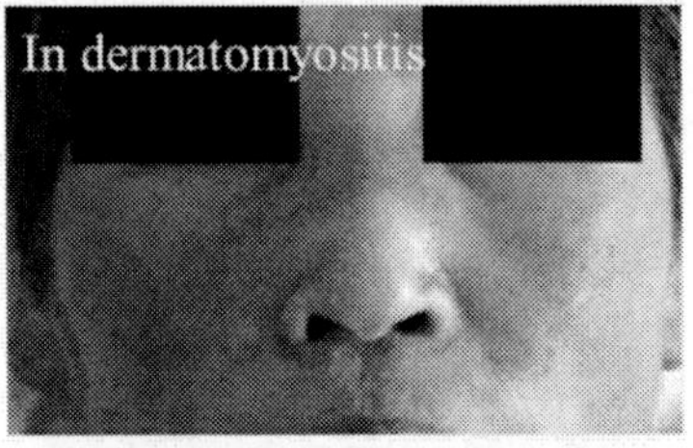

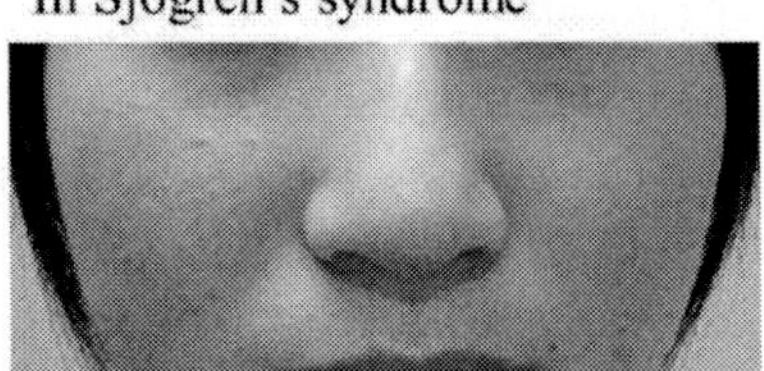

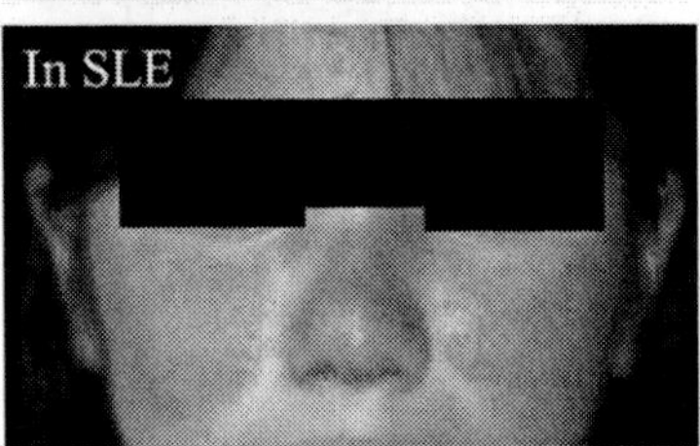

Figure 1. Malar rash (Butterfly rashes)

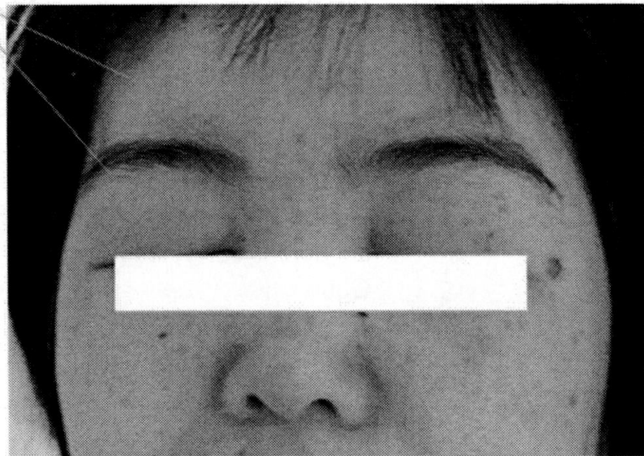

Figure 2. Dermatomyositis. Heliotrope.

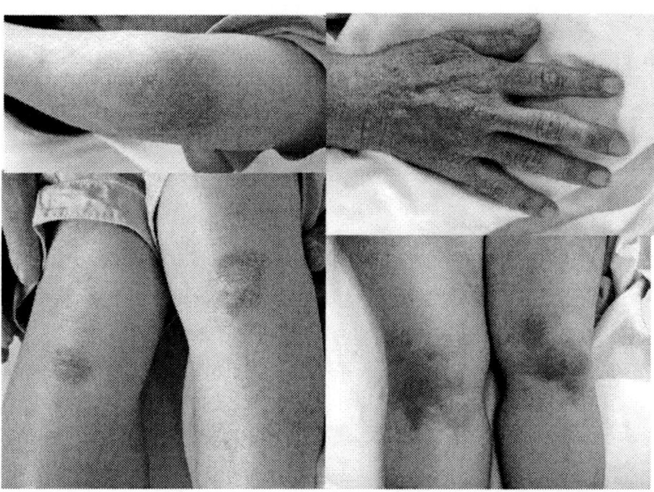

Figure 3. In dermatomyositis. Gottron's sign.

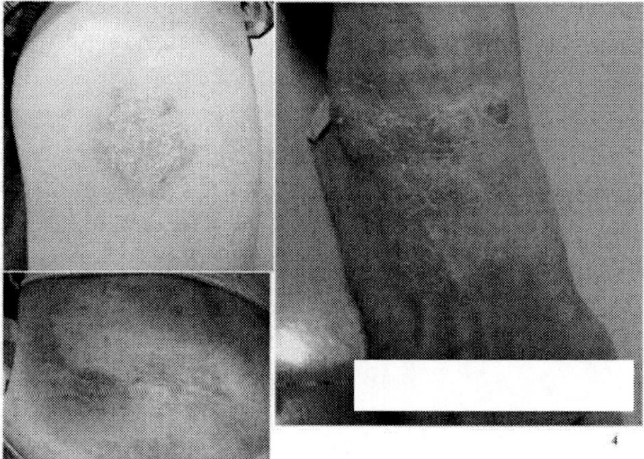

Figure 4. Plaques.

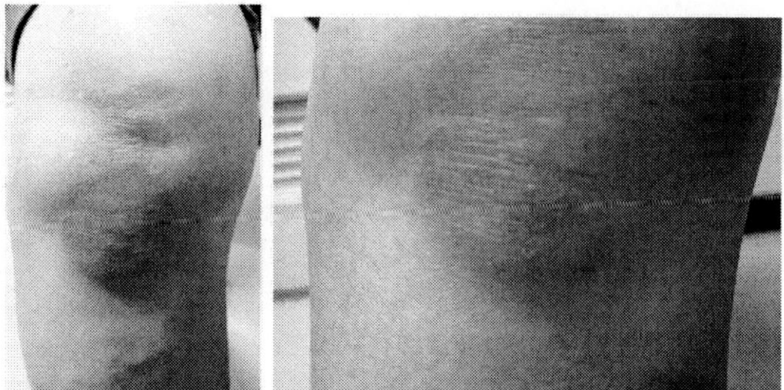

Figure 5. Plaques.

In patients with psoriatic arthritis.

Erythema nodosum (Figure 6).

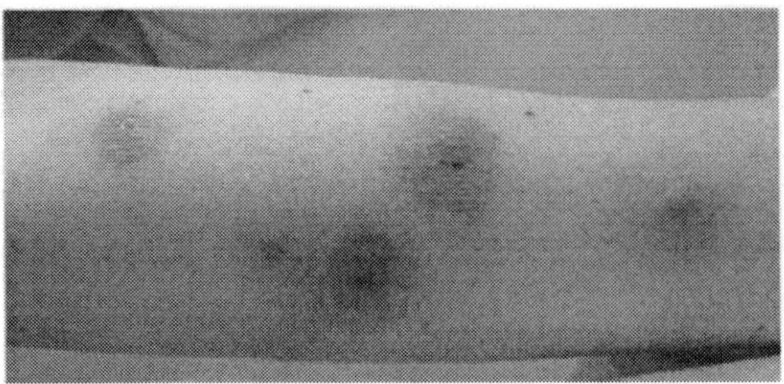

Figure 6. Behçet's disease

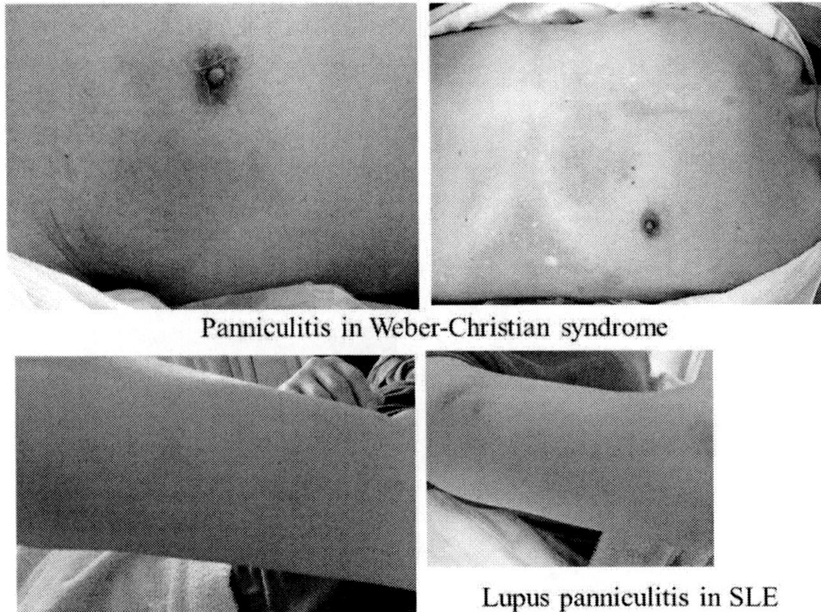

Figure 7. Panniculitis in Weber-Christian syndrome and Lupus panniculitis in SLE

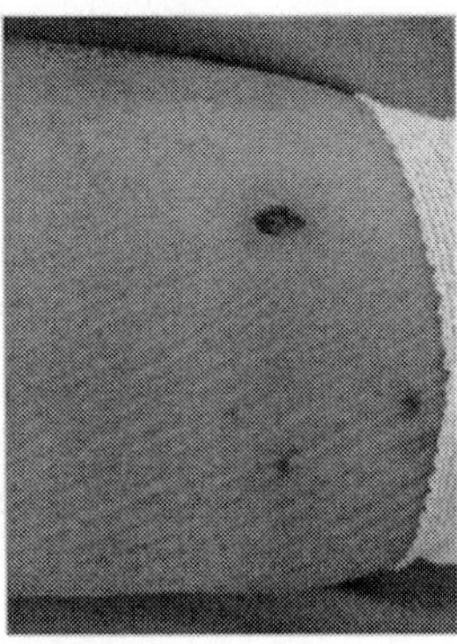

Figure 8. Skin ulcer and purpura. Microscopic polyangiiti.

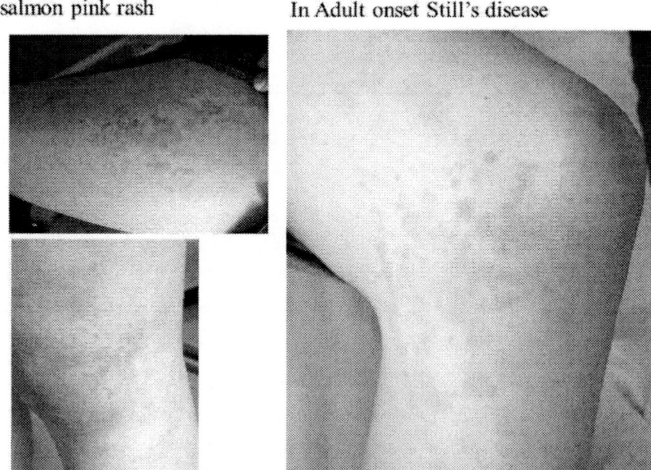

Figure 9. Salmon pink rash in Adult onset Still's disease.

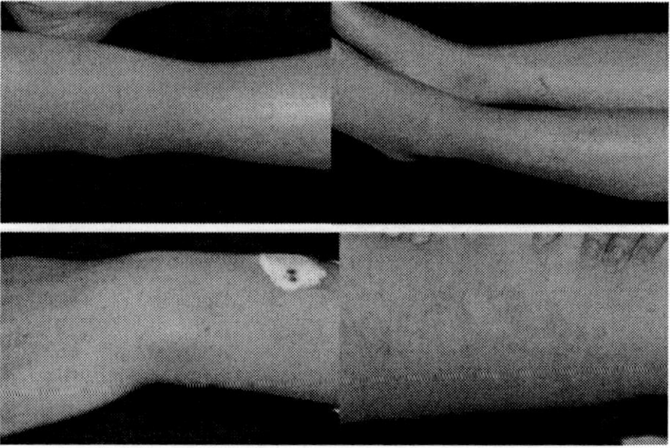

Figure 10. Salmon pink rash in Adult onset Still's disease.

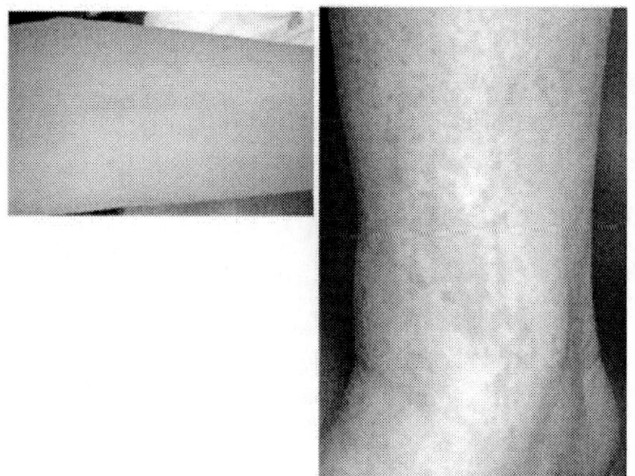

Figure 11. Salmon pink rash in Adult onset Still's disease.

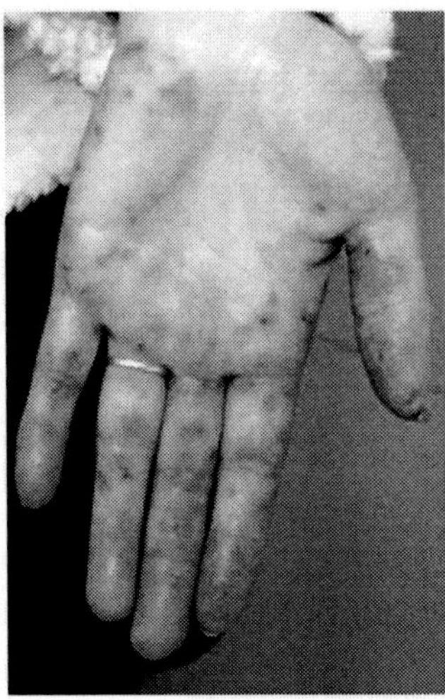

Figure 12. Lupus chilblain in SLE.

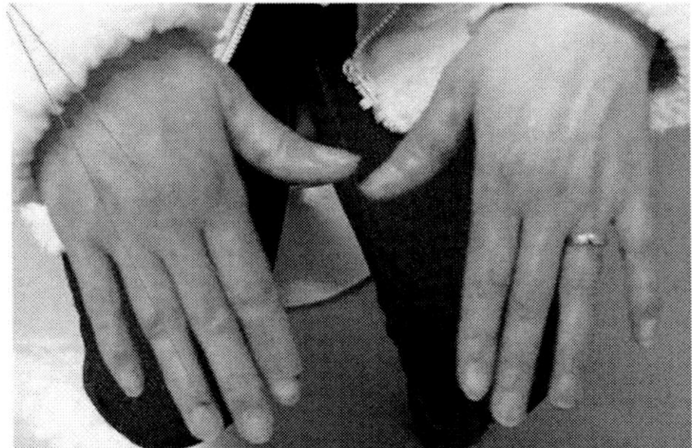

Figure 13. Perionychia in SLE.

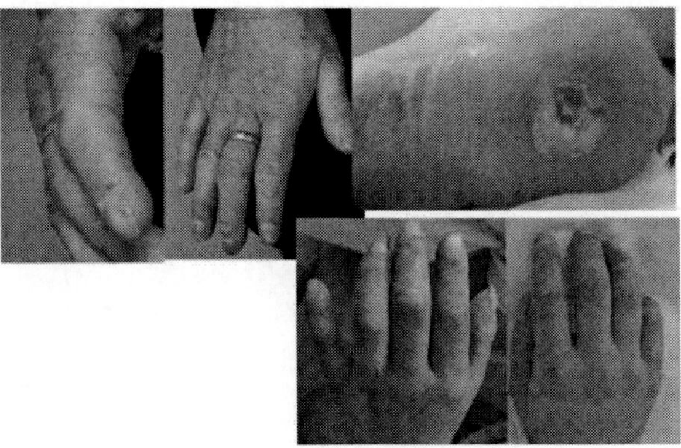

Figure 14. Sclerodactylia and skin ulcer in systemic sclerosis.

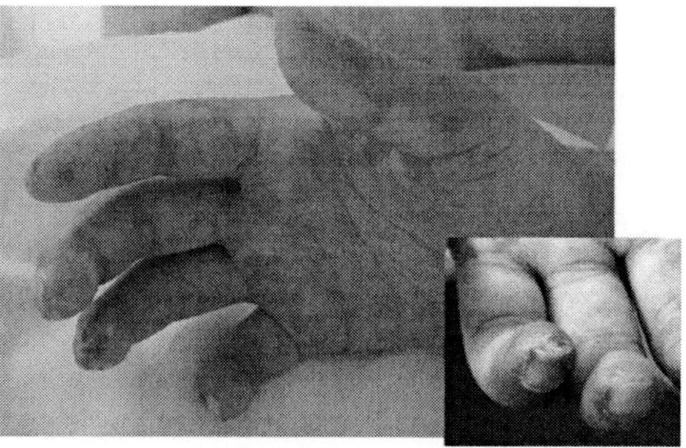

Figure 15. Finger tip ulcers in systemic sclerosis.

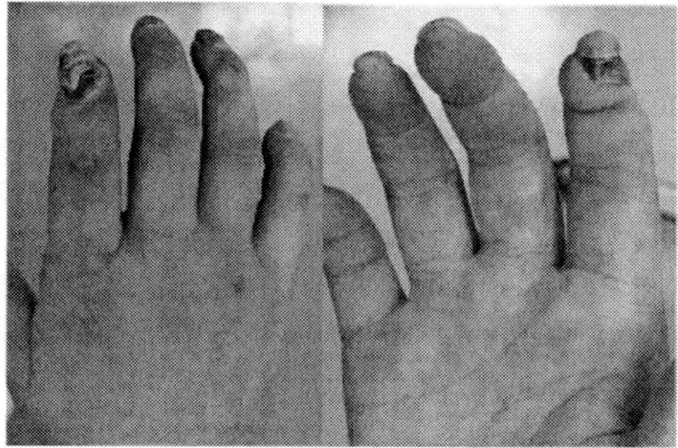

Figure 16. Necrosis of fingertip in systemic sclerosis.

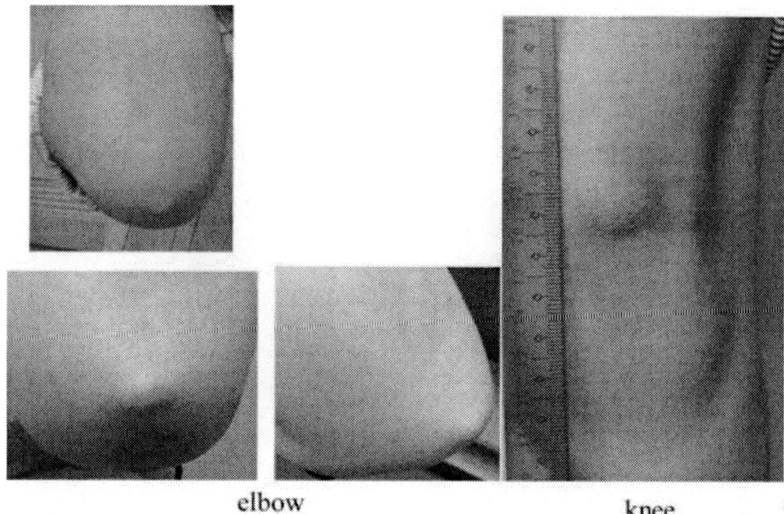

Figure 17. Rheumatoid nodule in RA

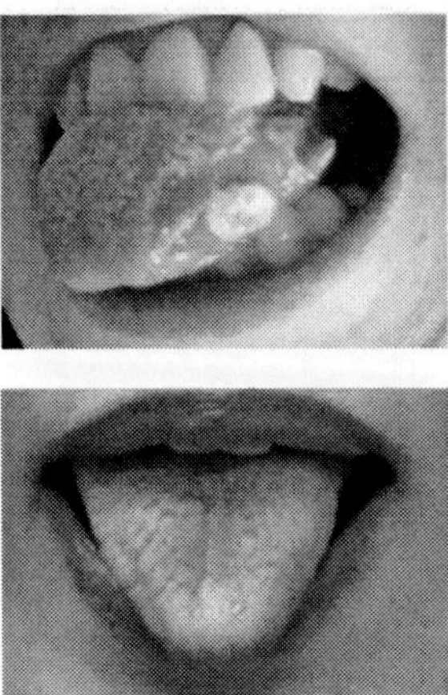

Figure 18. Oral ulcer in Behçet's Disease and glossitis in Sjögren's syndrome.

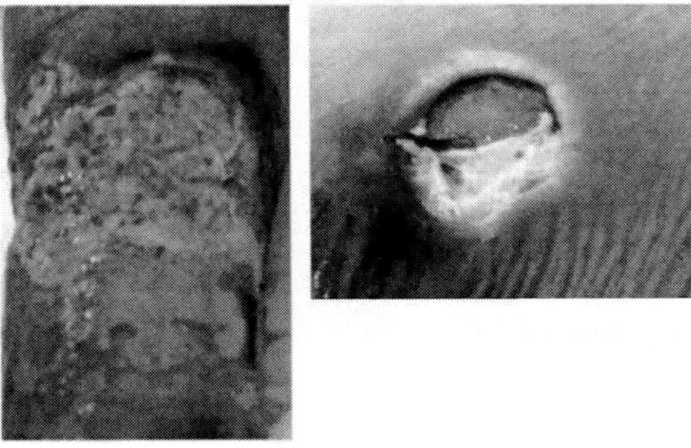

Figure 19. Skin ulcer in a patient with rheumatoid vasculitis.

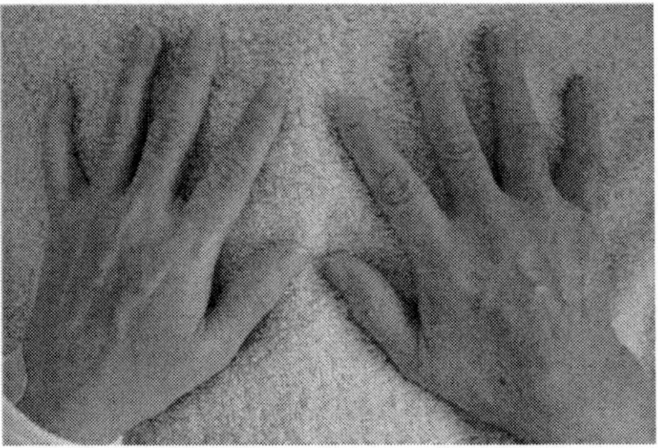

Figure 20. Mild swollen joints of the hand in PM.

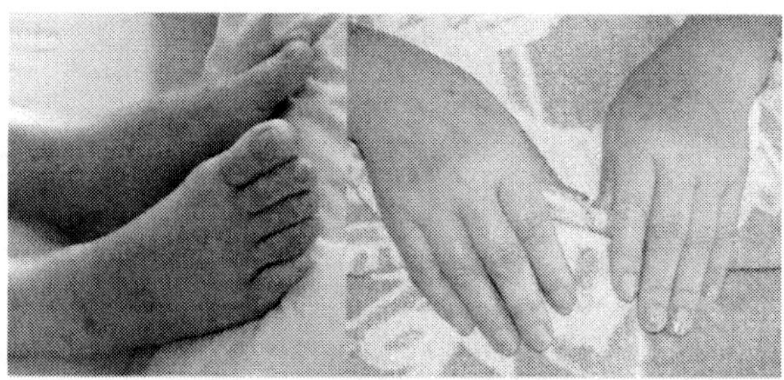

Figure 21. Primary RS3PE.

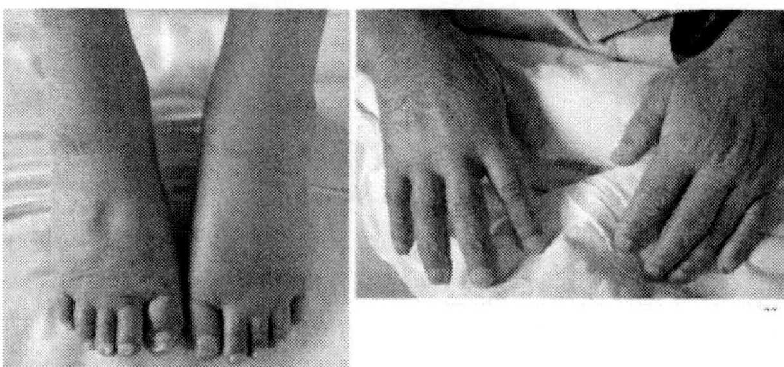

Figure 22. Secondary RS3PE (malignancy: lung cancer).

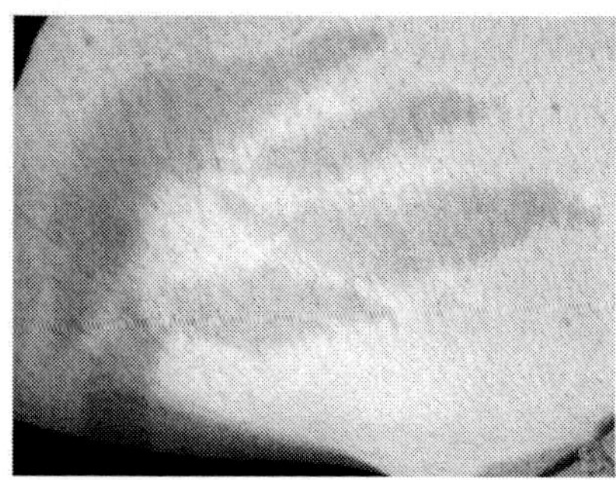

Figure 23. Striate cutis induced by glucocorticoid.

Eyes

Exophthalmus	Wegener's granulomatosis (Granulomatosis with polyangiits; GPA)*
Iritis or uveitis	Behçct's disease (hypopyon)*, Spondyloarthropathies, sarcoidosis, Wegener's granulomatosis (Granulomatosis with polyangiits; GPA)
Conjunctiviti	Spondyloarthropathies, SLE, GPA
Dry eyes	Sjögren's syndrome
Cytoid bodies (retinal exudates)	SLE
Scleritis	RA, relapsing polychondritis*
Ischemic optic neuritis	Giant cell arteritis, GPA

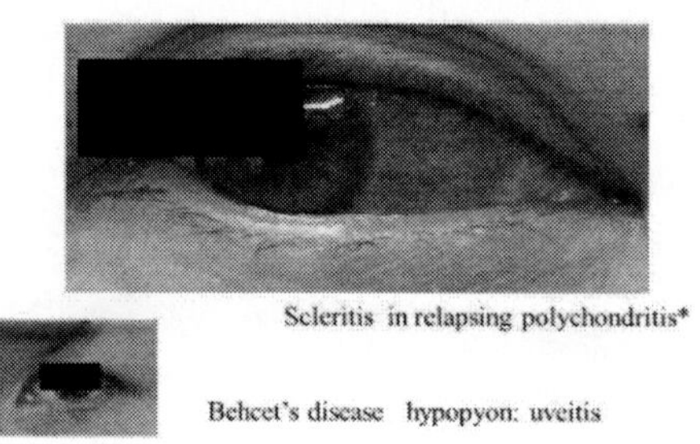

Figure 24.

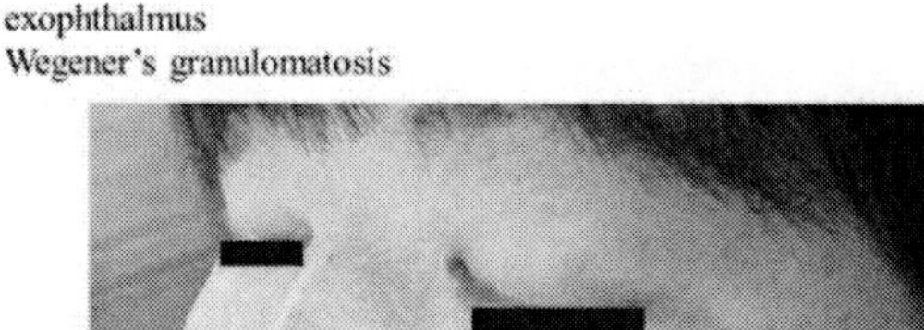

Figure 25.

Ears, Nose, and Throat

Parotid enlargement	Sjögren's syndrome, sarcoidosis
Macroglossia	Amyloidosis
Bloody or severe sinusitis	GPA
Inflammation of ear, sparing the lobe	Relapsing polychondritis*

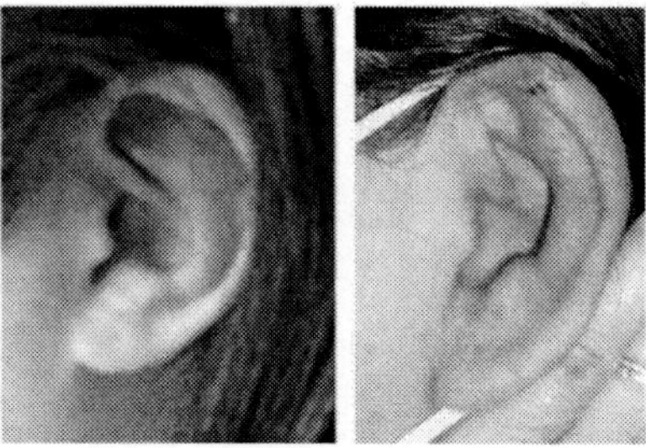

Figure 26. Inflammation of ear, sparing the lobe in Relapsing polychondritis.

SECTION 2. CARDIO-PULMONARY EXAMINATION

Chest radiograph and CT

Pleural effusion (pleuritis, serositis)	SLE, RA
Hematothorax	
Interstitial pneumonitis	RA, scleroderma, PM/DM
Early change	

Pulmonary fibrosis
Upper lobe fibrosis | Ankylosing spondylitis

Pulmonary hemorrhage
BOOP | SLE
Nodular lesion | RA, sarcoidosis, GPA
Pulmonary MALT Lymphoma | Sjögren's syndrome

Pericardial effusion
Pulmonary hypertension
Infections

Electrocardiogram
Right ventricular overloading | pulmonary hypertension
Atrioventricular block | Lyme disease, neonatal lupus, ankylosing spondylitis

Chest CT

To detect early change of interstitial pneumonia and nodular lesions due to rheumatic diseases.

To observe pulmonary lesions during diseases and evaluate efficacy of treatment.

To find pulmonary lesions of adverse effects due to treatment, infections, and malignacy.

Chest CT is a powerful modality for above purposes.

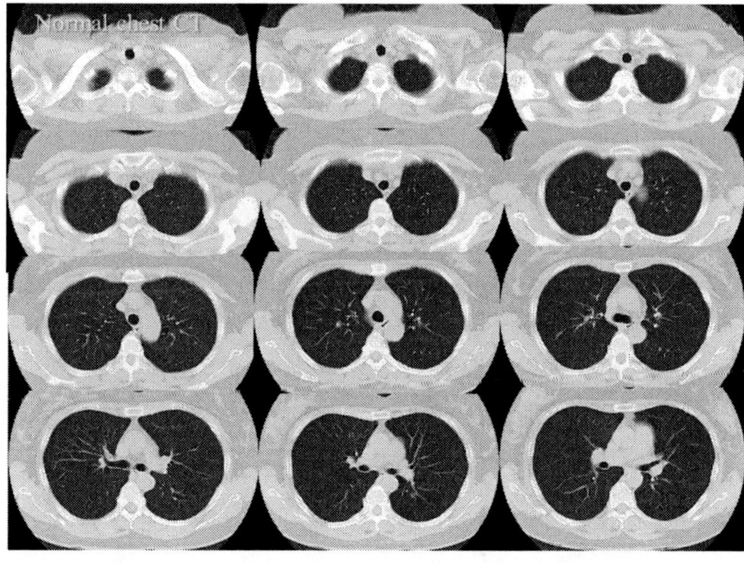

Figure 1. Normal chest CT.

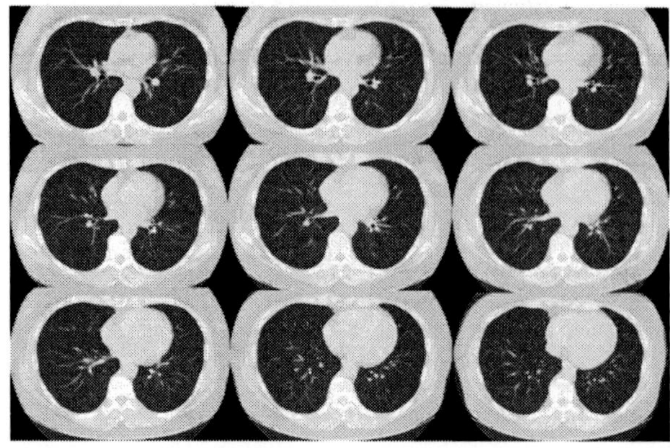

Figure 2. Normal chest CT.

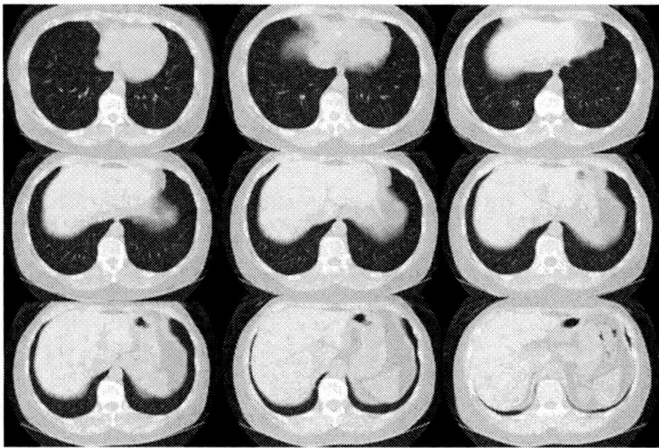

Figure 3. Normal chest CT.

Chest radiograph

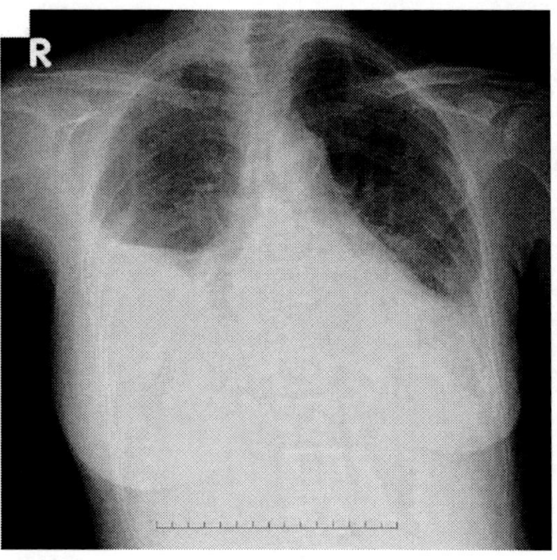

Figure 4. Pleuritis and effusion in a 64-year-old female with SLE.

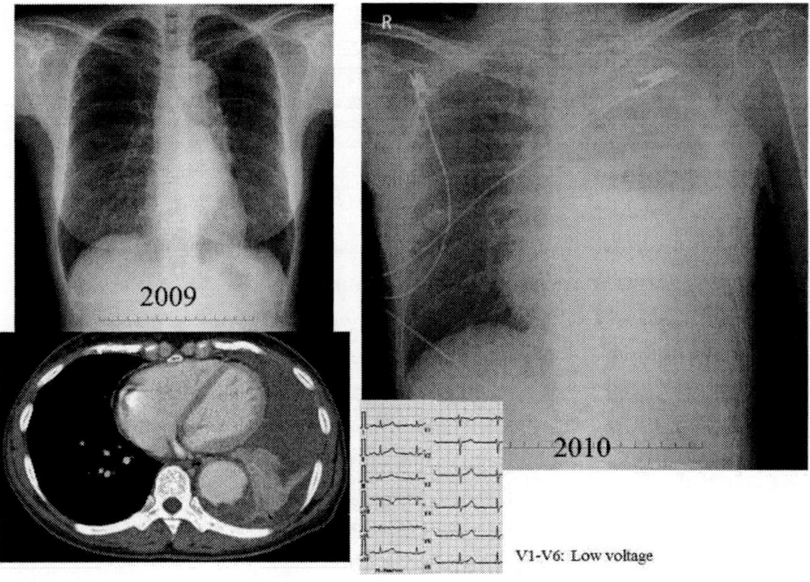

Figure 5. Rupture of aorta.

41-year-old Female with Behçet's disease.

Interstitial pneumonitis

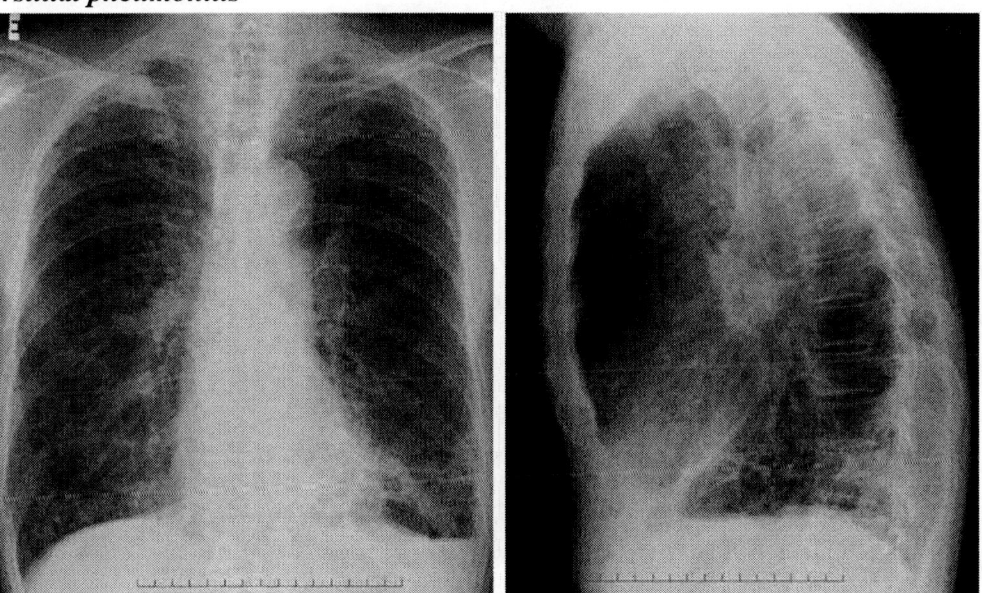

Figure 6. RA lung.

In some cases, interstitial pneumonia follows by rheumatic disease.

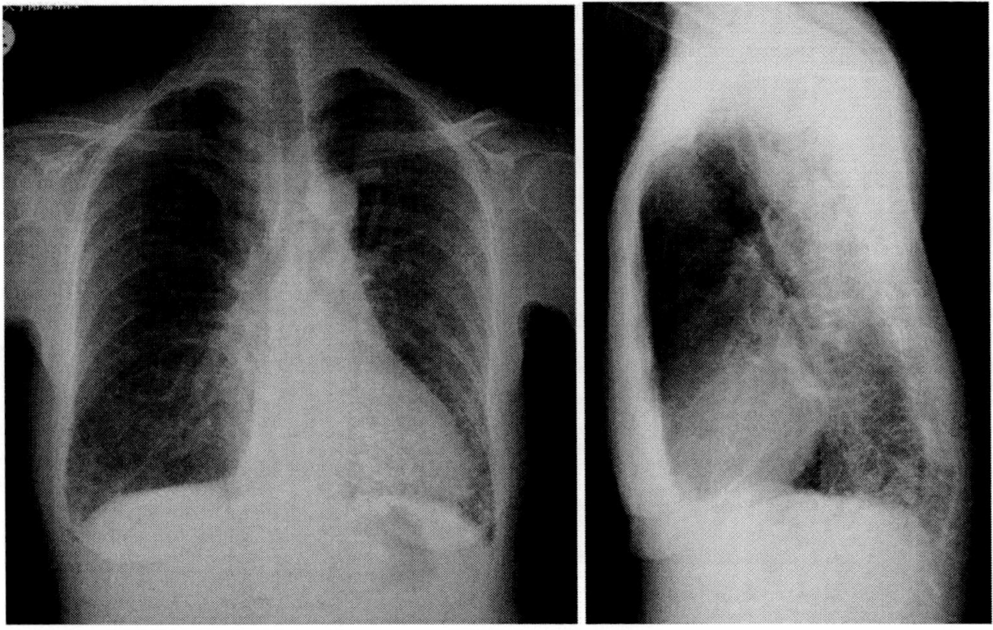

Figure 7. Interstitial pneumonitis. A 66-year-old female with polymyositis.

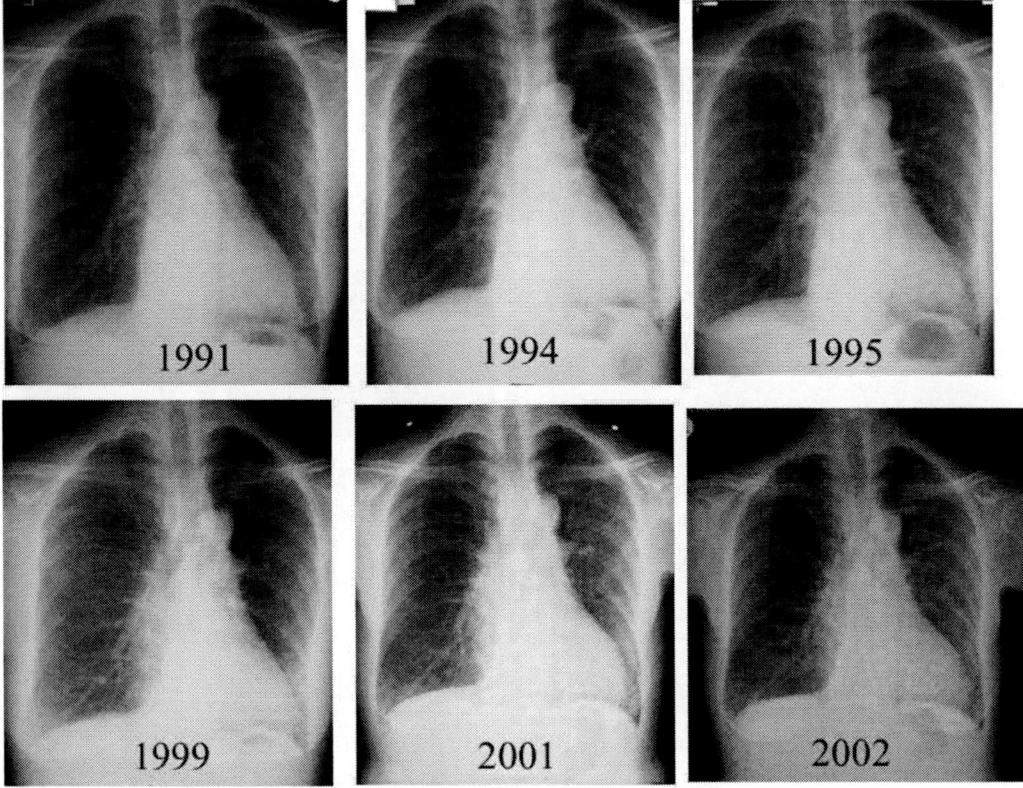

Figure 8. Pulmonary fibrosis in a DM patient: slowly progression.

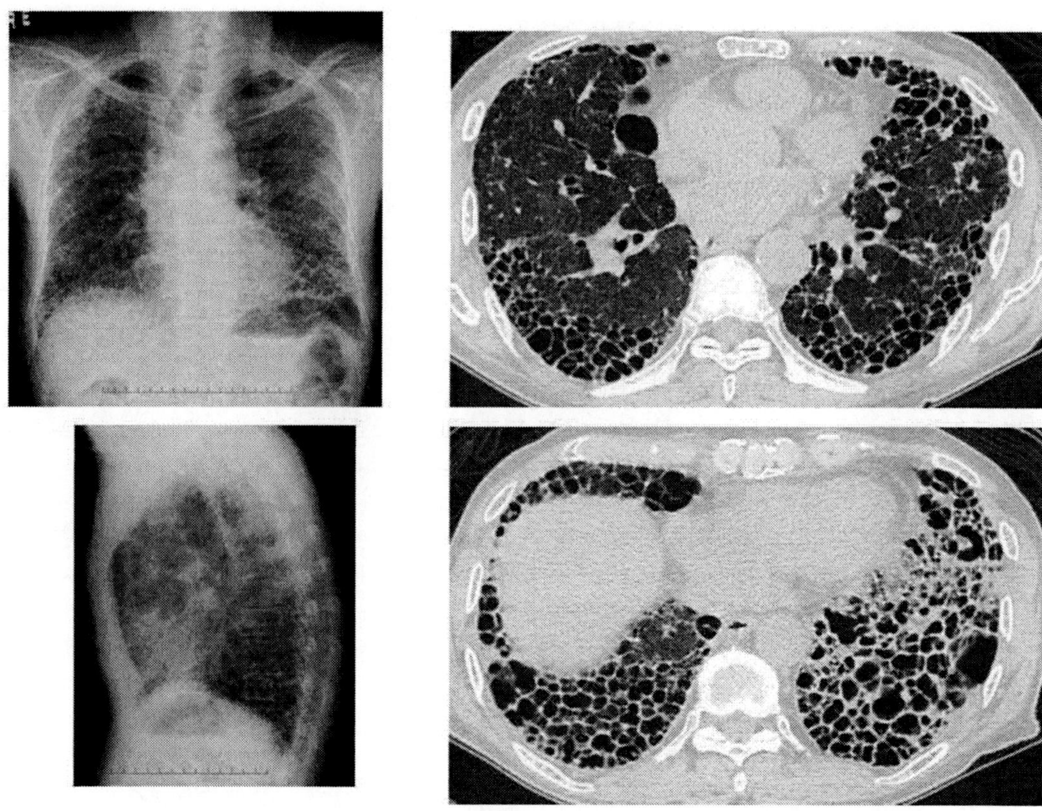

Figure 9. Honey comb lung in mPA patients.

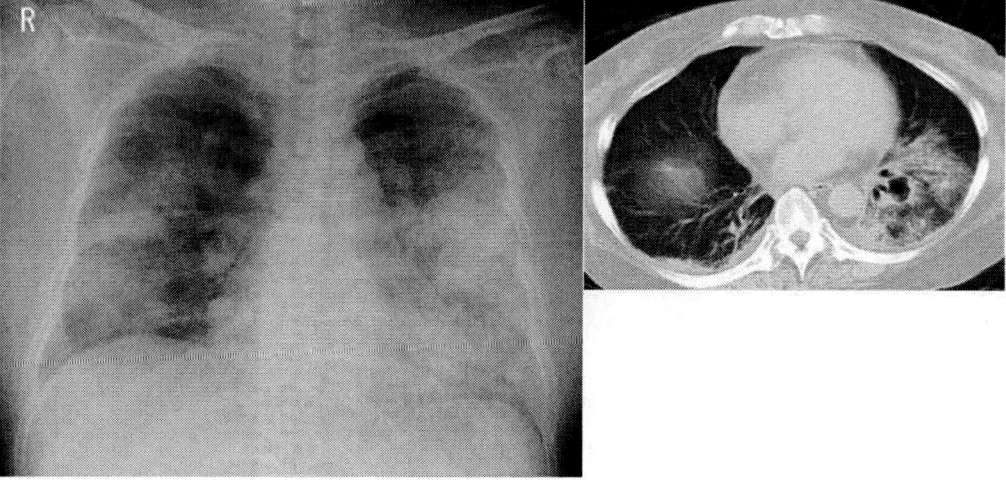

Figure 10. Pulmonary hemorrhage, severe in mPA.

Cherry-blossom like appearance
Pulmonary hemorrhage may occur in SLE,mPA, WG

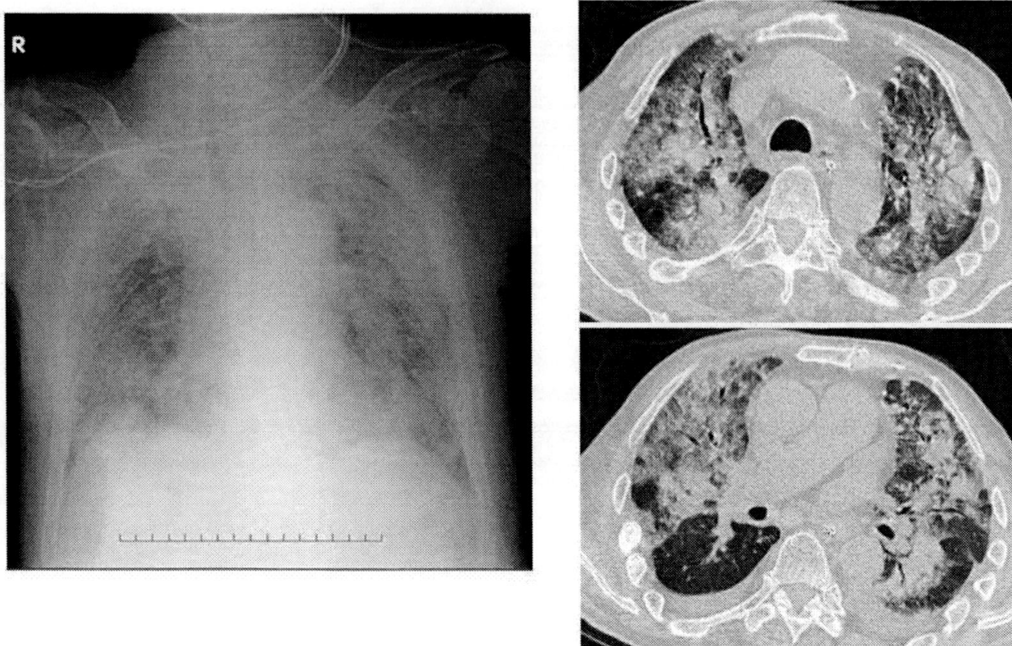

Figure 11. Pulmonary hemorrhage, severe in WG.

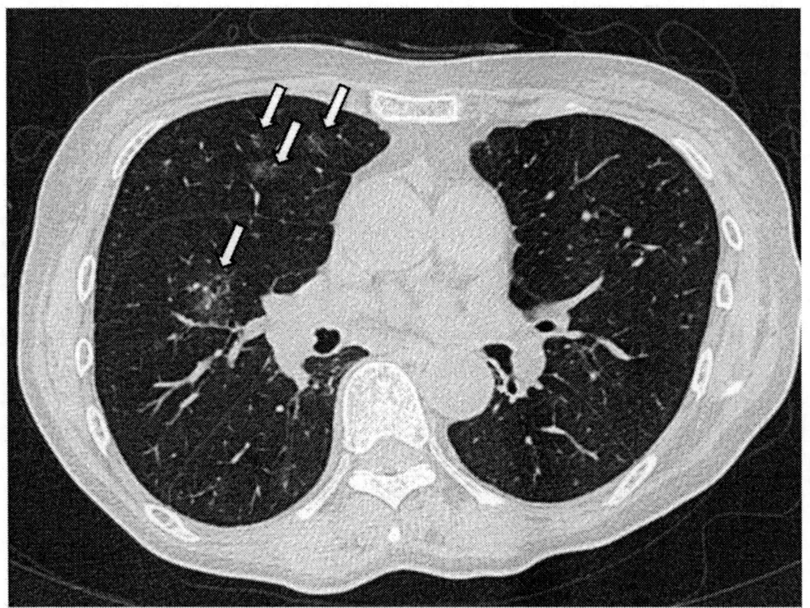

Figure 12. Early stage of Pulmonary hemorrhage in mPA.

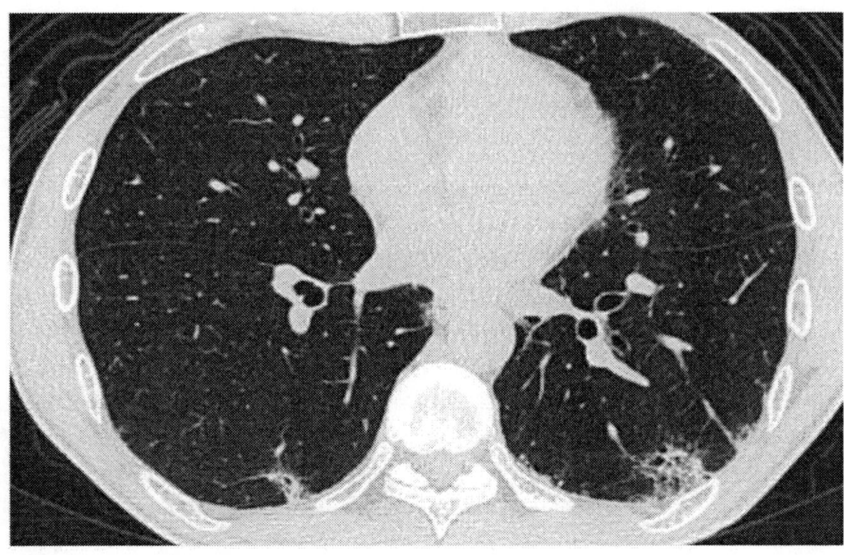

Figure 13. BOOP type pneumonitis in amyopathic DM patient.

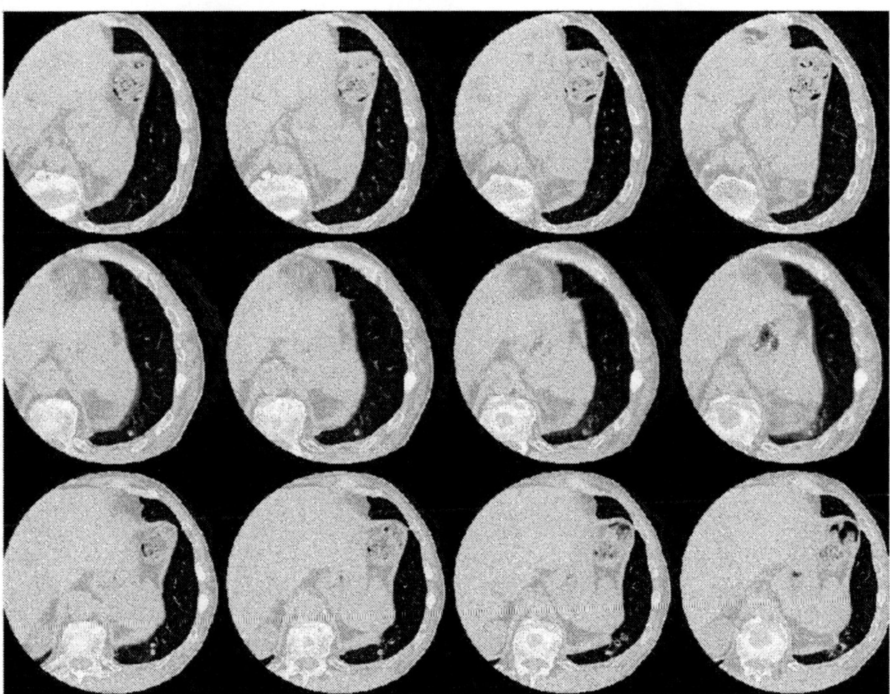

Figure 14. Early nodular lesion in WG.

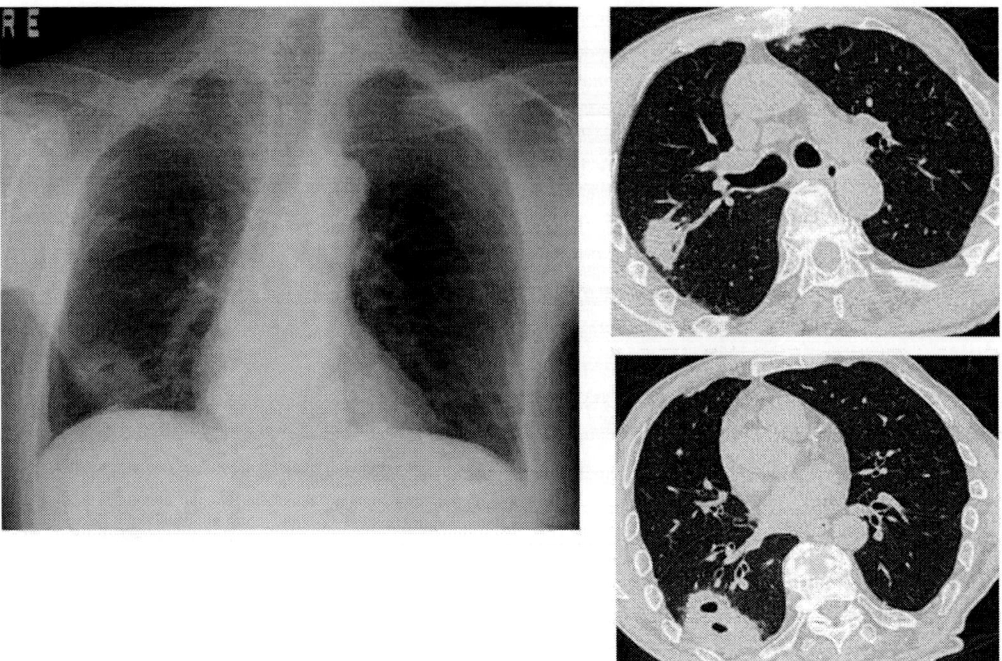

Figure 15. Lung granuloma in WG.

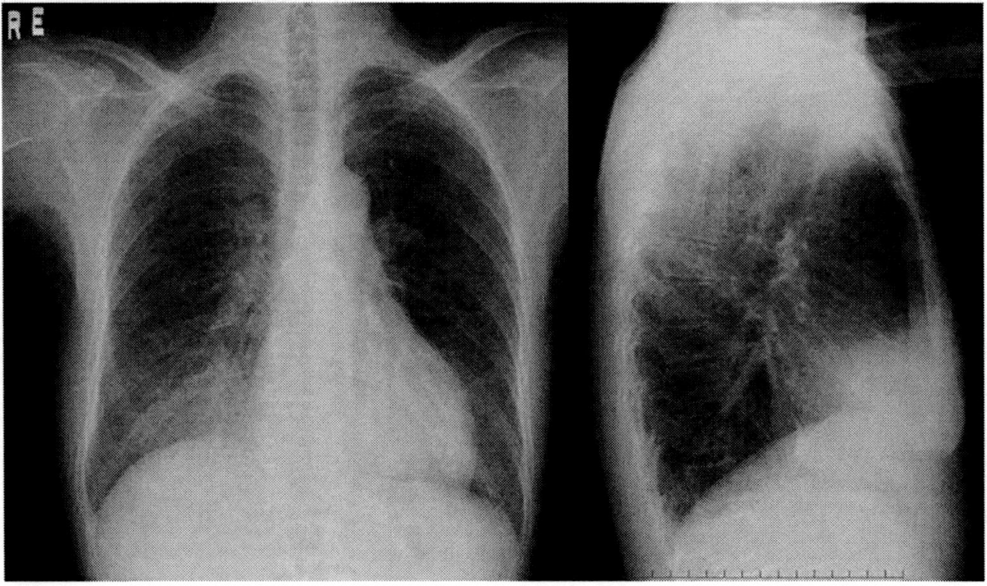

Figure 16. A 60 –year-old female Pulmonary MALT Lymphoma in Sjögren's syndrome.

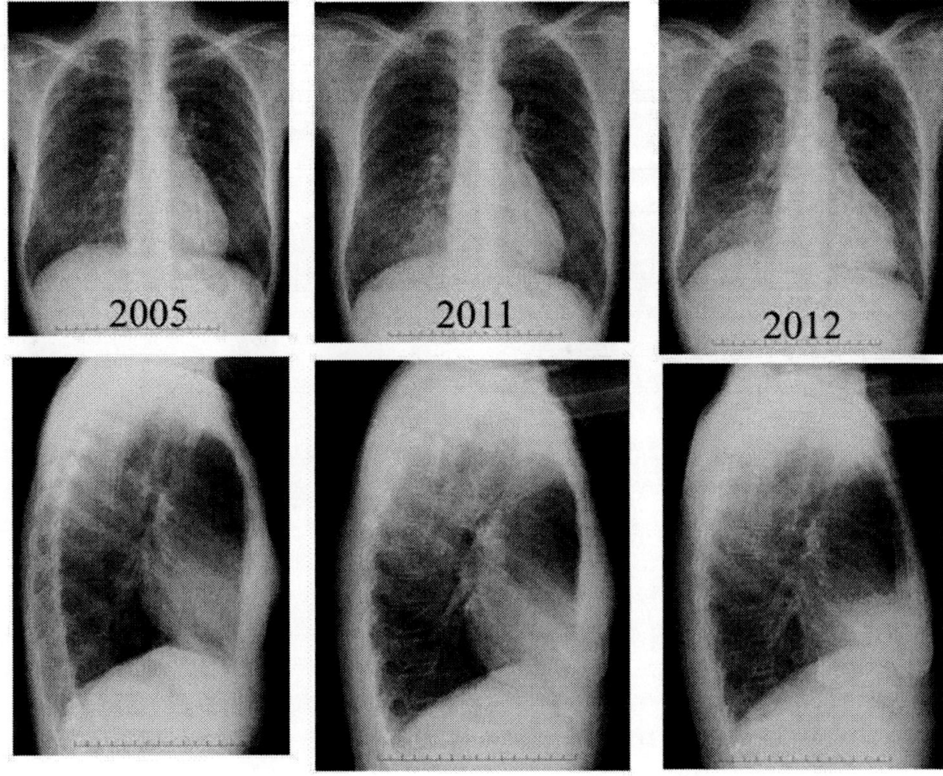

Figure 17. Series of chest X-ray.

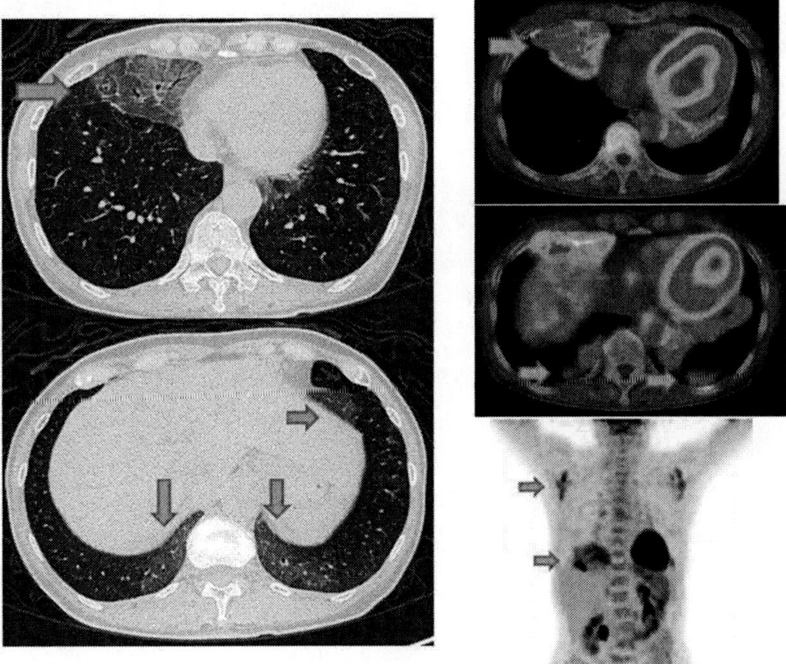

Figure 18. Chest CT and PET. Uptake at lungs and lymph nodes.

Lung biopsy

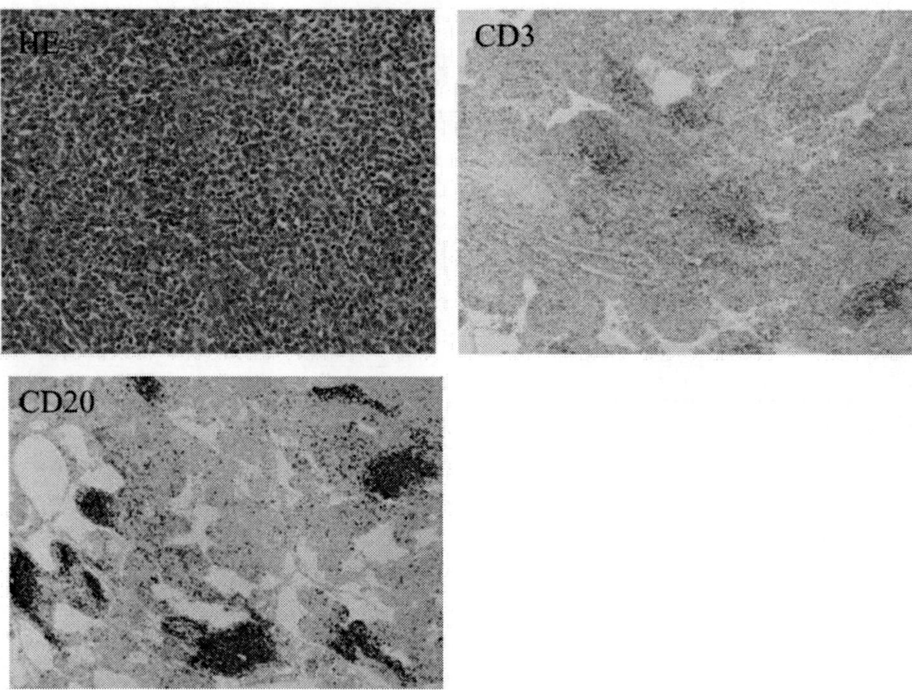

Figure 19. Infiltrating CD20+ lymphocytes.

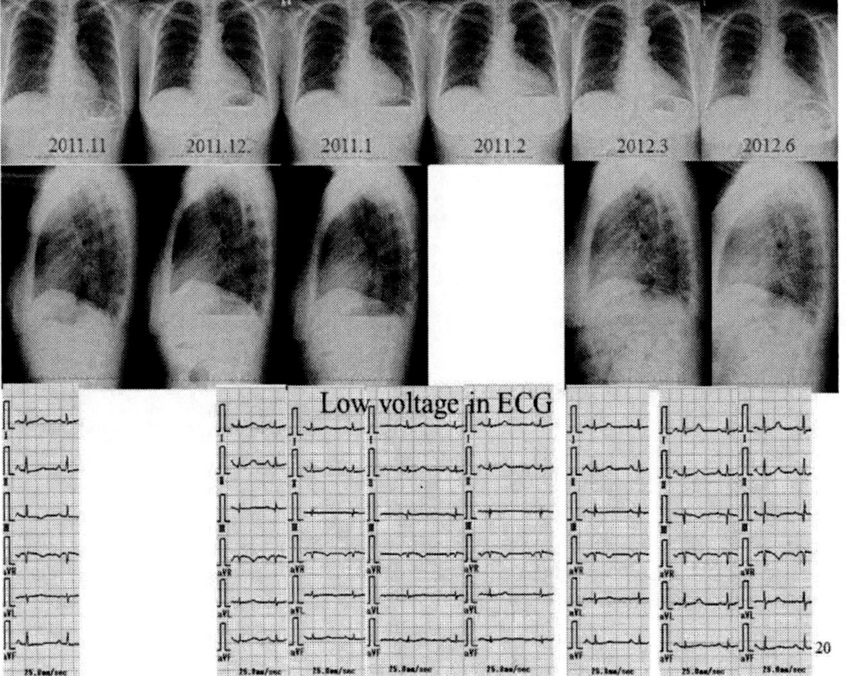

Figure 20. 49-year-old Female. Pericariditis in PM patient.

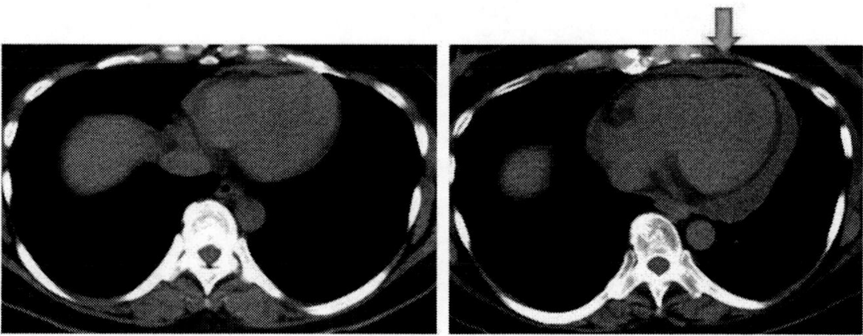

Figure 21. Pericardial effusion in CT.

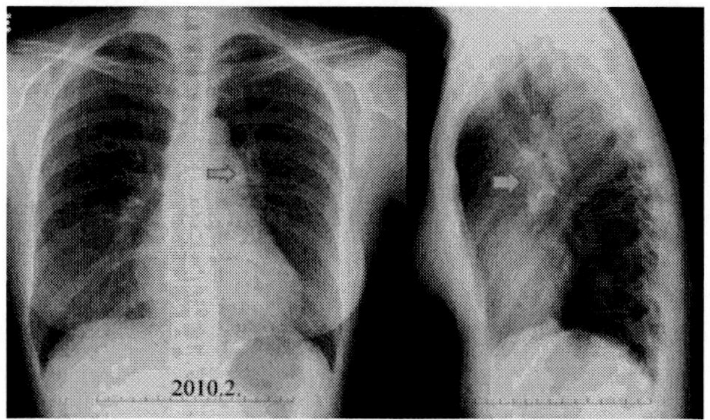

Figure 22. Pulmonary hypertension in SLE patient.

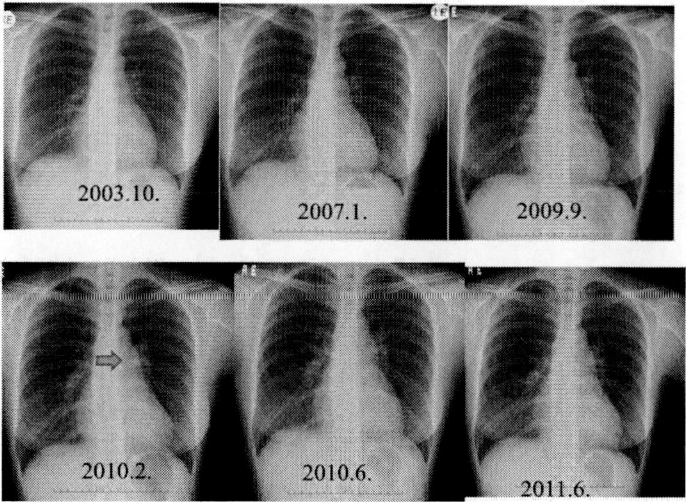

Figure 23. Pulmonary hypertension in a 30-year-old female with SLE.

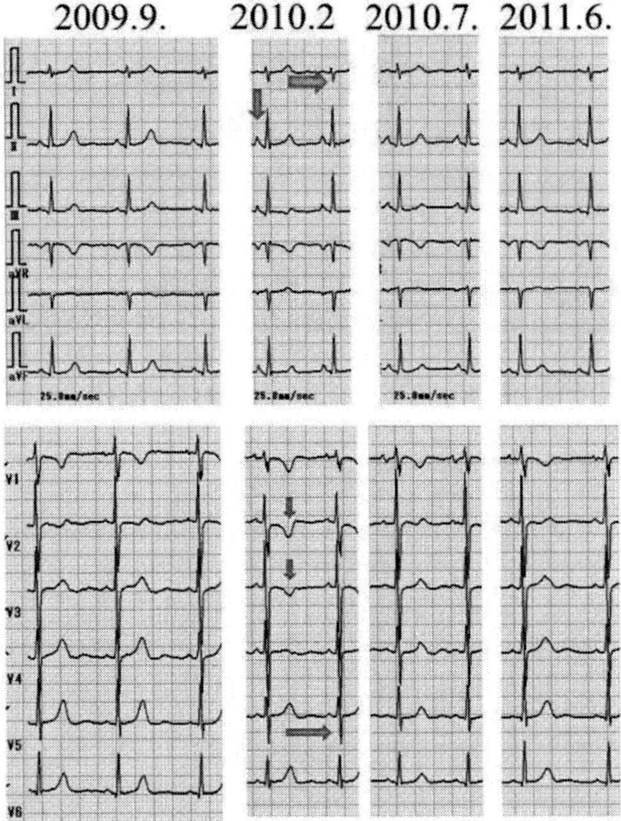

Figure 24. Pulmonary hypertension in SLE patient.

PH: SLE, SSc, MCTD, PM/DM, Sjögren's

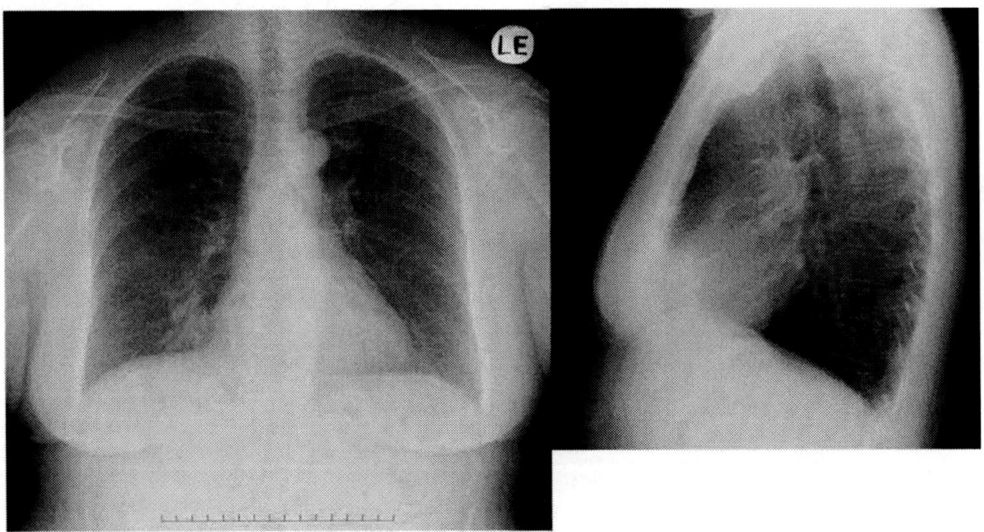

Figure 25. Pneumonia in RA patient treated with biological agent.

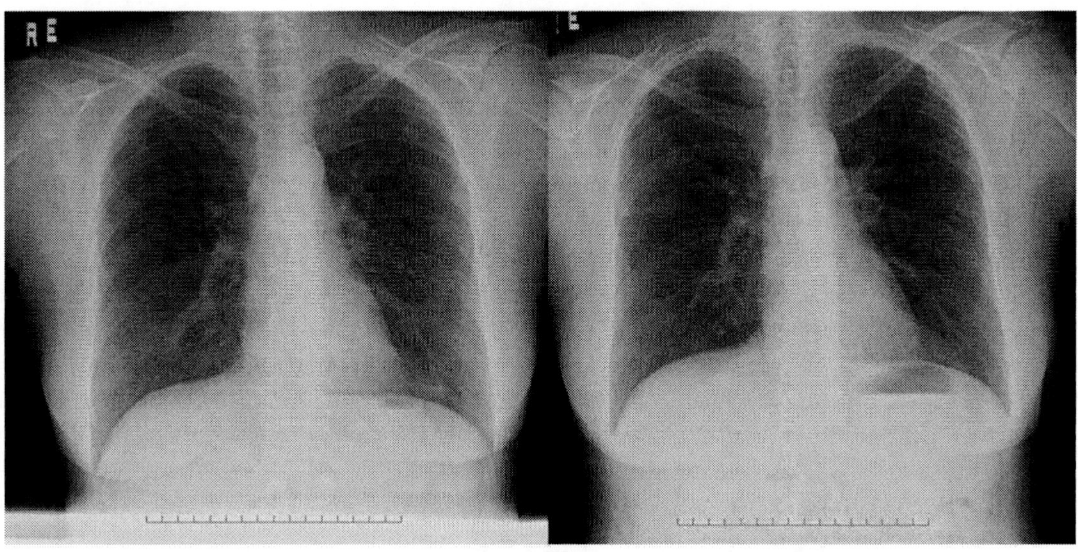

Figure 26. Bacterial pneumonia after treatment with cyclophosphamide in SLE patient.

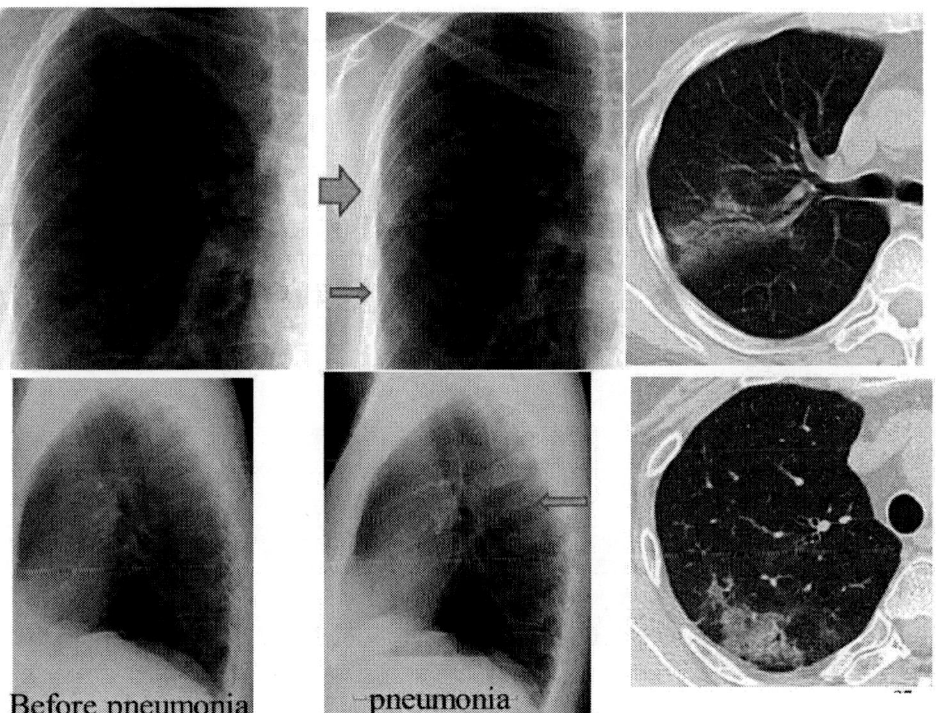

Figure 27. Bacterial pneumonia after treatment with cyclophosphamide in SLE patient.

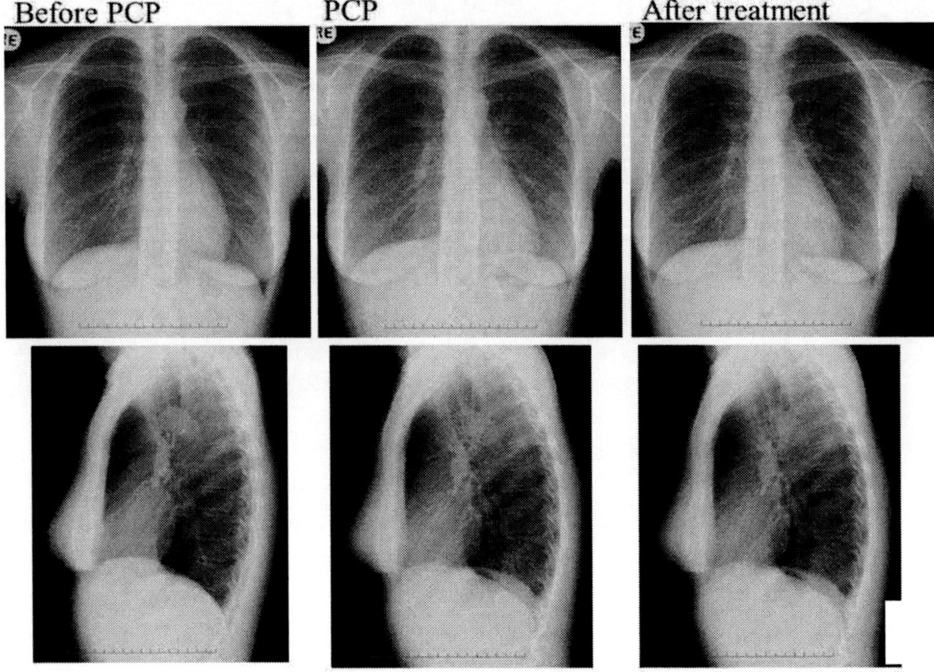

Figure 28. Pneumocystis pneumonia.

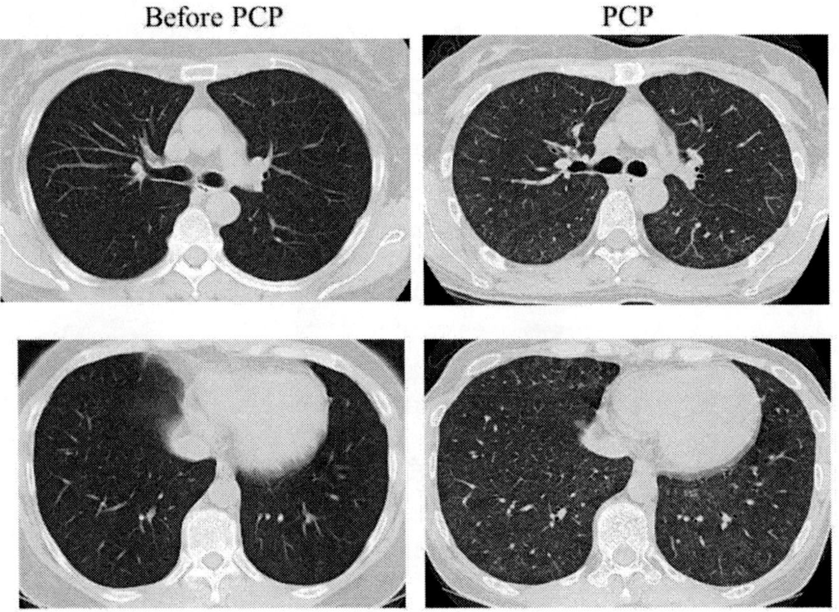

Figure 29. Pneumocystis pneumonia.

A 30-year-old Female with SLE

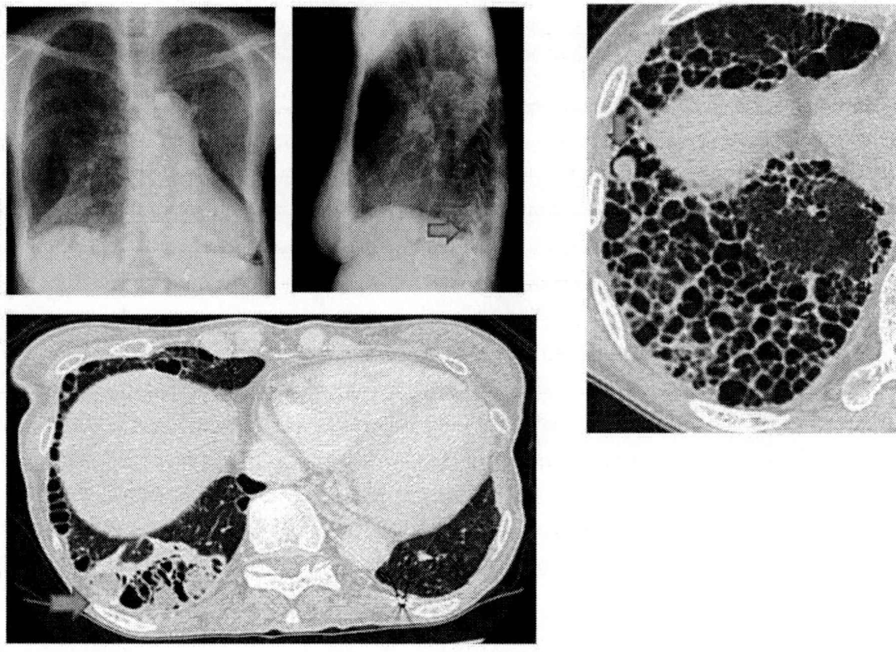

Figure 30. Pulmonary aspergillus in SLE.

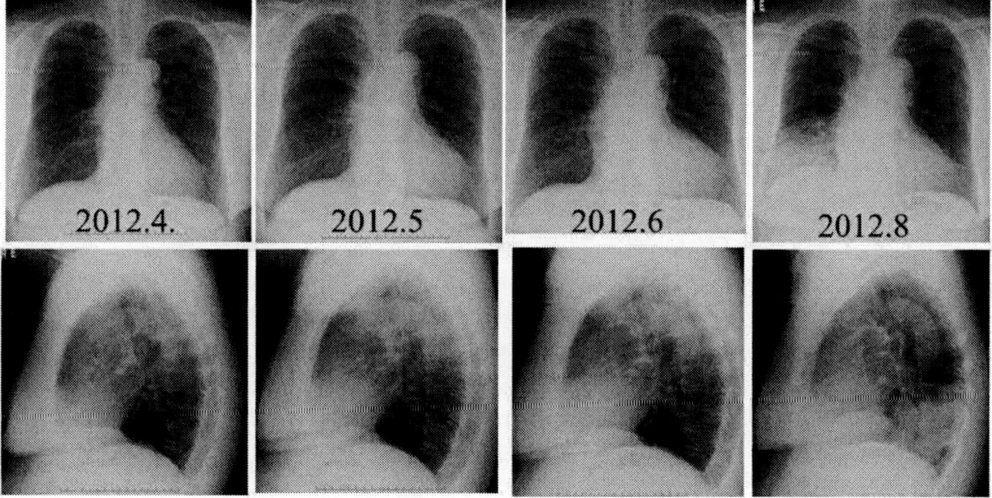

Figure 31. Pulmonary cryptococcosis in WG.

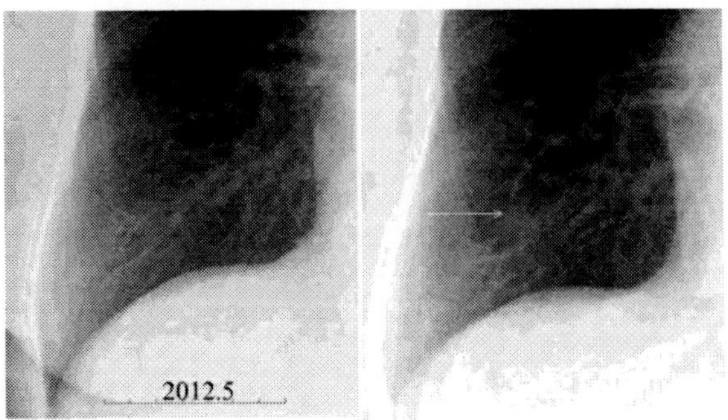

Figure 32. Pulmonary cryptococcosis in WG.

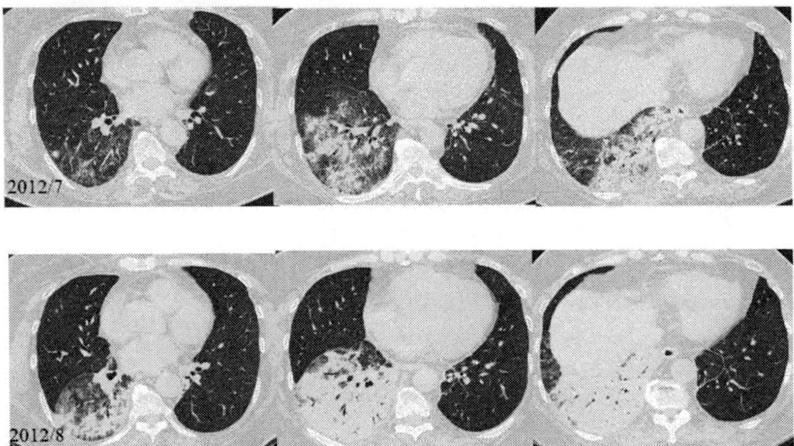

Figure 33. Pulmonary cryptococcosis in WG.

Pulmonary tuberculosis in SLE

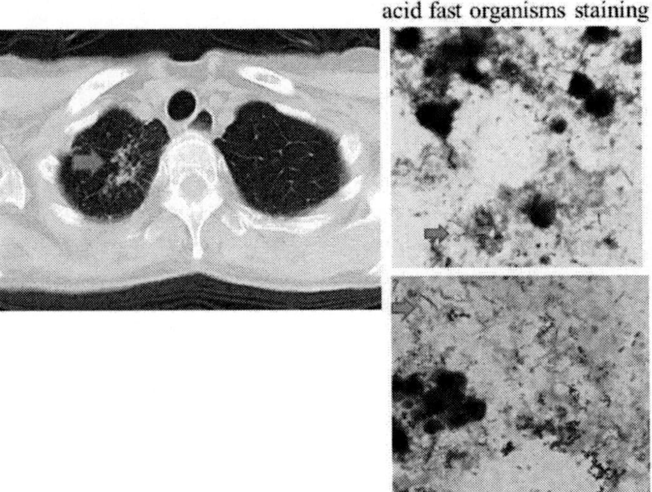

Figure 34. A 65-year-old female with SLE.

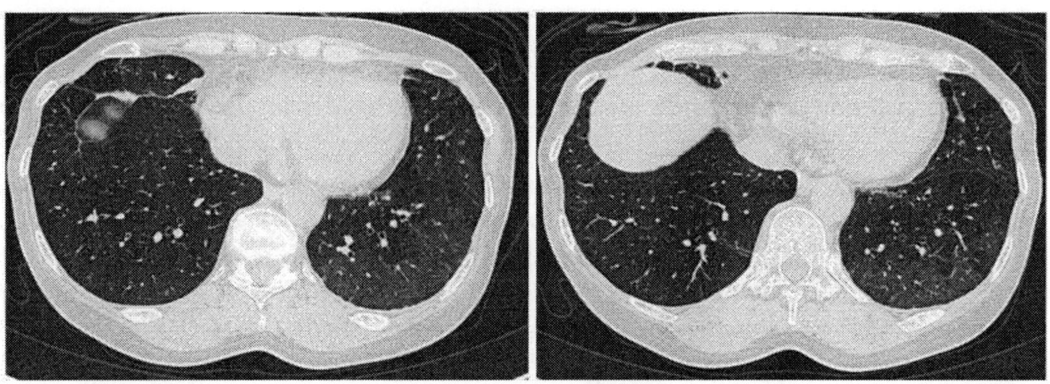

Figure 35. MTX lung in RA patient.

SECTION 3. ULTRASONOGRAPHY

- Grey scale and Doppler signals (red color)
- Synovitis
- Joint effusion
- Bone erosion
- Osteophyte

Ultrasonography is more sensitive for the detection of erosions

The synovitis

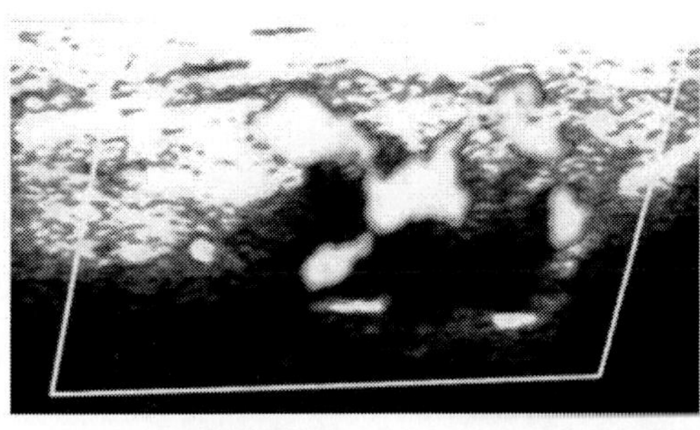

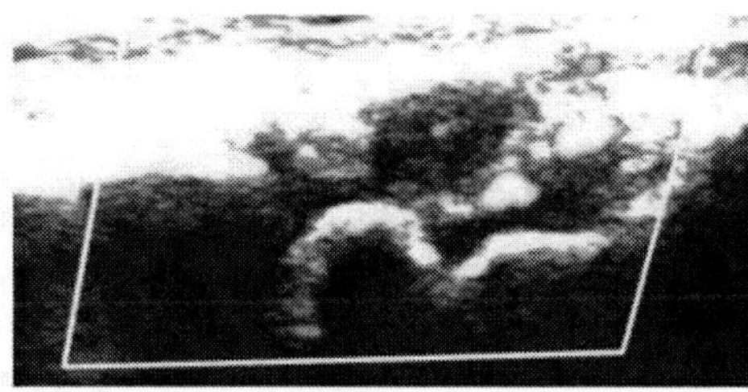

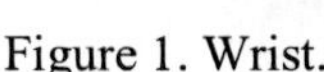

Figure 1. Wrist.

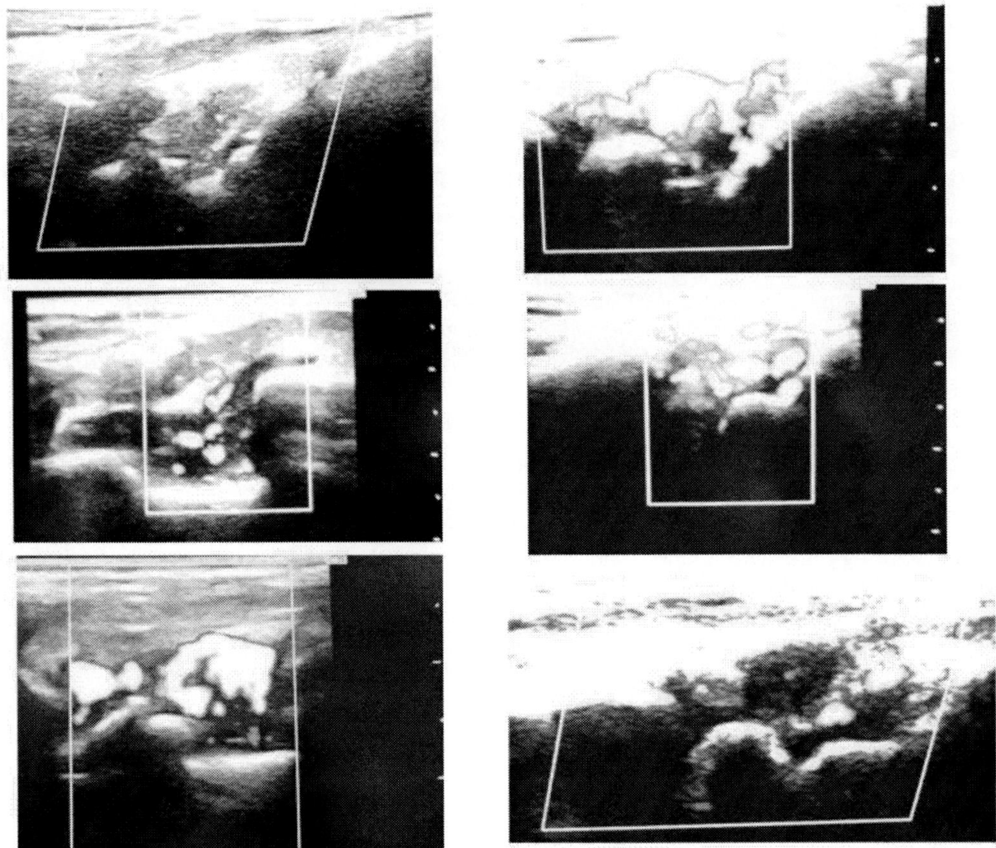

Figure 2. Synovitis of the radiocarpal and midcarpal joints of the wrist in RA patients is observed in the dorsal longitudinal view. Doppler signals (red color) are in the thickened synovium.

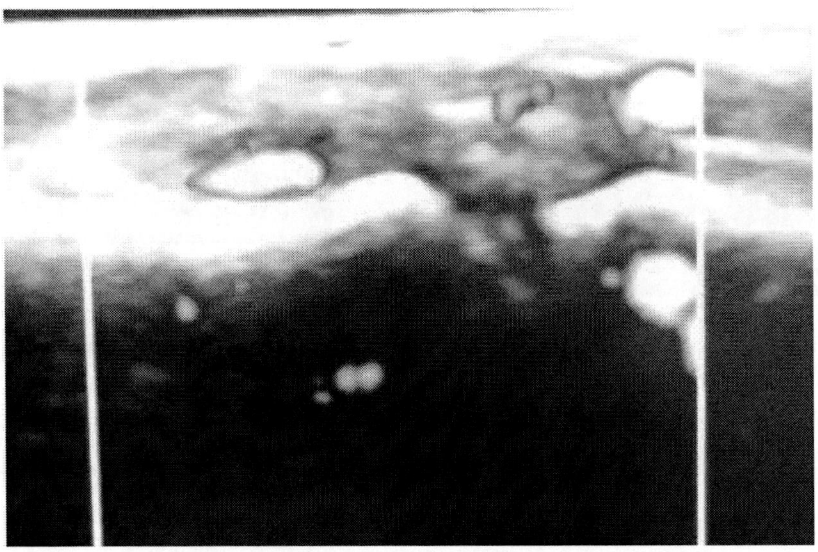

Figure 3. The PIP joint. Doppler signals (red color) are found even in the small joint.

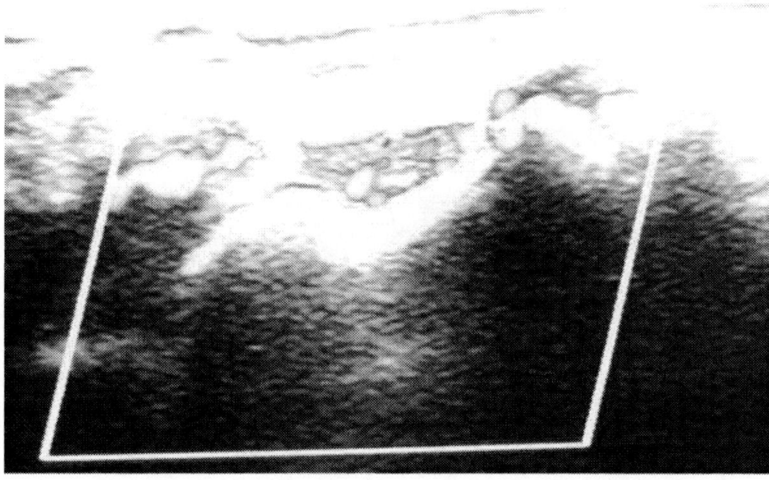

Figure 4. The Elbow. Synovitis in RA.

The Knee

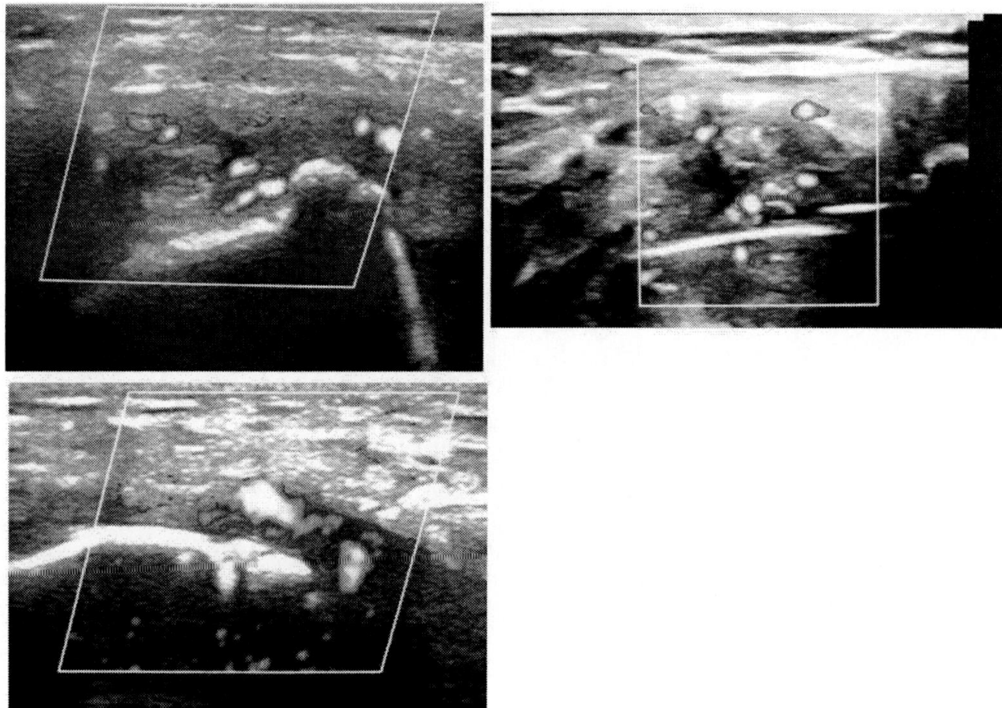

Figure 5. Synovitis in RA.

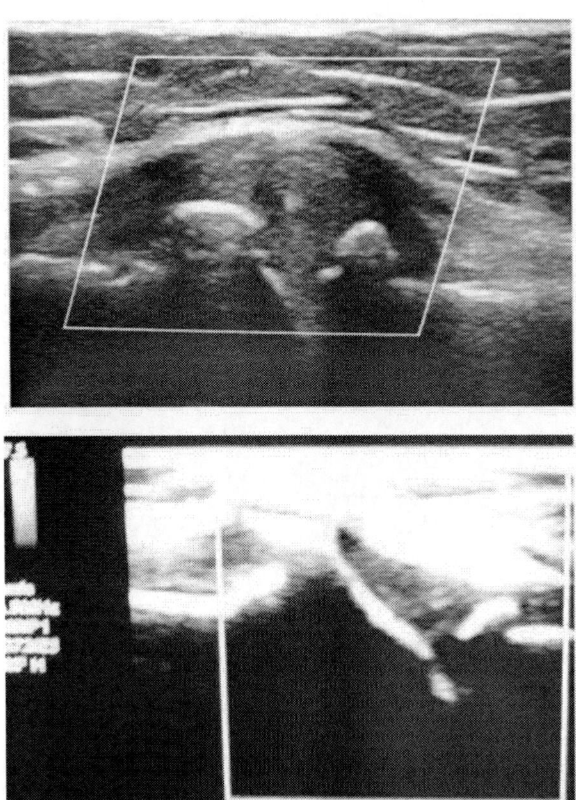

Figure 6. OA.

Thickness Synovium and joint effusion (+)
No Doppler signal

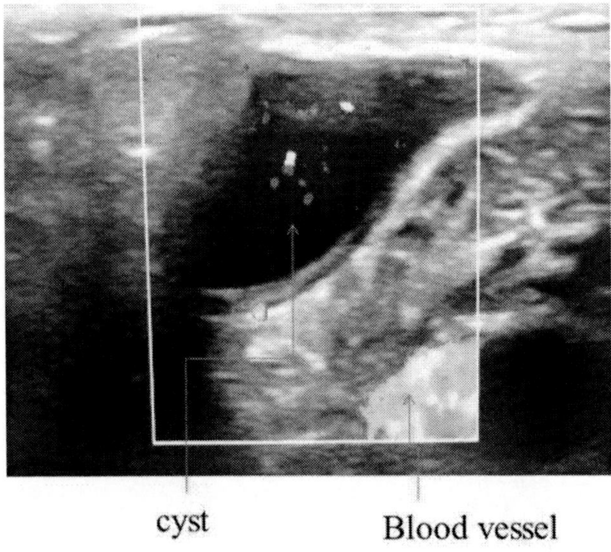

Figure 7. Baker's cyst at the knee of a RA patient.

SECTION 4. MRI

Magnetic resonance imaging (MRI) is one of the most important tools in diagnosis of rheumatic disease.

MRI is more sensitive for the detection of early changes than plain radiography. In very early stage of RA, only MRI can detect bone edema.

Moreover, bone erosions, synovitis, and joint fluid can be detected, that have not been seen in a plain radiography.

Especially, to study the soft tissue, MRI shows inflammatory myositis and edematous change in angiitis exclusively compared with other tools. In the surveying the patient with angiitis, MR-angiography is a non-invasive and powerful tool.

MRI findings of Typical RA

- Multiple erosions
- Synovitis
- Joint effusion
- Bone marrow edema (osteitis)
- Tenosynovitis

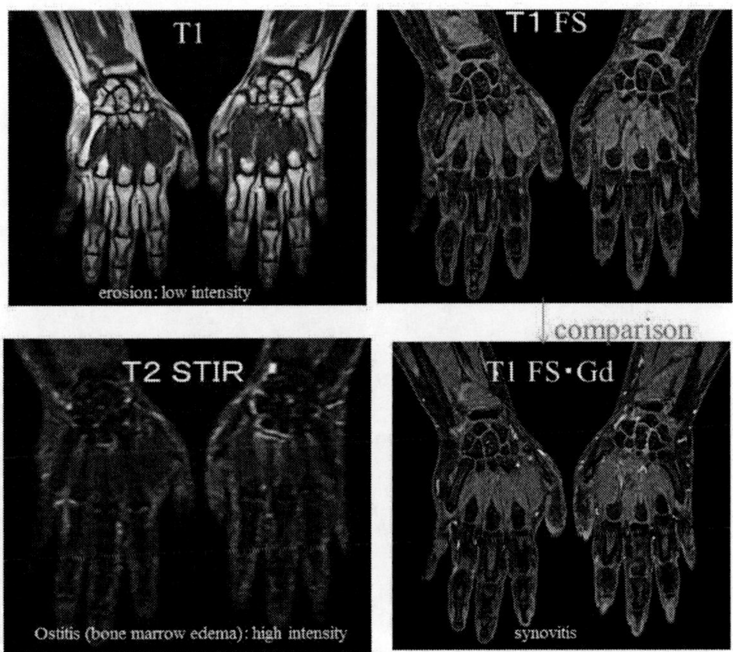

Figure 1. Very Early RA.

Very mild Ostitis (bone edema) and mild synovitis

Early RA (Figure 2)

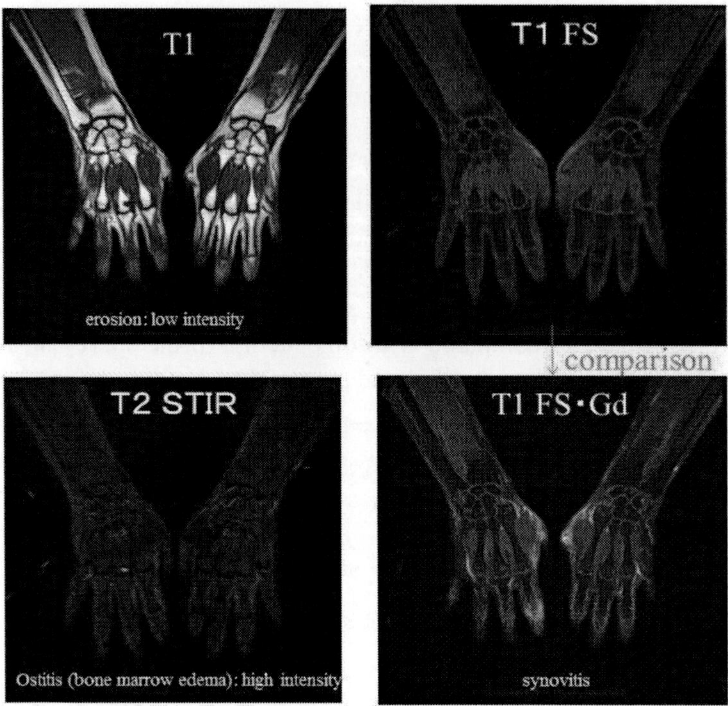

Figure 2. Ostitis (Bone edema) and mild synovitis.

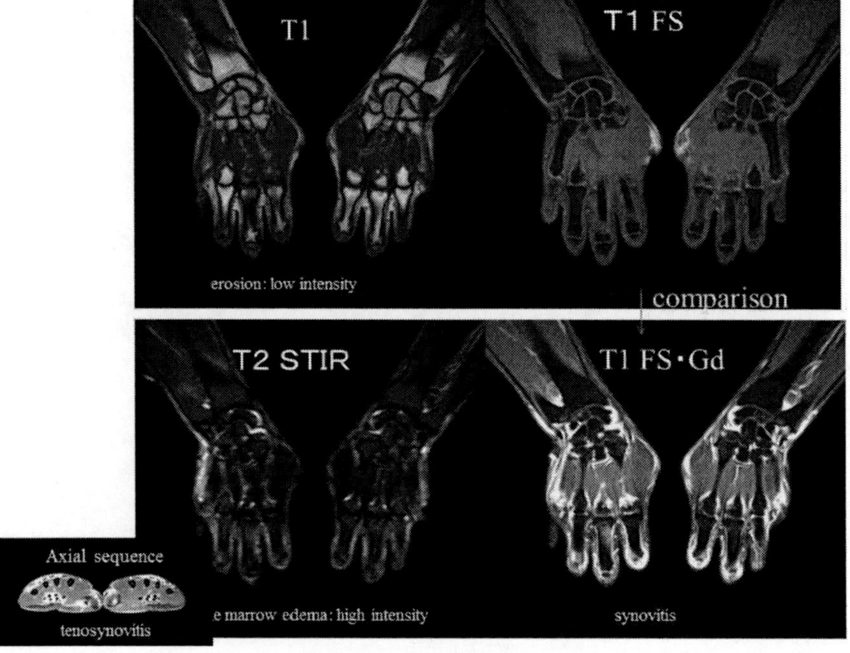

Figure 3. Early but Severe synovitis and tenosynovitis in RA.

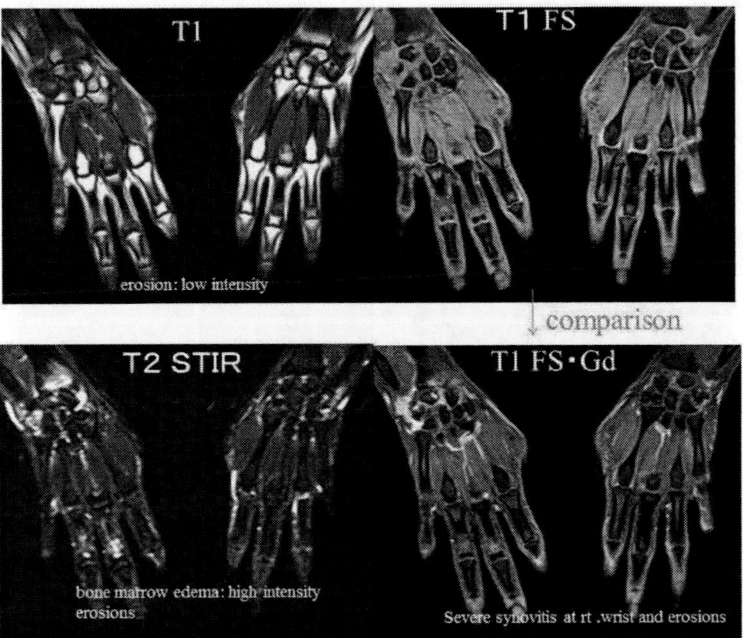

Figure 4. Complain mono-arthralgia at right wrist in early RA.

Severe synovitis at rt. wrist, however, lt. hand also shows arthritis with multiple small erosions.

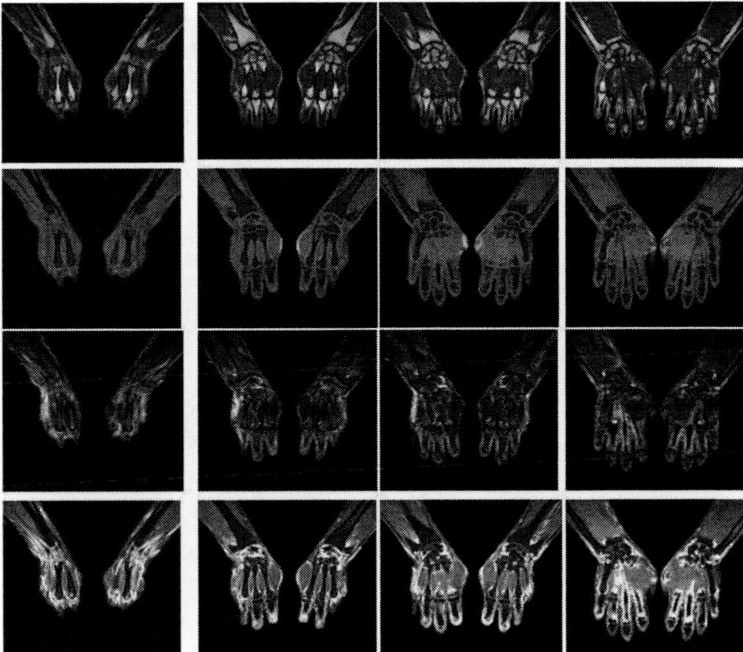

Figure 5. Coronal sequence.

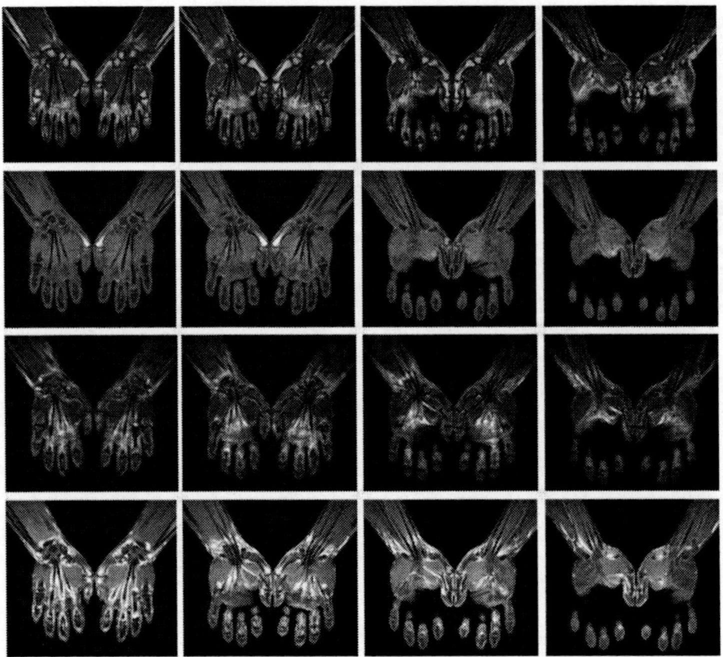

Figure 6.Coronal MRI of the hands can detect synovitis of the wrists, metacarpophalangeal joints and proximal interphalangeal joints in RA.

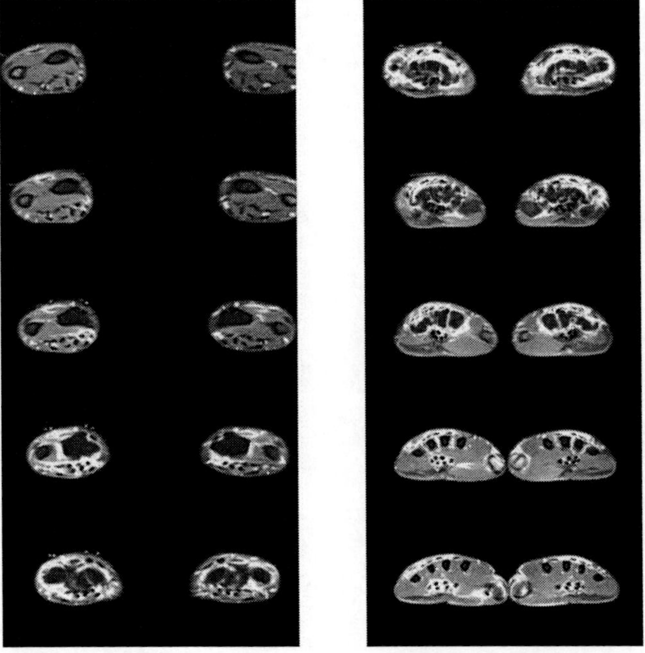

Figure 7. Axial sequence.

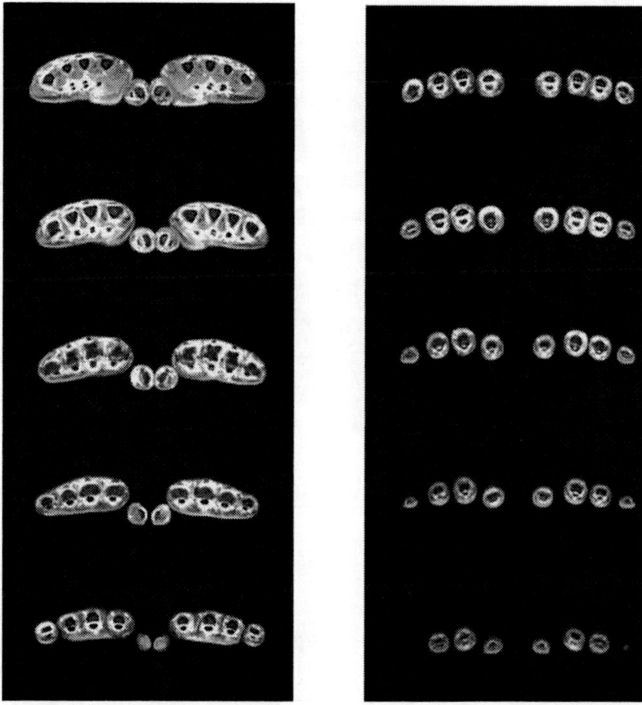

Figure 8. Axial sequence of hand MRI shows synovitis of the wrists, metacarpophalangal joints and proximal interphalangeal joints. Moreover, tenovitis of the extensor and flexor tendons in the bilateral hands was remarkable in this series.

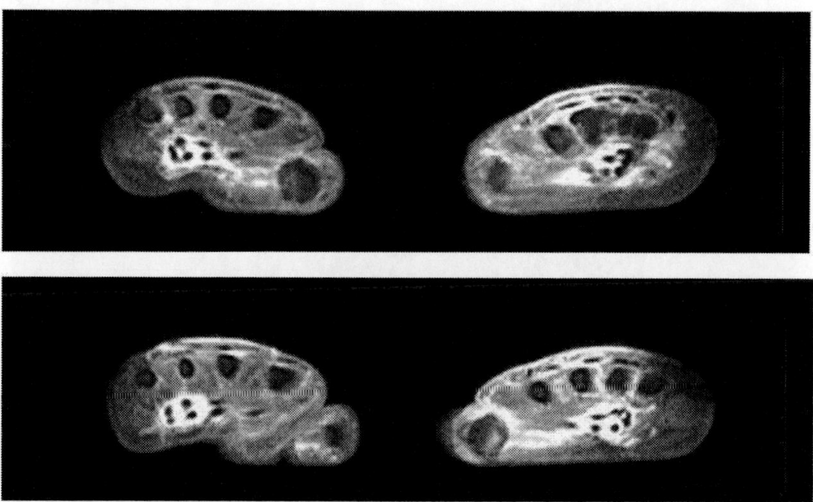

Figure 9. RS3PE syndrome.

MRI of the hands detects synovitis, tenosynovitis and subcutaneous edema of the dorsum.

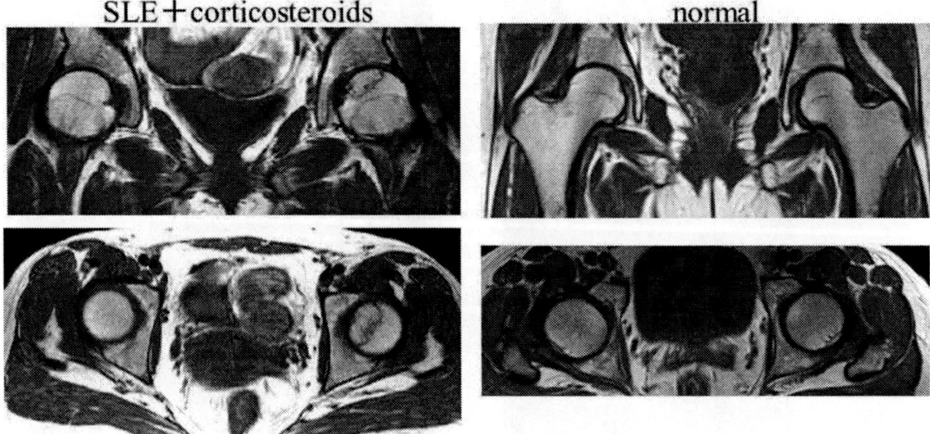

Figure 10. Osteonecrosis of femoral head (ONF) in SLE.

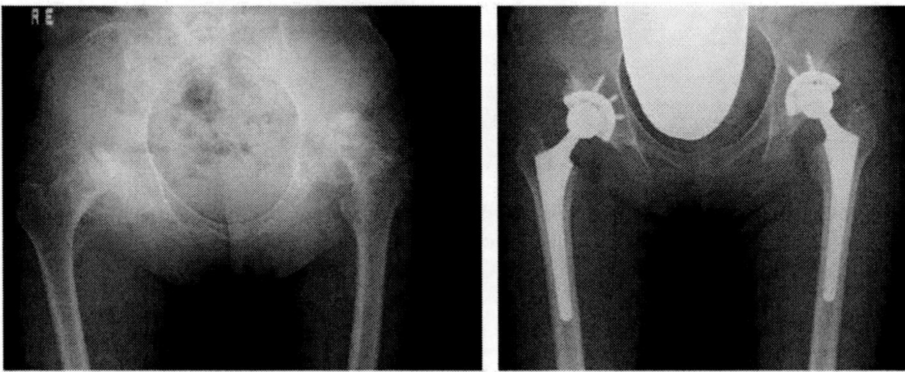

Figure 11. ONF in a 28-year-old female with SLE.

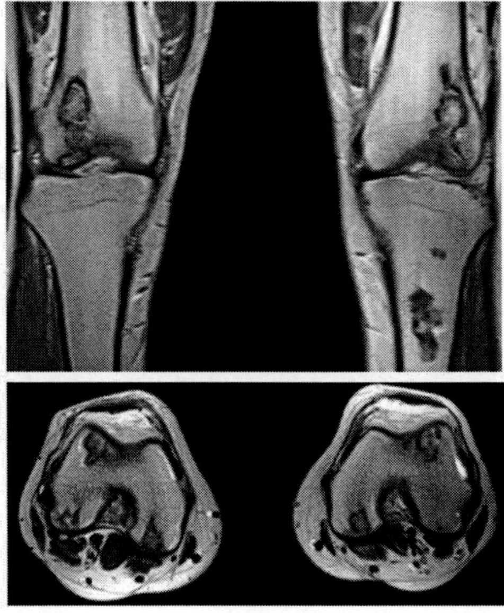

Figure 12. A 40-year-old male with SLE. Osteonecrosis of the knee in SLE.

MRI of both knees in a patient with SLE. Osteonecrosis is observed in both femoral condyles.

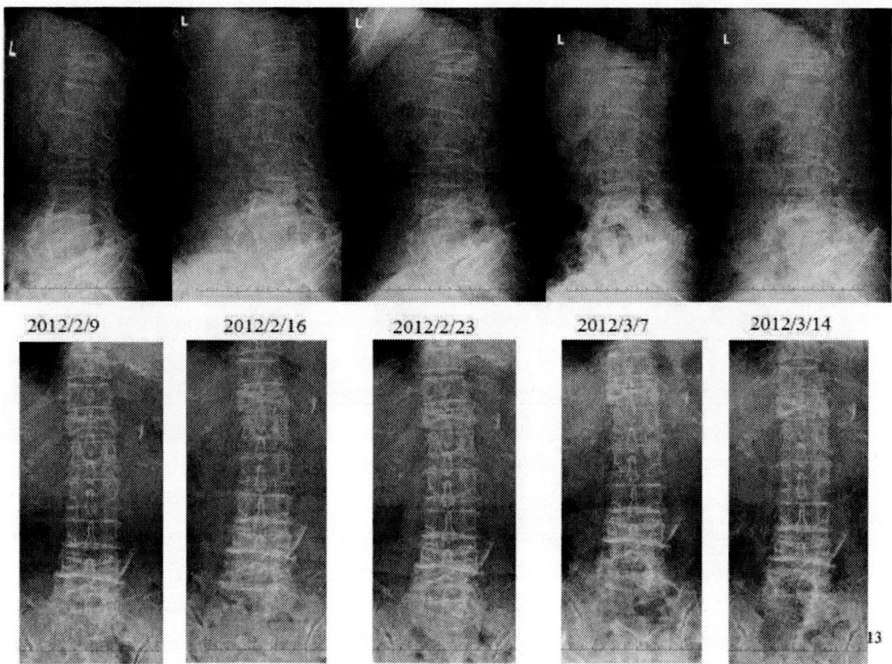

Figure 13. Fracture of spine.

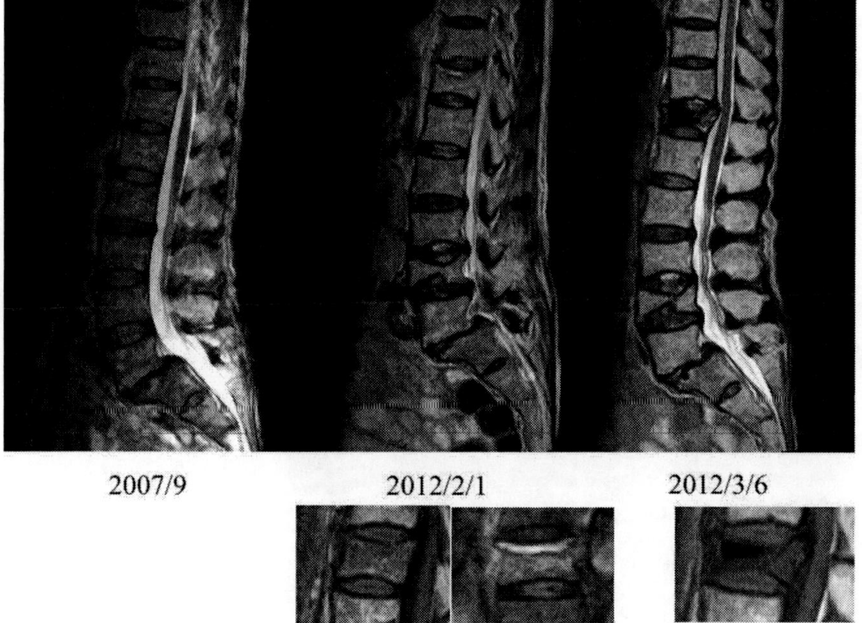

Figure 14. Fracture of spine.

 Syuichi Koarada and Yoshifumi Tada

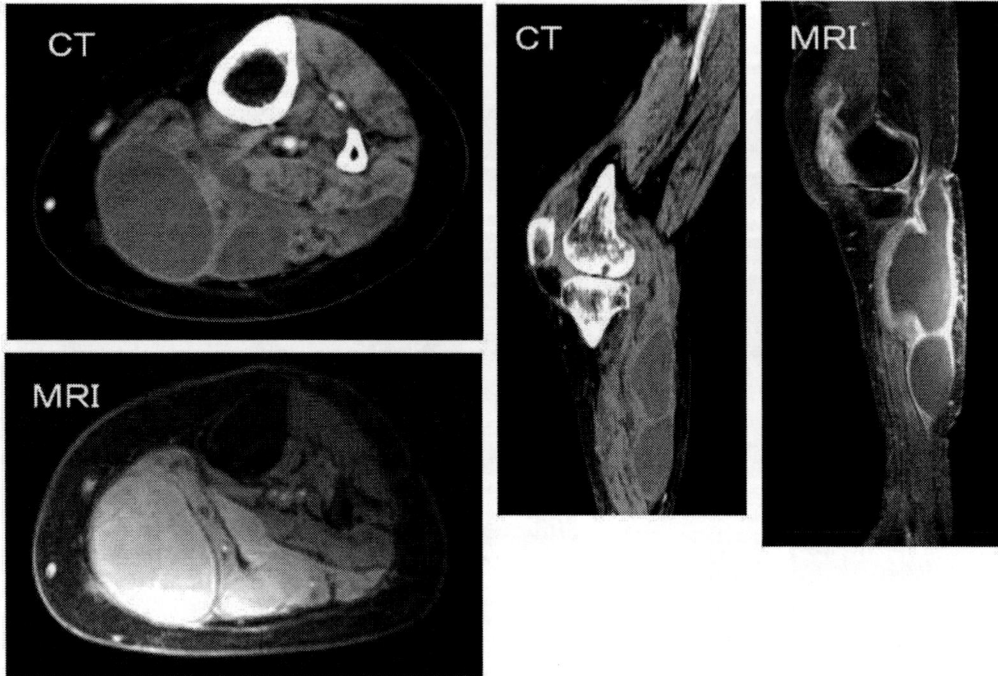

Figure 15. Baker's cyst.

Takayasu arteritis

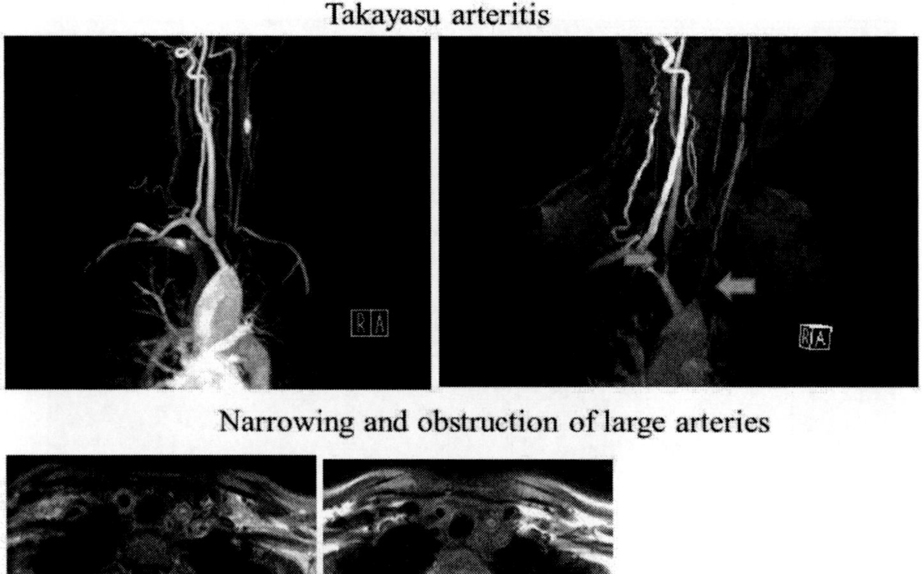

Narrowing and obstruction of large arteries

Figure 16. Takayasu arteritis.

SECTION 5. SCINTIGRAPHY

Bone Scintigraphy

To know the distribution of arthritis and rule out bone metastasis of malignancy

Gallium67 (Ga) Scintigraphy (Gallium Imaging)

The gallium scan was used for cancer diagnosis and staging. It was replaced by positron emission tomography using fludeoxyglucose, Gallium scintigraphy is still useful to image inflammation and chronic infections. Also, it still sometimes finds unsuspected tumors. Therefore, in rheumalogy, it is used for distribution of arthritis, tumor-associated arthritis, and screening of FUO (fever of unknown origin).

Scintigraphy of the salivary glands with technetium-sodium pertechnetate (99mTc).

Scintigraphy of the major salivary glands is useful for the routine investigation of patients with Sjögen's syndrome.

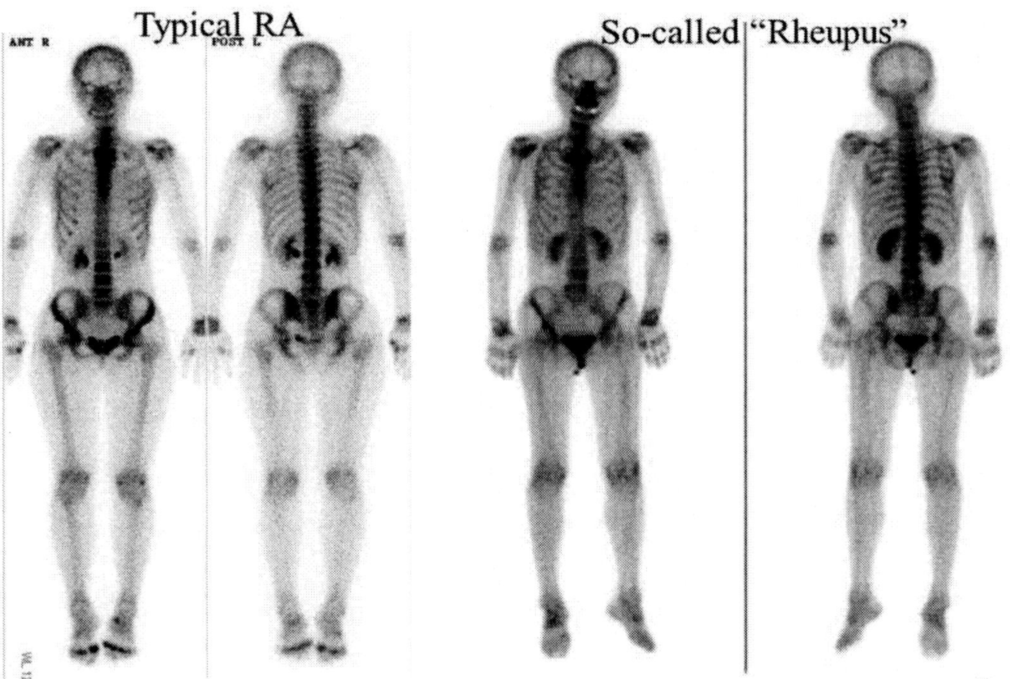

Figure 1. RA and "rheupus".

(left) Ga-67 scintigraphy showed symmetrical multiple increased uptakes in the joints of the extremities, including hand and feet.

(right) In a patient with RA and SLE, bilateral symmetrical uptake including joints of hand and feet like as typical RA.

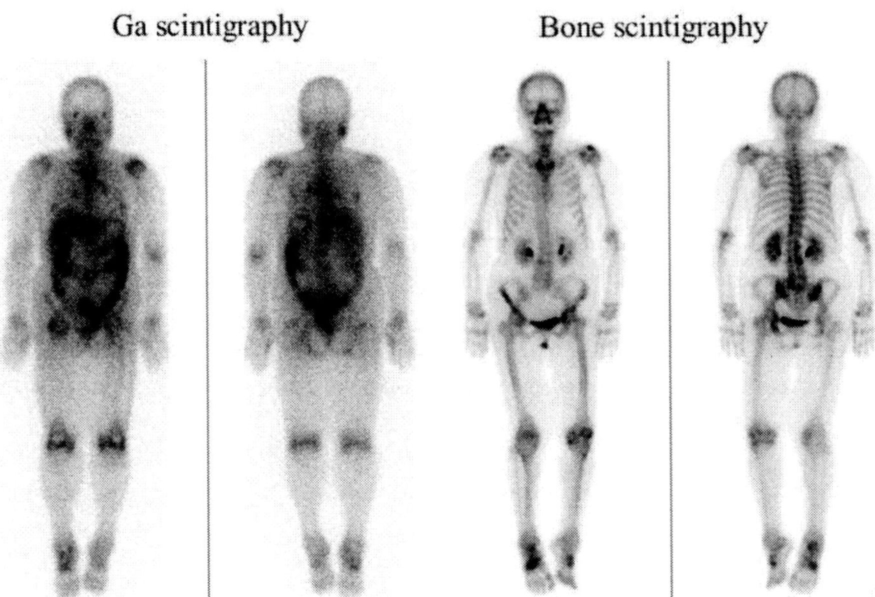

Figure 2. Elderly onset rheumatoid arthritis (EORA).

Sometimes, in elderly onset rheumatoid arthritis, Ga-67 scintigraphy shows asymmetrical multiple increased uptakes predominantly in the large joints including knees, shoulders, ankles and hips.

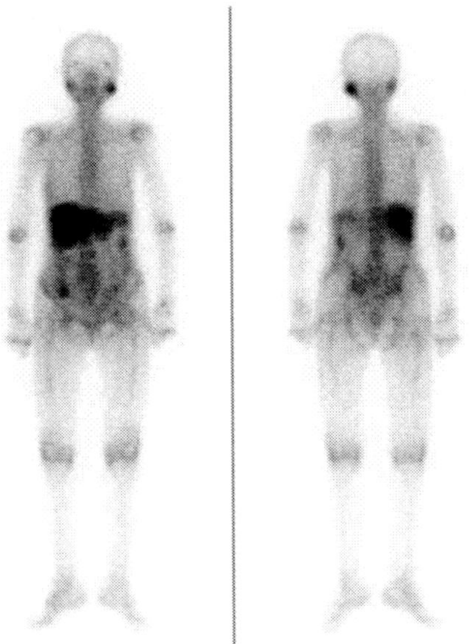

Figure 3. A 71-year-old female. Rheumatoid vascutitis.

In vasculitis with rheumatoid arthritis, Ga-67 scintigraphy shows symmetrical increased uptakes in the large and small joints including the hands, wrists, elbows, shoulders, knees, ankles feet, and hips. This figure shows increased uptakes of bone marrow and salivary glands.

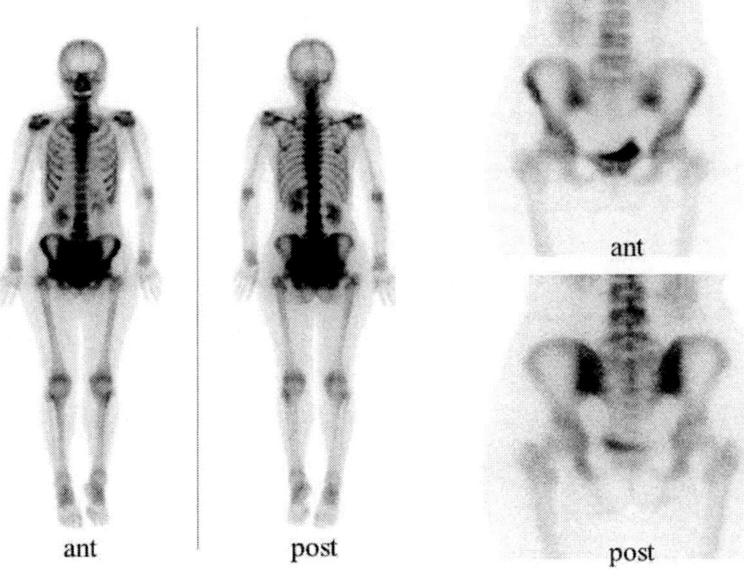

Figure 4. Ankylosing spondylitis (AS).

Bone scintigraphy

A 48-year-old female. In the pelvic view, increased uptakes at the sacroiliac joints suggest a possible sacroiliitis. Also, in large joints increased uptakes are found.

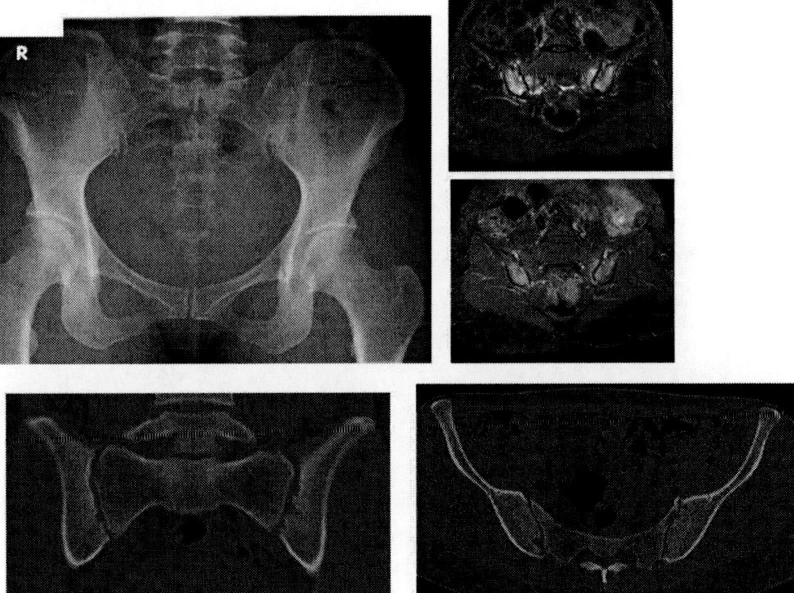

Figure 5. Sacroiliitis in pelvic view and CT and MRI.

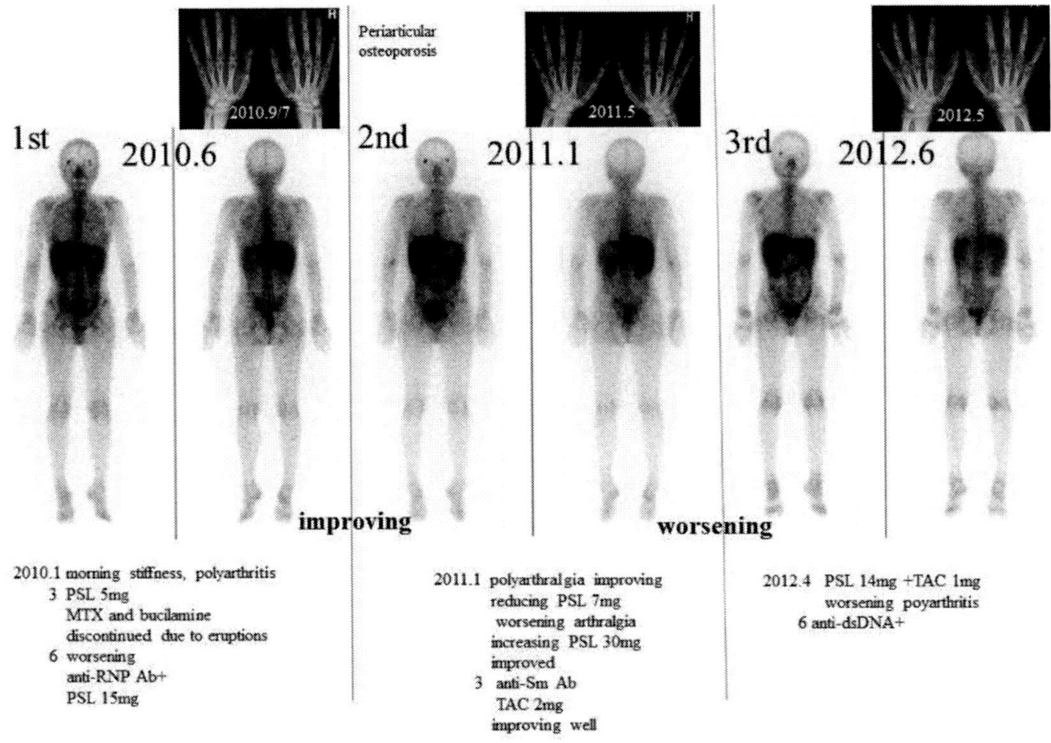

Figure 6. Serial analysis of Ga scintigraphy in a SLE+RA patient.

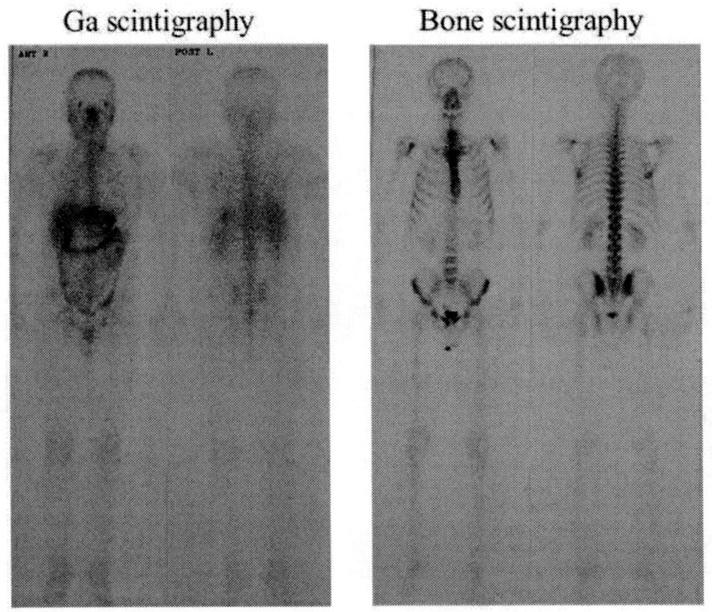

Figure 7. SLE. A 37-year old male with SLE had polyarthralgia.

Ga-67 scintigraphy showed symmetrically multiple but mild increased uptakes in the joints of the extremities.

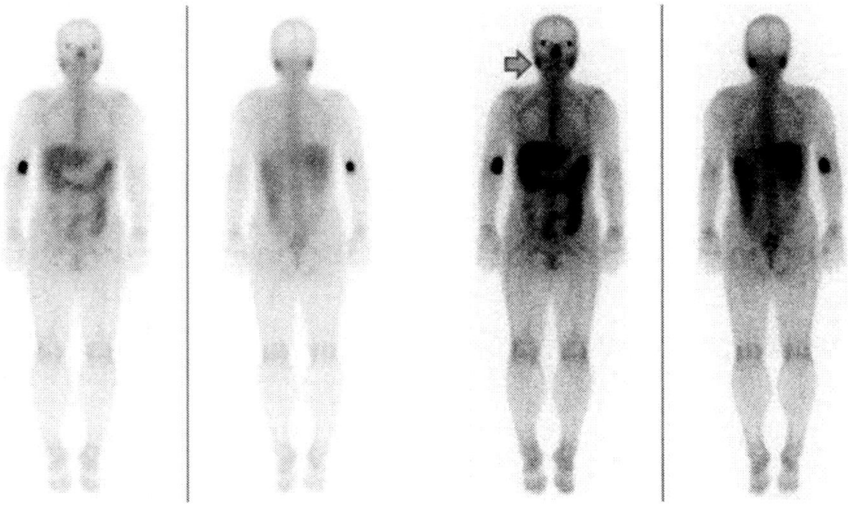

Figure 8. Sjögen's syndrome.

Ga scintigraphy

Ga-67 scintigraphy of a patient with Sjögen's syndrome showed symmetrical mild uptakes in the joints of the extremities and marked increased uptakes in salivary glands

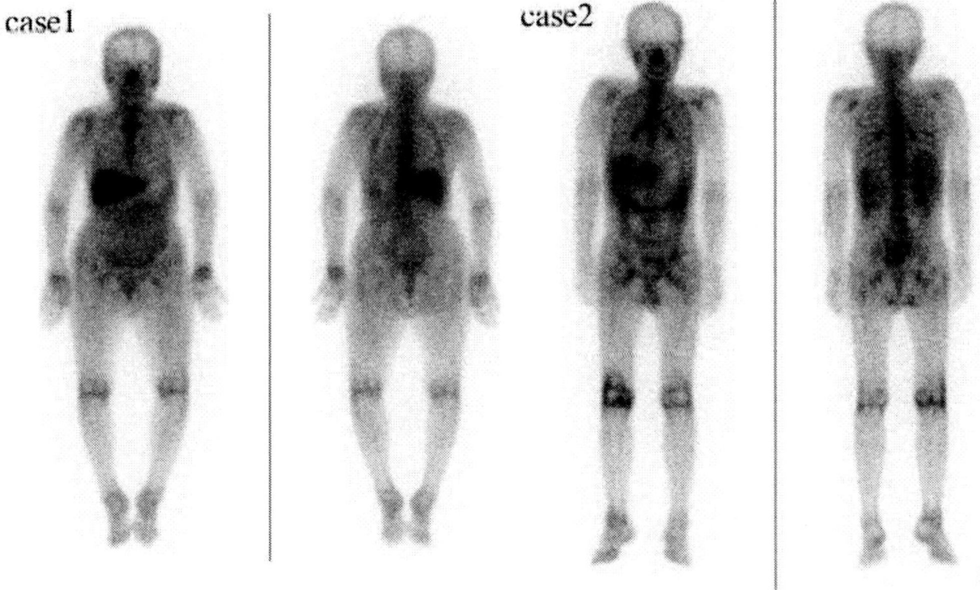

Figure 9. Calcium pyrophosphate dehydrate (CPPD).

Ga scintigraphy

Ga-67 scintigraphies of two elder patients showed multiple increased uptakes in the joints.

Linear uptakes in knees was found and no uptake in fingers.

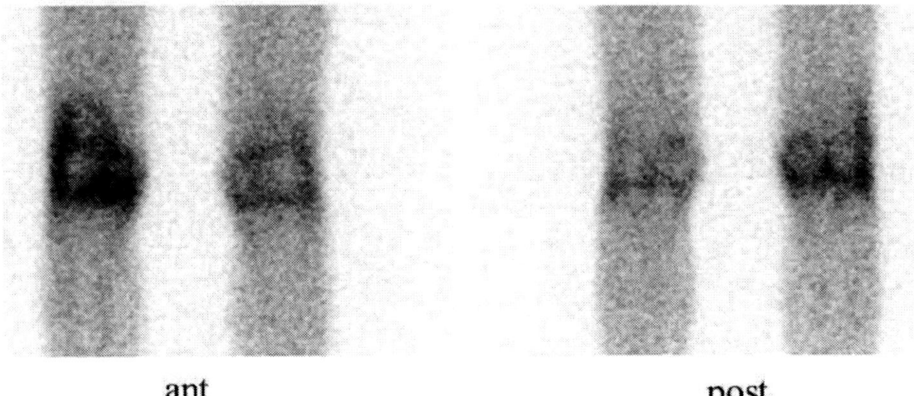

Figure 10. At the knees.

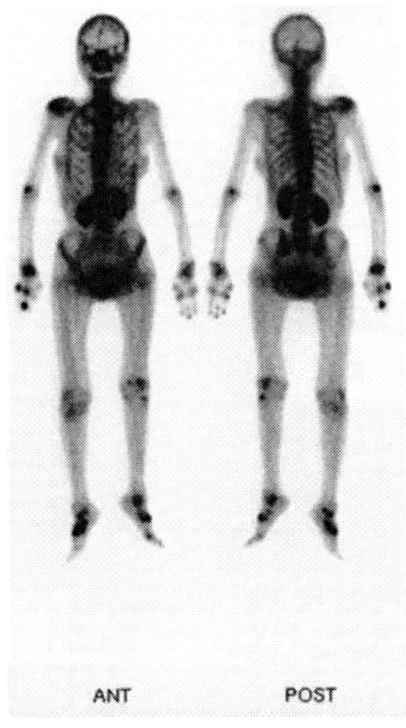

Figure 11. ONF in a 28-year-old female with SLE.

Bone scintigraphy

Uptakes including large and small joints but non-symmetrical

HADD (hydroxyapatite deposition disease) (Figure 12)
Uptakes in large joints

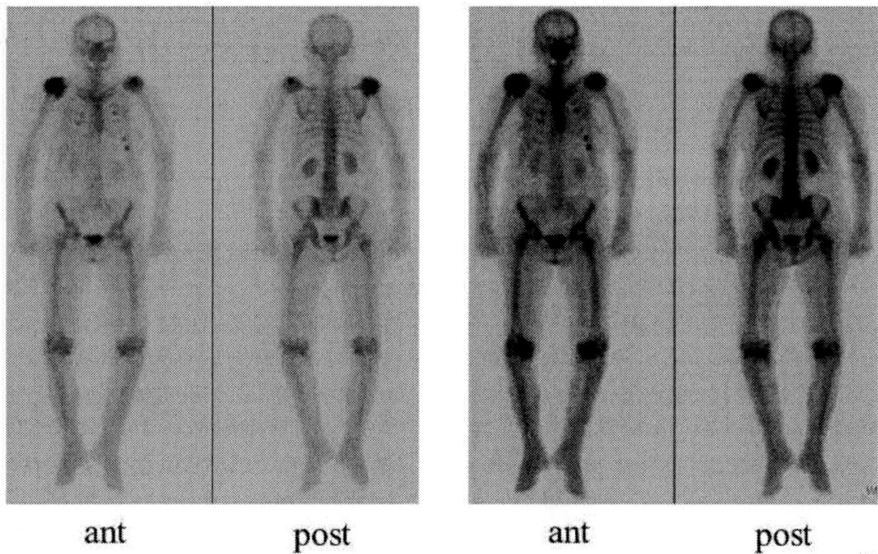

Figure 12. HADD (hydroxyapatite deposition disease).

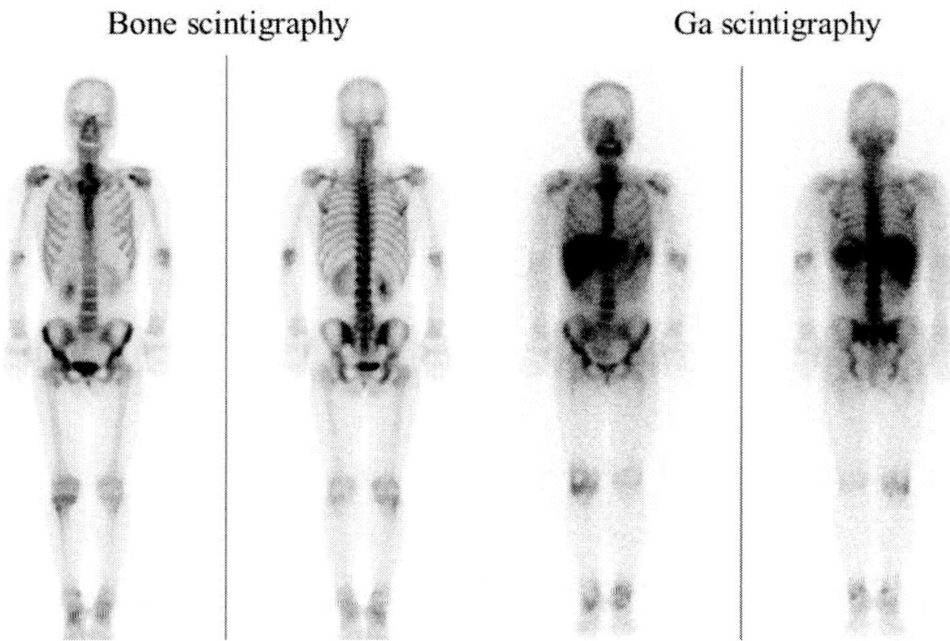

Figure 13. Relapsing polychondritis.

Uptakes including large joints and non-symmetrical distribution.

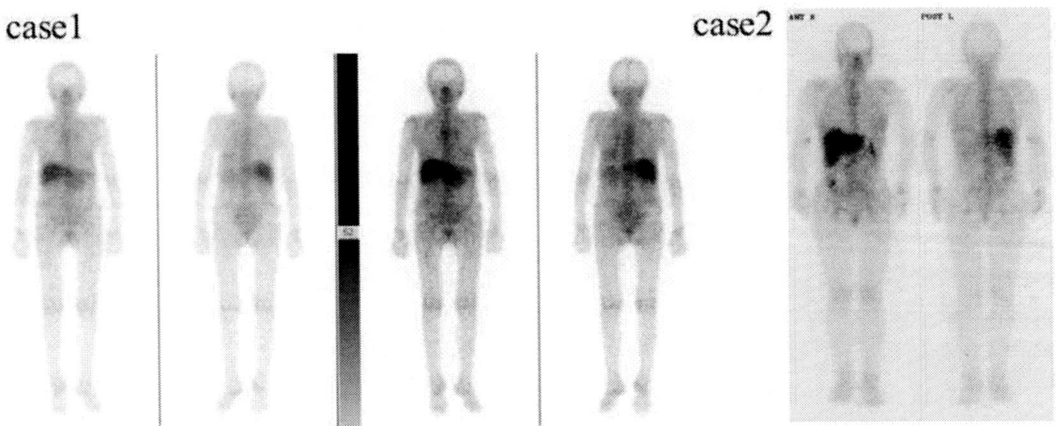

Figure 14. SSc.

Ga scintigraphy

Mild uptakes including large and small joints

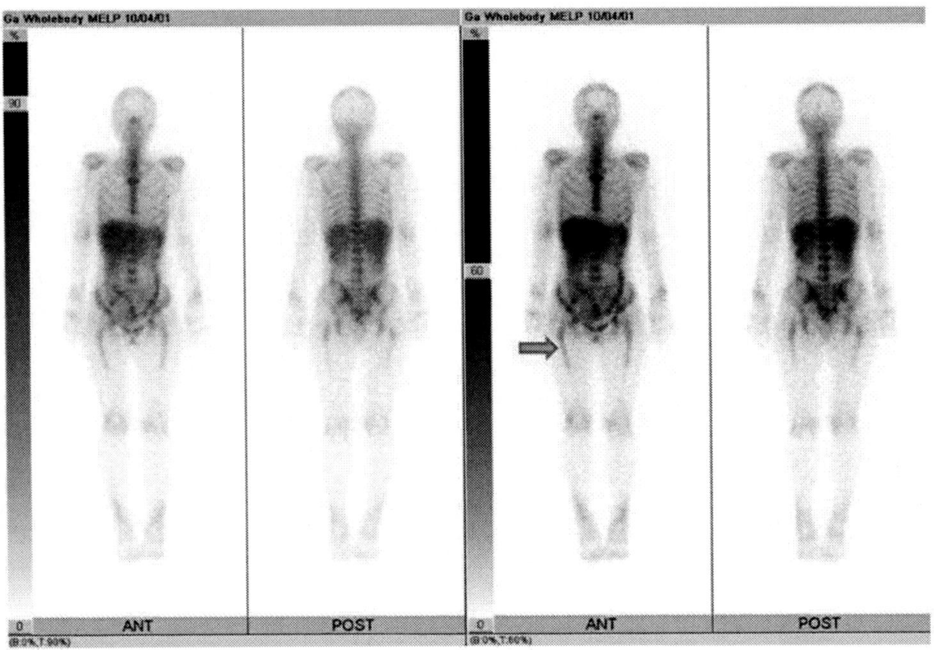

Figure 15. AOSD.

Ga scintigraphy

Uptakes of joints and bone marrow in the shaft of the femur

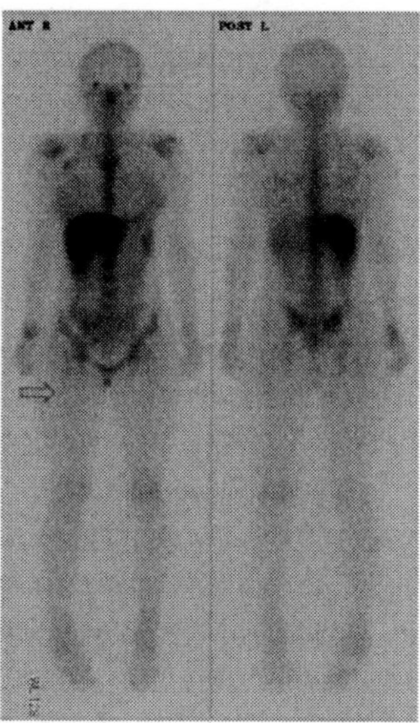

Figure 16. Ga scintigraphy.

A 24-year-old female with AOSD
Uptakes of joints and bone marrow in the shaft of the femur

Interstitial pneumonitis (IP)
Ga scintigraphy (Figure 17) uptakes in lungs

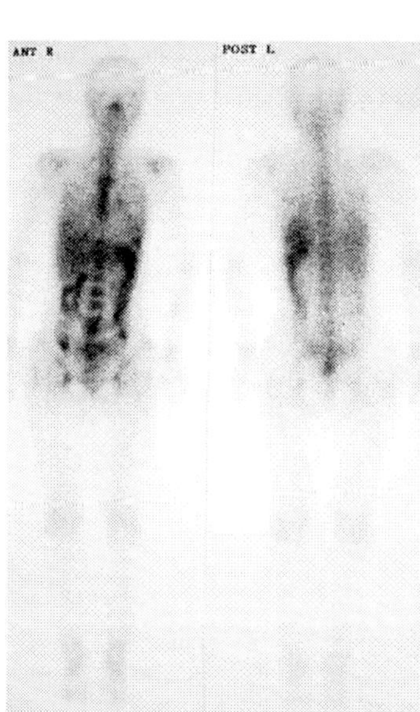

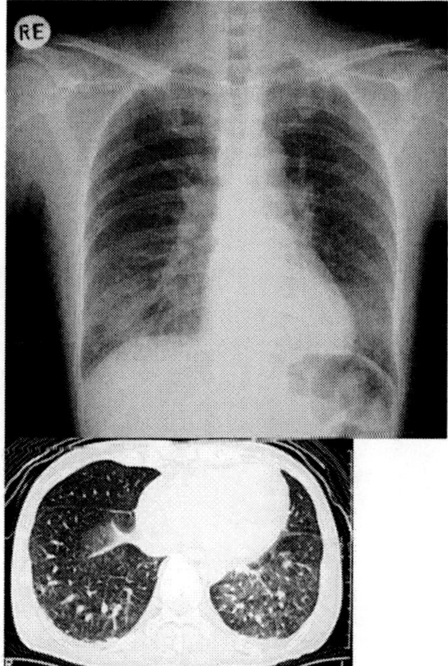

Figure 17. Ga scintigraphy uptakes in lungs in a patient with DM and IP.

Salivary Gland Scintigraphy

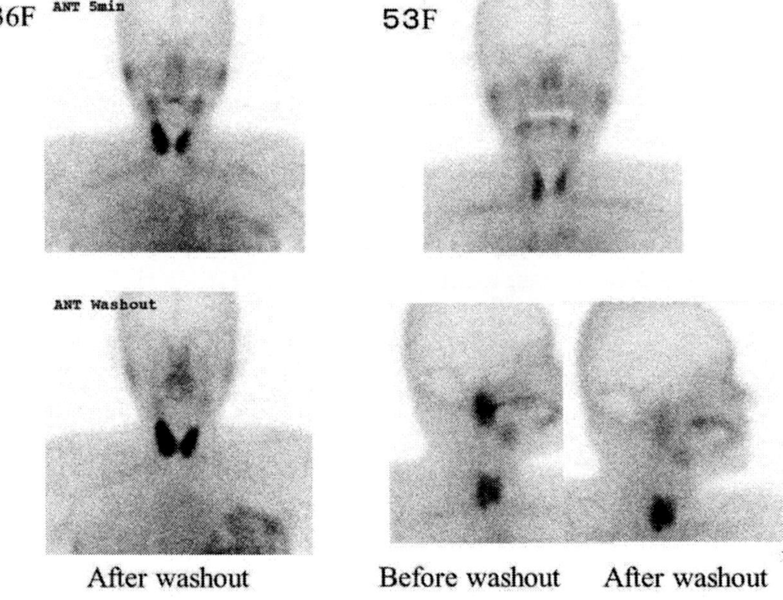

Figure 18. Salivary Gland Scintigraphy.

Sjögren's syndrome
Decreased uptakes at salivary glands

SECTION 6. OTHER INFORMATION

Gastrointestinal Imaging

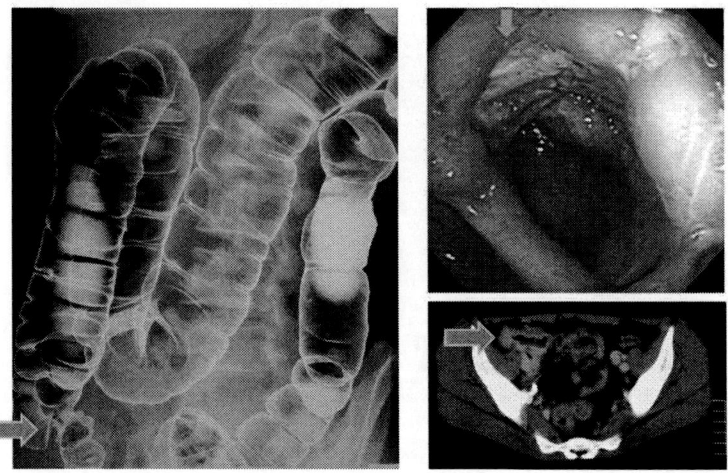

Figure 1. Ulcers in Behçet's Disease with arthritis.

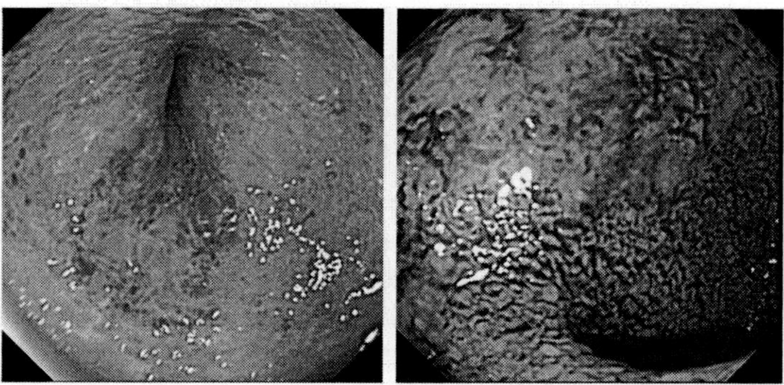

Figure 2. Ulcers in ulcerative colitis with arthritis.

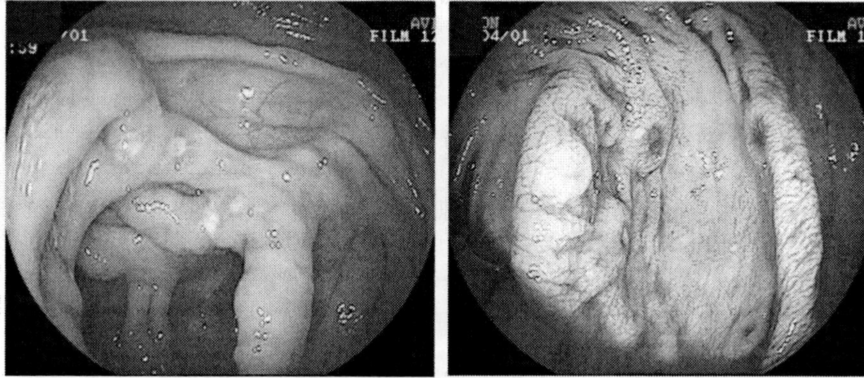

Figure 3. Small ulcers, non-specific, in Sweet's disease with arthralgia.

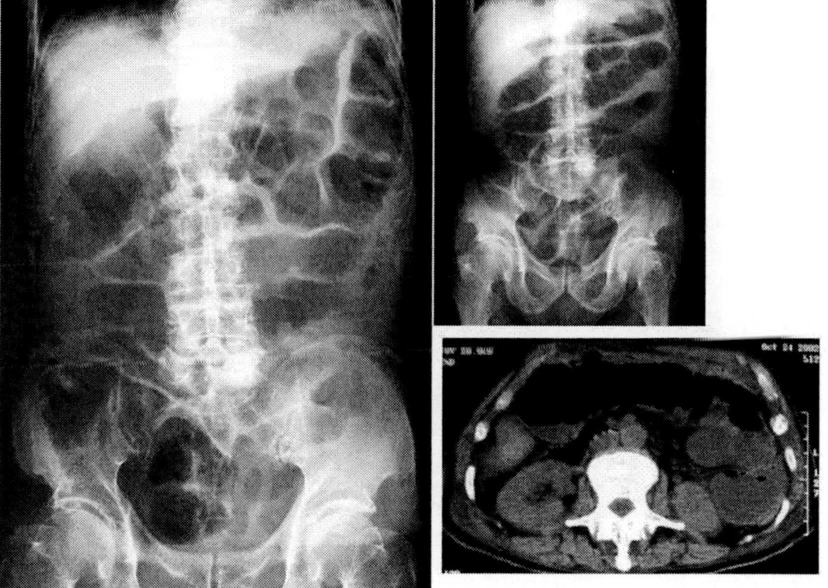

Figure 4. Ileus in mPA.

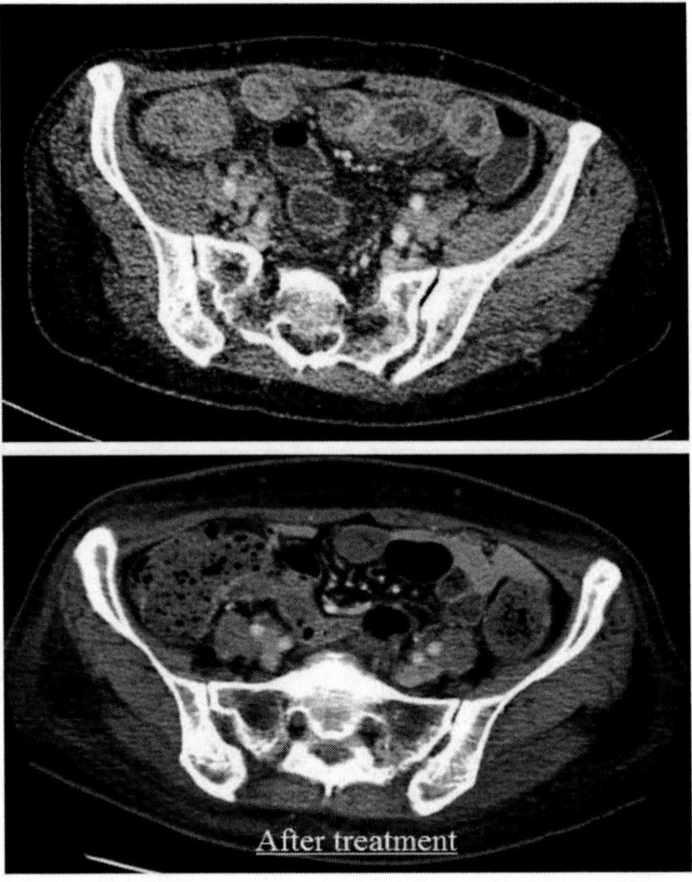

Figure 5. Lupus enteritis. A 61-year-old female Edematous change of small intestine.

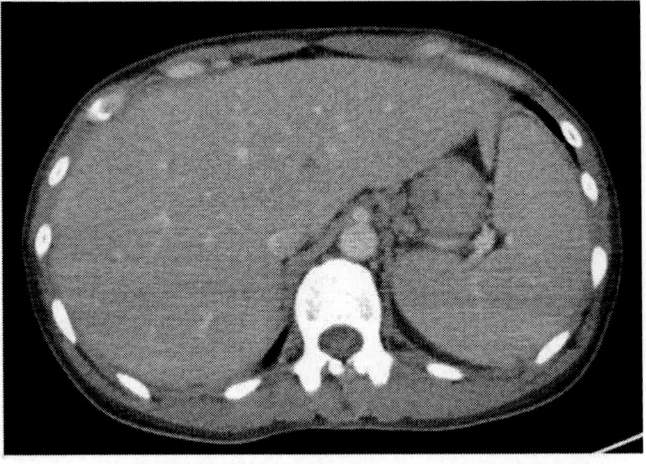

Figure 6. Splenomegaly in AOSD patient.

Neurological Imaging

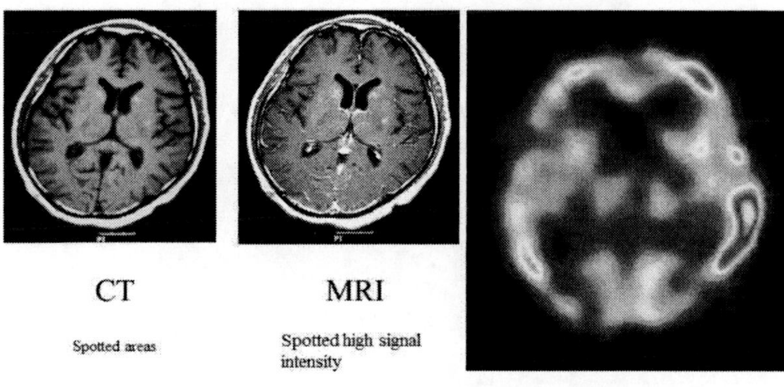

Figure 7. CNS lupus.

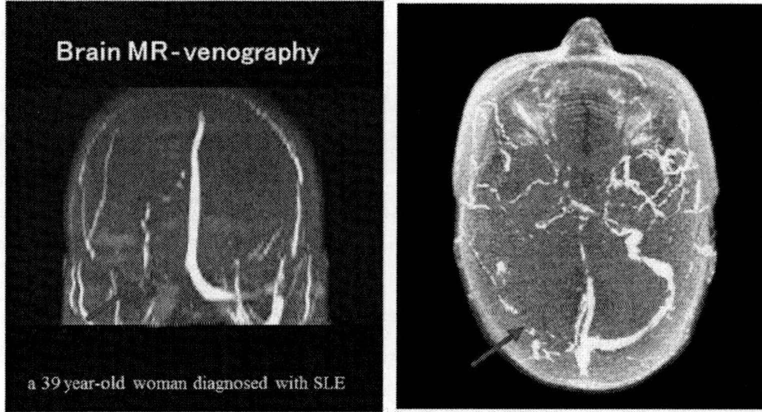

Figure 8. CNS lupus complicated by right transverse sinus thrombosis.

The patient was admitted with headache and nausea. Neurological abnormalities were unremarkable. Coagulation time was nearly normal, while complement levels were remarkably decreased. An assay for antinuclear antibodies was positive, but anti-dsDNA, anti-Sm, anticardiolipin antibodies, and lupus anticoagulant assays were non-reactive. A lumbar puncture were unremarkable. T2 weighted brain magnetic resonance imaging (MRI) scans showed multiple lesions with high signal intensity and Dawson's finger sign. The results of her MR -venography(MRV) suggested right transverse sinus thrombosis. She was successfully treated with oral betamethasone (5 mg/day), intravenous cyclophosphamide, and anticoagulant therapy (heparin and warfarin potassium). Her symptoms improved and the findings of second MRV showed recanalization of the right transverse sinus. Radiological examinations including MRV are useful in diagnosing complication with cerebral venous sinus thrombosis in patients with SLE complaining of strong headache without abnormal neurological signs.

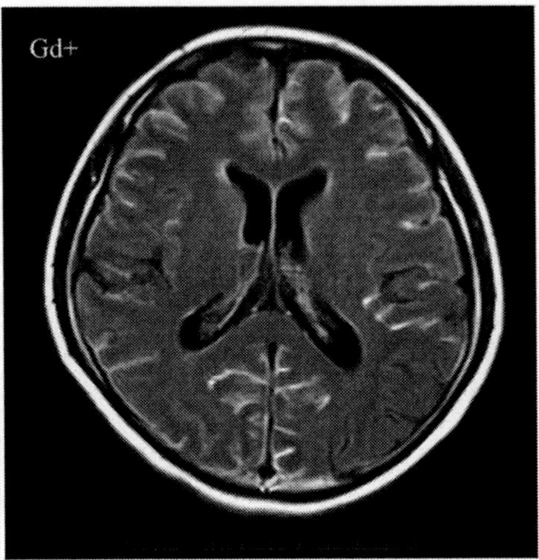

Figure 9. Meningitis due to lupus.

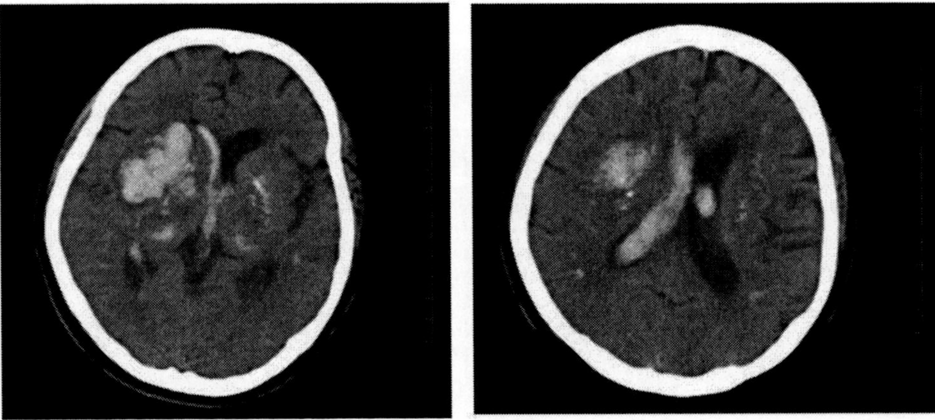

Figure 10. Cerebral hemorrhage in APS.

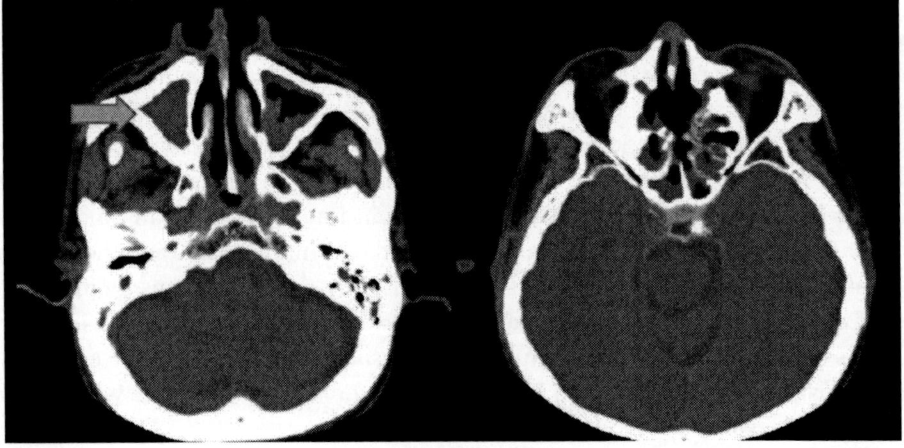

Figure 11. Wegener's granulomatosis (Granulomatosis with polyangiits; GPA).

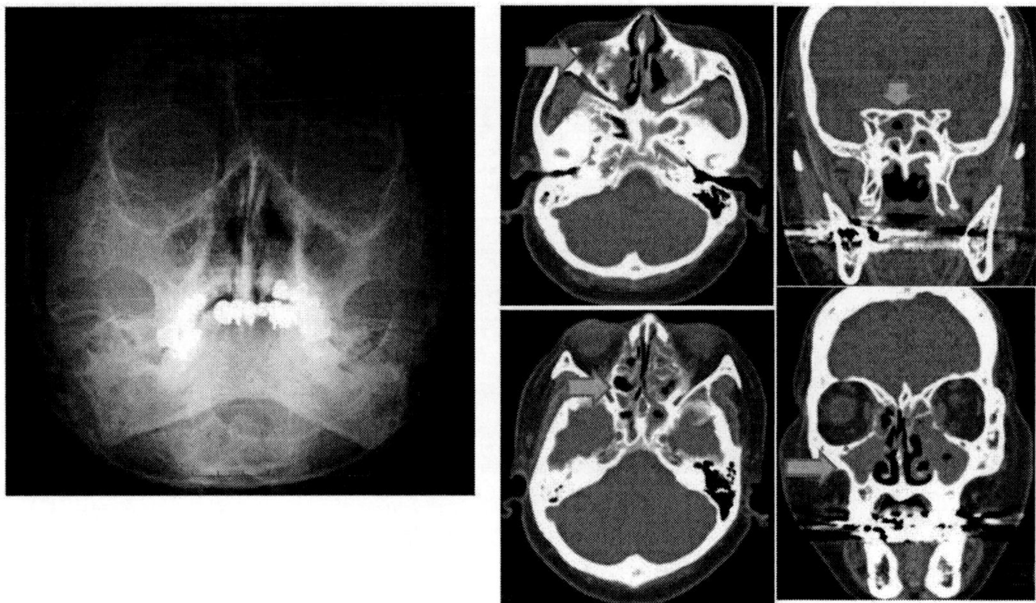

Figure 12. Wegener's granulomatosis (Granulomatosis with polyangiits; GPA).

Extensive soft tissue opacification of the nasal cavities.

Vascular Imaging

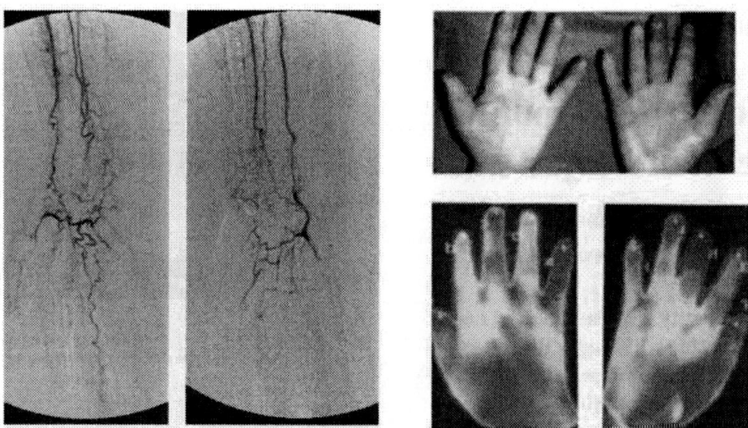

Figure 13. Polyangiitis. A 66-year-old female with angiitis.

Angiography of the hands shows occlusions of bilateral ulnar arteries at the portion of the wrist and most of the proper palmar digital arteries.

Photographs of the hands shows the 2nd and 3rd finger tip ulcers.

Thermographic image of the hands shows reduced temperature of the right 2nd and 3rd fingers.

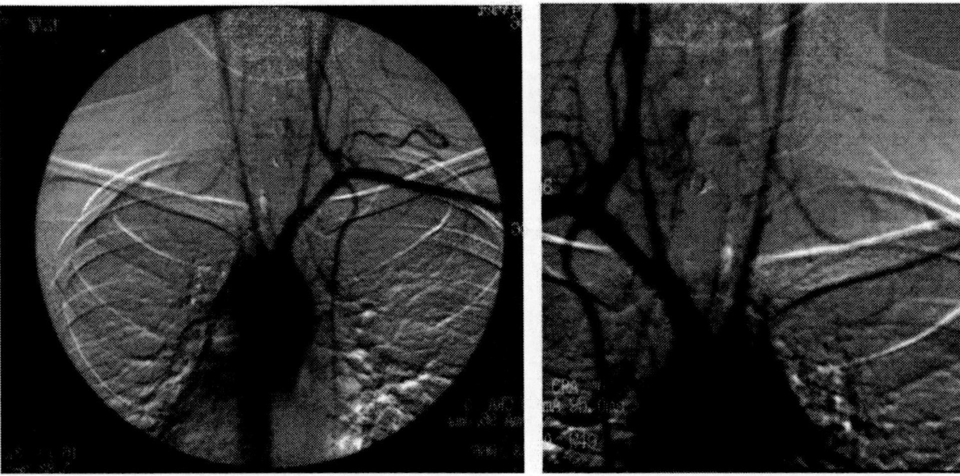

Figure 14. Takayasu Arteritis.

Immunological Research and Studies

Immunoglobulin subsets
    IgA
    IgD
    IgE
    IgG
        IgG4:   IgG4-related disease

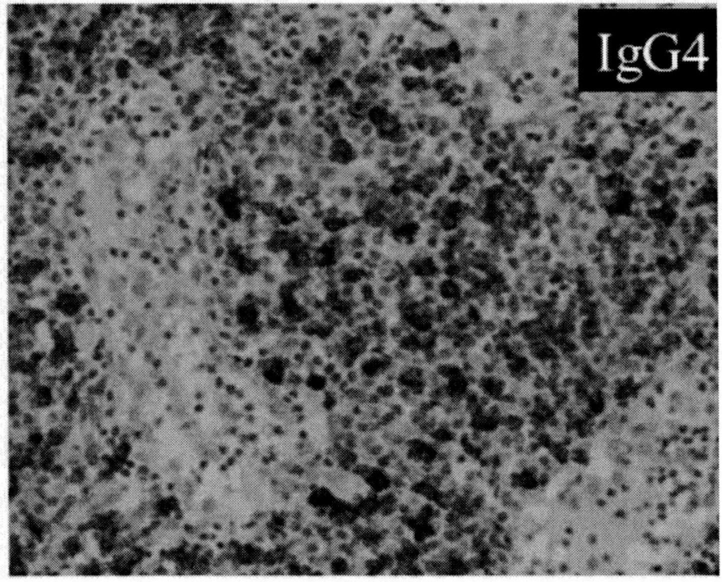

IgG4+/IgG=50%

Figure 15. Immunohistochemistry.

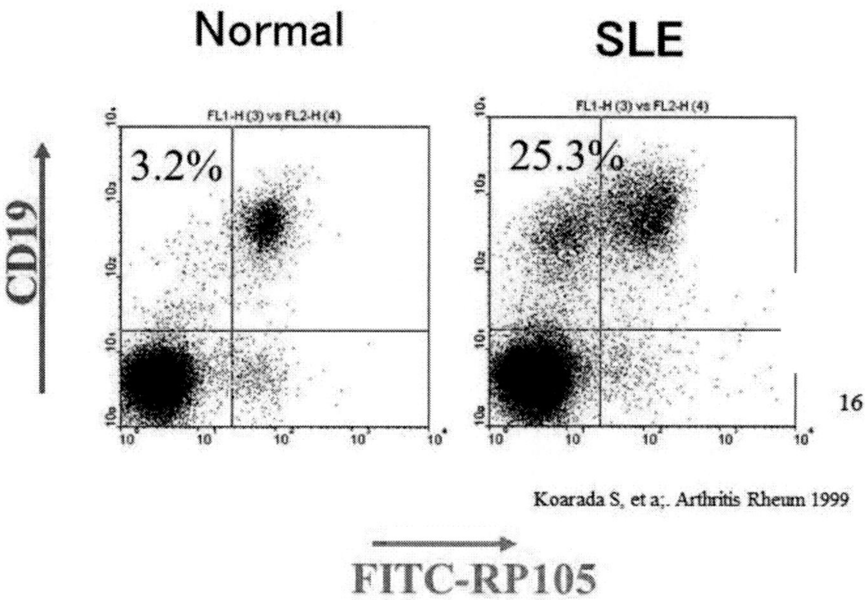

Figure 16. Flow cytometry Surface antigens.

Expression of RP105 on peripheral B cells from a normal person and a patient with systemic lupus erythematosus (SLE). Peripheral blood mononuclear cells were stained with monoclonal antibody against RP105 and CD19 and analyzed using a flow cytometry.

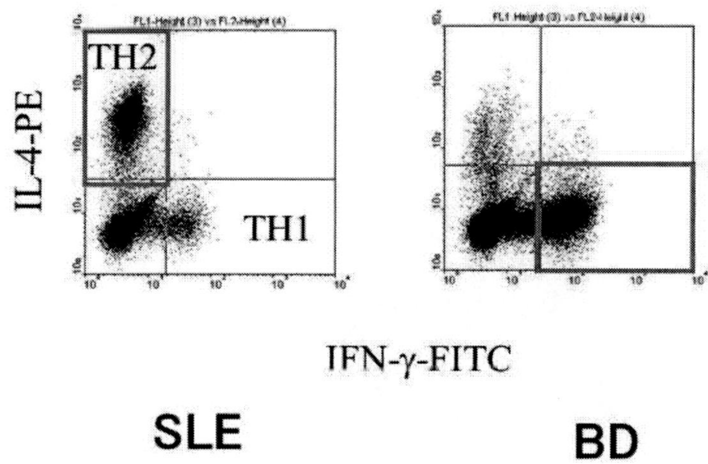

Figure 17. Intracellular cytokines.

Intracellular IFN-γ and Il-4 production in Con A-PMA-ionomycin-stimulated CD4+ T cells form a patient with SLE. Peripheral mononuclear cells were cultured with Con A and then re-stimulated with PMA-ionomycin and assayed for cytokine production by intracellular cytokine analysis using flow cytometry plus staining for CD4 expression. One representative result suggests increased IL-4 (Th2 dominance) in SLE compared with Behçet's disease.

Histological Findings

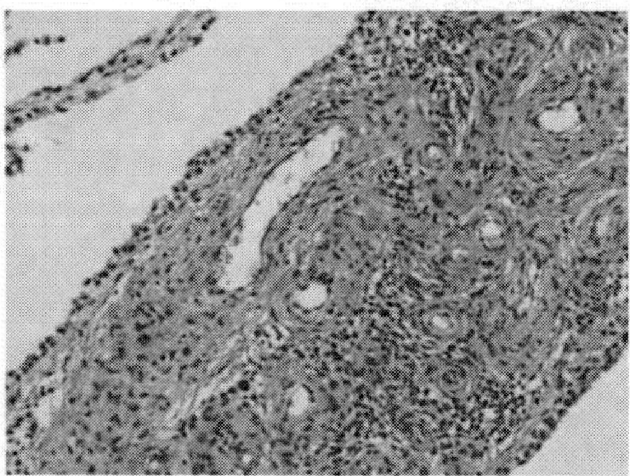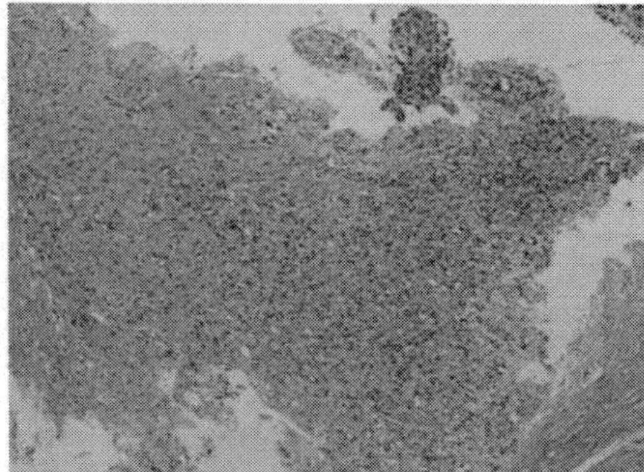

Figure 18. RA joint.

Infiltration of plasma cells and germinal center formation in synovium

In histological examination, the synovium form RA patients shows infiltration by plasma cells and lymphocytes with/without lymphoid follicles and fibrin deposits often seen close to the synovial lining or within the stroma [Rosai J. Bone and joints. In: Rosai J, ed. Ackerman's surgical pathology, 8th ed. St. Louis, MO: Mosby,1996: 1991-1996].

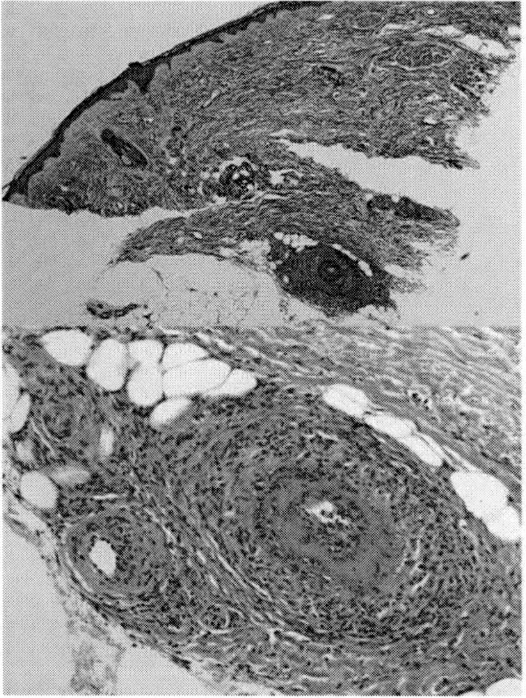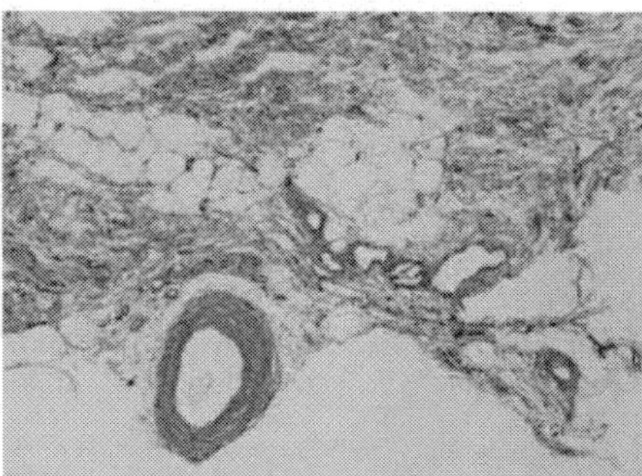

Figure 19. Rheumatoid vasculitis. Biopsy of skin shows vasculitis in RA patients.

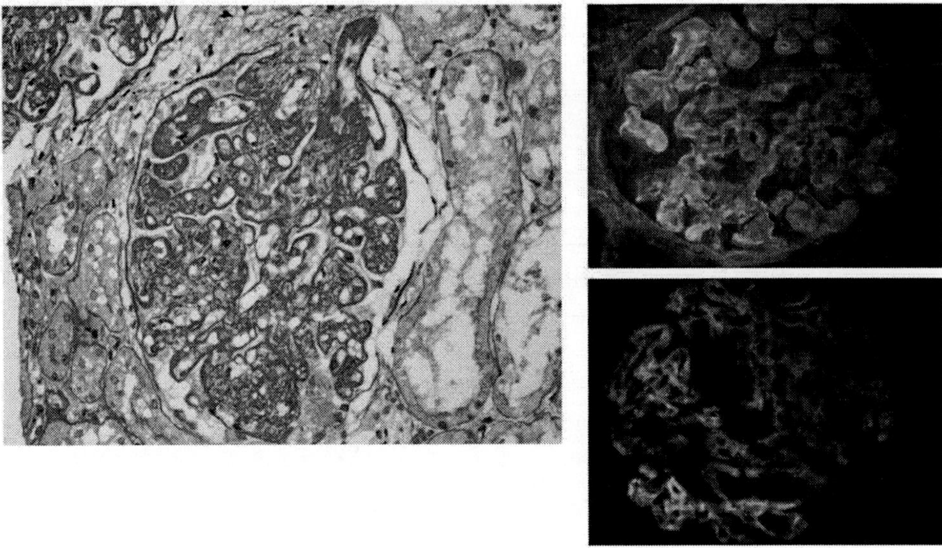

Figure 20. Renal Biopsy: lupus nephritis.

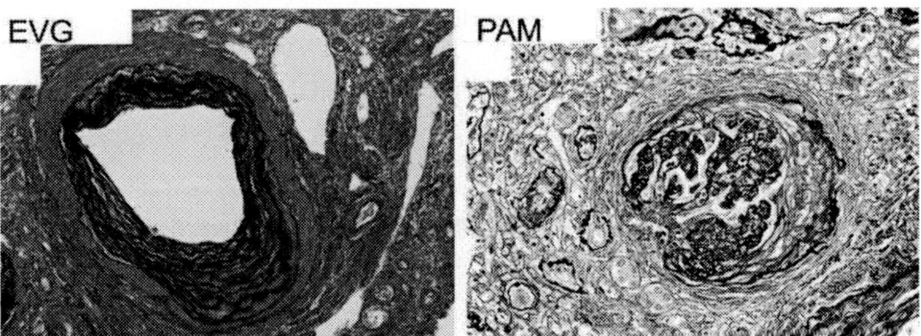

Figure 21. mPA.

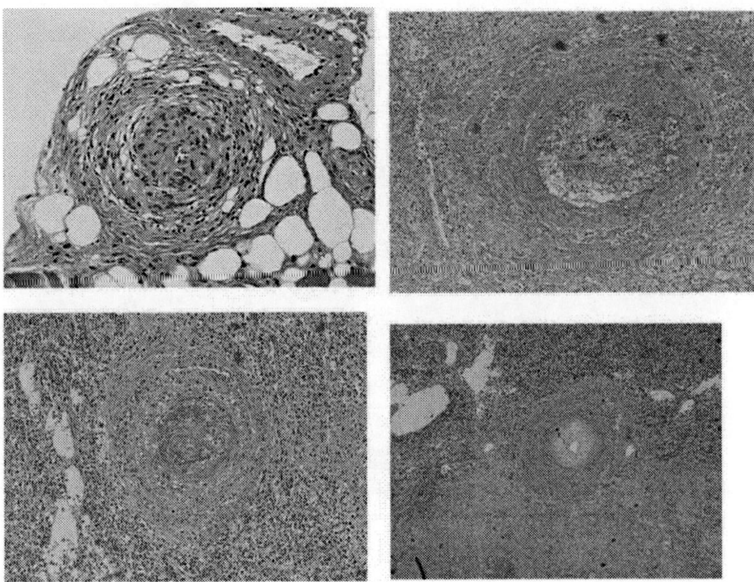

Figure 22. mPA.

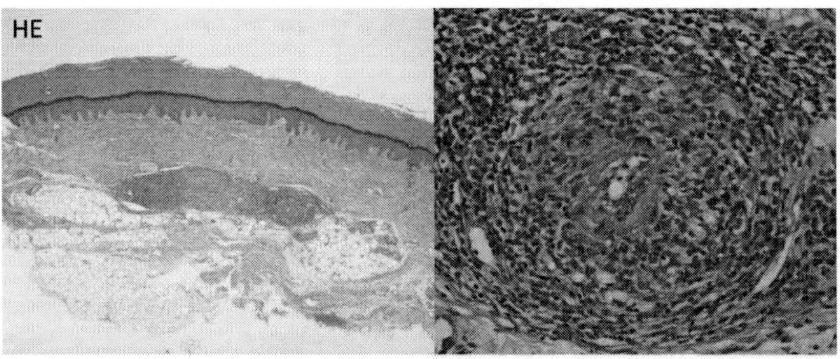

Figure 23.mPA.

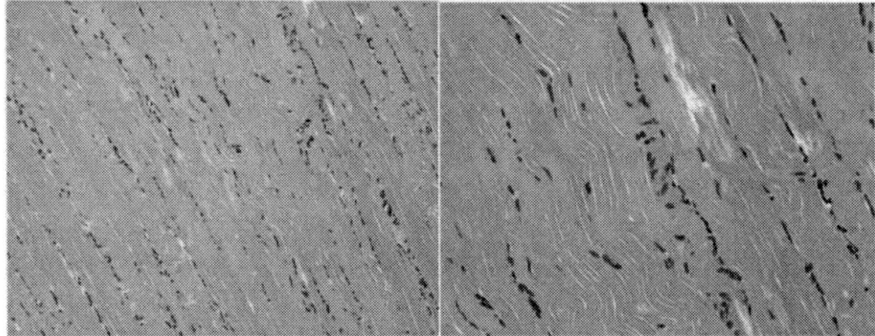

Figure 24. Polymyositis (PM).

Mononuclear cells infiltrate into a large muscle fiber. (hematoxylin-eosin, high power)

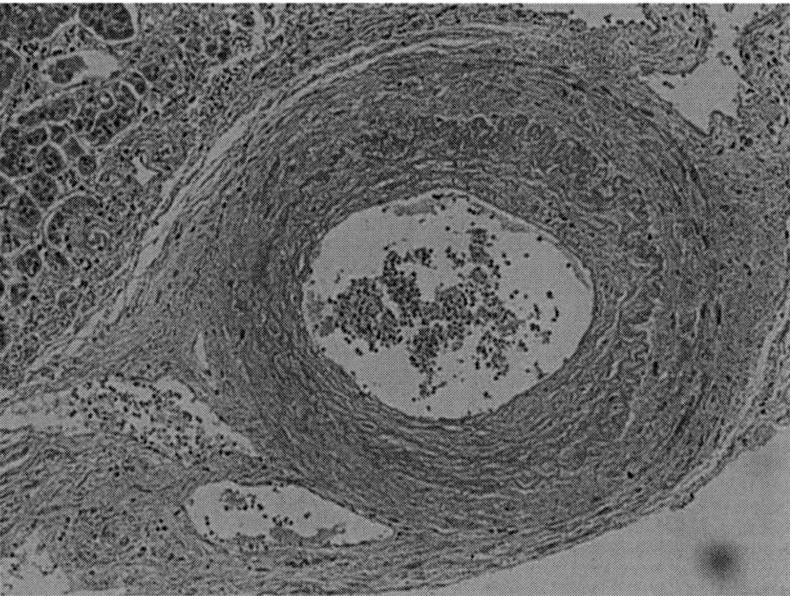

Figure 25. PN.

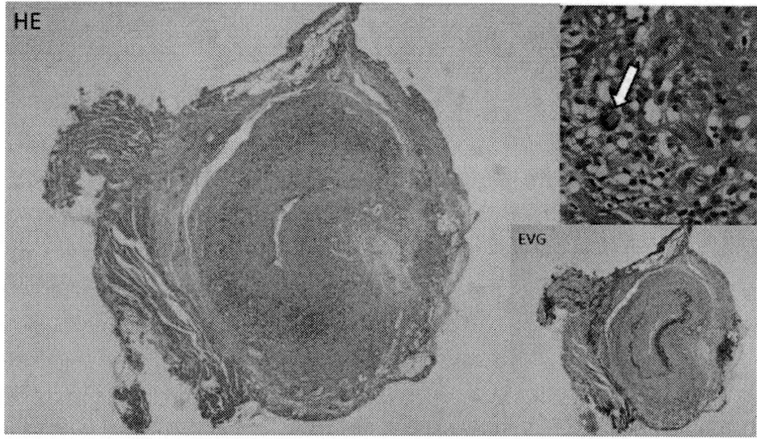

Figure 26. Giant cell arteritis.

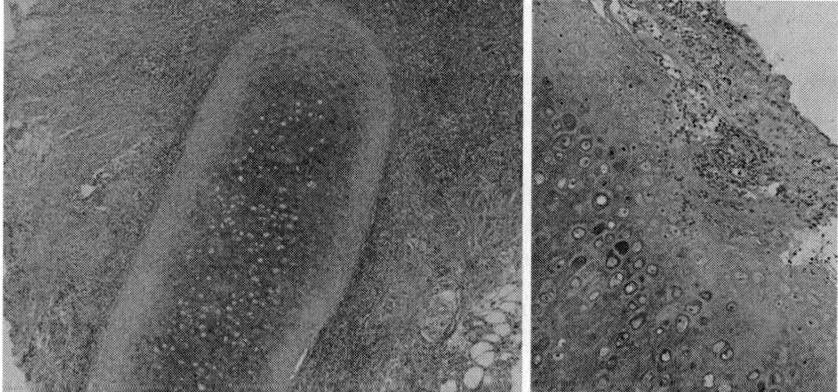

Figure 27. Relapsing polychondritis.

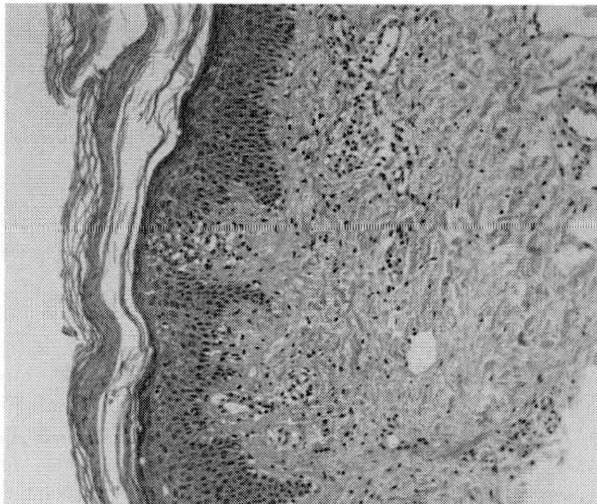

Figure 28. Psoriatic arthritis.

Laboratory Findings

CBC (Complete blood count)
WBC

Leukopenia	SLE	50%
	(RA)	
	Felty's syndrome	
	Sjögren's syndrome	
	Human parvovirus B19 infection	
lymphocytopenia	SLE	75%
Leukocytosis	RA	
	AOSD	
	Behçet's disease	
	Vasculitis	
	Reactive arthritis	
	Infection	

RBC

Anemia	Many inflammatory arthritides
	Especially SLE
	RA
	IBD
	Human parvovirus B19 infection

PLT

Thrombocytopenia	SLE	20%
	Human parvovirus B19 infection	
Thrombocytosis	Acute-phase reaction	
	Active RA	
	Vasculitis	
	Infection	

Eosinophilia

SLE, RA, IBD, sarcoidosis, dermatomyositis, scleroderma, Churg-Strauss syndrome (EGPA), PAN, eosinophilic fasciitis, cholesterol emboli, HES (hypereosinophilic syndrome)

Tests with low specificity
Frequently positive in the general population

Rheumatoid factor (RF)
Non-specific finding

Healthy persons	up to 20%
RA	70%
Sjögren's syndrome	
SLE	
Sarcoidosis	
Reactive arthritis	
PMR	
Polymyositis	

Psoriatic arthritis
Endocarditis
Chronic infections and tuberculosis
Cancer
Chronic liver disease
Many other causes

Negative for AOSD, RS3PE syndrome

Antinuclear antibody   (ANA)

One of the most frequent evaluation in rheumatic diseases
However, non-specific finding

ANA-associated rheumatic diseases
    SLE   99%
    Scleroderma >   95%
    Sjögren's syndrome
    Polymyositis
    Dermatomyositis
    MCTD   100%

ANA-non-associated rheumatic diseases
    Vasculitis
    RA

Medications
Many nonrheumatic causes
    Thyroiditis
    Chronic hepatitis

Healthy persons   (5% positive)

Negative for
    Seronegative spondyloarthropathies
    PMR
    Behçet's disease
    AOSD

Tests with high specificity
Specific autoantibodies

Anti-Double-stranded DNA	SLE, especially lupus nephritis	70%
Anti-Sm	SLE, especially CNS lupus	30%
Anti–SS-A (anti-Ro)	Sjögren's syndrome	
	SLE	
	healthy persons	

Anti–SS-B (anti-La) antibodies   Sjögren's syndrome
Anti-U1RNP   MCTD
Anti-Jo-1   polymyositis

False-positive VDRL   SLE
                                        anticardiolipin antibody syndrome
Antineutrophil cytoplasmic autoantibody
    Cytoplasmic (c-ANCA)   GPA
    p-ANCA   mPA, CSS

Inflammatory markers
    elevated erythrocyte sedimentation rate(ESR) or C-reactive protein (CRP)
            Infection
            most inflammatory arthritides
                        SLE   elevated ESR but low CRP
                        RA
            advanced age
            PMR
            giant cell arteritis
            cancer, anemia, pregnancy; menses
    no inflammatory markers
            fibromyalgia
            osteoarthritis

Decreased C3   SLE   65%
Decreased CH50   SLE

Hepatic transaminase
    elevated aspartate transaminase or alanine transaminase (AST, ALT)
        SLE
        AIH (autoimmune hepatitis)
        PAN
        sarcoidosis
        hemochromatosis
        Sjögren's syndrome
        infectious hepatitis
        polymyositis
        drug-induced

    elevated alkaline phosphatase (AL-P)
        Bone metastases, Paget's disease, osteomalacia, PMR, ankylosing spondylitis,
        hyperparathyroidism

Elevated uric acid (UA)
        Gout, psoriatic arthritis, Paget's disease; healthy persons

Elevated creatinine (Cr)
      SLE, GPA, vasculitis

Elevated creatine kinase (CPK)
      Polymyositis, dermatomyositis, hypothyroidism, drug-induced

Elevated calcium
      Hyperparathyroidism, cancer, sarcoidosis

Synovial Fluid by Joint aspiration

Gram staining and Culture	Infection
Crystals	Gout
	pseudogout

White blood cell count

Normal	0- 200 per mm3
	(0 to 0.2 × 109 per L)
non-inflammatory	Osteoarthritis
	internal derangement
	myxedema
Inflammatory	2,000 - 50,000 per mm3
	(2 to 50 × 109 per L)
	Rheumatoid arthritis
	psoriatic arthritis
	pseudogout
	Neisseria gonorrhoeae infection
Septic	Probable > 50,000 per mm3 (50 × 109 per L)
	usually > 100,000 per mm3 (100 × 109 per L)
	Septic arthritis (primary concern)
	occasionally, gout
	pseudogout
	reactive arthritis
	Lyme disease

Polymorphonuclear neutrophilic leukocytes

Normal and non-inflammatory	< 25% (0.25)
Inflammatory	>75% (0.75)
Septic	> 90% (0.90)

Lymphocytes

Urinalysis

Hematuria	SLE,	GPA, PAN
Proteinuria	SLE	50% ; GPA, amyloidosis

HLA-B27	Healthy persons; spondyloarthropathies, reactive arthritis
HLA-B51	BD
HLA-B52	Takayasu
and so on	

Chapter 8

GOAL AND FUTURE PURPOSES

"G"; GOAL AND FUTURE PURPOSES

Diagnosis and Treatment by the information "A" to "F"
Research of pathophysiology in the disease
Establishment a new therapy for the disease

Final goal of this process is the making diagnosis, and establishing the clinical and immunological approach to the future treatment and management for the patients.

Arthritis is one of the most interesting diagnostic challenge for general physicians and rheumatologists, because the extensive differential diagnosis, including about or more than 200 diseases and conditions. It is sometimes difficult to solve initially, however, the step-by-step diagnosis using "A" to "F" tools helps to narrower differential diagnosis.

Even though, not all patients with arthritis reach a definitive diagnosis at the first visit. Therefore, a series of visits over time again and again may be important to reach a proper diagnosis in some cases. However, it may not be possible to establish a definitive diagnosis in even several cases. There may be still unknown diseases defined well presently.

There are a lot of radiographic and clinical signs and laboratory findings including immunological examination. Although they may not directly suggest the diagnosis, the physician should consider more common causes first and interpret the decision comprehensively in the clinical context.

More importantly, while the physicians engage the daily management of the patients in their clinic, they should remind always to participate in development the medicine for the patients even when they work in a remote area and send a scientific message to the public in any form with high aspiration. These small developments make the great progress of rheumatology now and tomorrow.

Chapter 9

CASE STUDIES OF RHEUMATIC DISEASES

RHEUMATOID ARTHRITIS (RA)

Definition

Rheumatoid arthritis (RA) is a chronic systemic inflammatory autoimmune disease characterized by mainly appendicular joint inflammation and destruction, affecting about 1% of the population [Winalski CS, Palmer WE, Rosenthal DI, Weissman BN. Magnetic resonance imaging of rheumatoid arthritis. Radiol Clin North Am 1996; 34:243-258]. However, etiology has been still unknown.

In RA, erosions induce the aggressiveness of the arthropathy and disability.

Prominent characteristic of arthritis is symmetric polyarthritis and various extra-articular manifestations are found in many patients.

Therefore the presentation at onset and clinical features are extremely heterogeneous.

A
alignment of fingers:
    Subluxations or deviations
        at the MCP joints
        the proximal phalanges: ulnarly and palmarly
RC joint:
    Radial deviation and so on

B
Juxta-articular osteoporosis progressing to generalized osteoporosis
    The earliest changes
    nonspecific but suggesting an inflammation
Lack of bone formation (osteosclerosis is rare)

C
Uniform loss of joint space
    the cartilages are lost and joint space narrowing uniformly
Very early erosions: very subtle

Loss of the continuity of the white cortical line
PA view
      in the heads of the metacarpals
      at the margins of the PIP joints

the Nørgaard, or semisupinated oblique view of the hands
erosions on the radial aspect of the base of the proximal phalanges

Marginal erosions progressing to severe erosions of subchondral bone
      The marginal erosions progress to large subchondral erosions

Synovial cyst formation

D
In the joints
Erosions occur in the bare areas of the bone.
In the joint fibrous capsule, cartilage does not cover the bone, or marginal areas, where synovium directly touches bones

In the hand
MCP and/or the PIP joints
In the wrist
      all carpals

In the body
symmetrical arthritis of the appendicular skeleton, sparing the axial skeleton except for the cervical spine
Bilateral symmetrical distribution
Distribution in hands, feet, knees, hips, cervical spine, shoulders and elbows in decreasing order of frequency

E
Periarticular symmetrical soft tissue swelling around PIP and MCP joints and wrist
      The earliest change
nonspecific but suggesting an inflammation
rheumatoid nodules

F
      MRI
      Ultrasonography
      Gallium and bone scintigraphy

Very early RA
Plain radiography   normal
                    possible periarticular osteoporosis
                    and

| | Periarticular symmetrical soft tissue swelling around PIP and MCP joints and wrist |
| MRI | bone marrow edema (osteitis) |

Case 1. A 59-year-old female, stage I, early RA

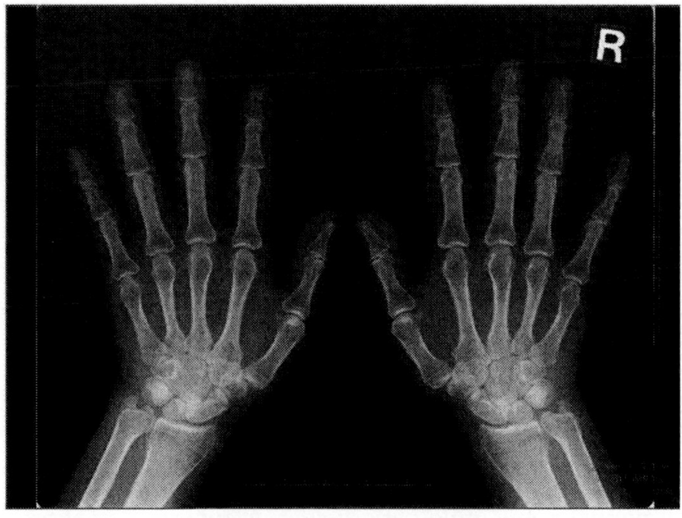

Figure 1. Hand and wrist pain, morning stiffness for four weeks.

History

A 59-year-old woman with symmetric hand and wrist pain and prolonged morning stiffness for four weeks would seem to have rheumatoid arthritis

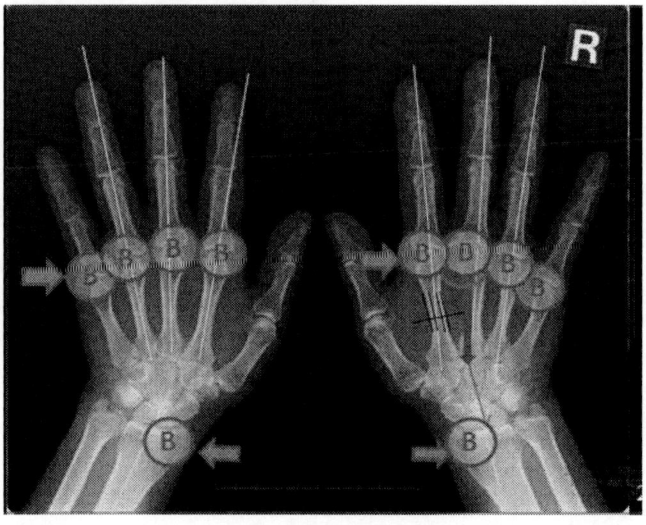

Figure 2.

A. fingers: maintained
   RC joints: maintained
   height of carpal: normal
       (B/A＝0.56)
B. mineralization:
   II metacarpal within normal range
   possible periarticular osteoporosis at MCPs and RC joints
C. joint spaces: DIP, PIP, MCP: maintained
                    carpals: maintained
   erosions: DIP, PIP, MCP, carpals: none
   rt. 3MCP: early erosion suspected
   osteophytes: none
   calcification: none
D. bil. PIPs, bil. RC joints
E. distal soft tissues: normal
   no swelling of joints
F. none
G. tentatively diagnosis: possible early RA

Conventional radiography is almost normal except the 3rd MCP.

It may be with normal range, mild periarticular osteoporosis is observed at PIP and RC joint. The finding may suggest very early RA, but it is difficult to diagnose the disease in this plain radiography. Further information is required.

Therefore we suspected early RA and MRI showed erosions for 2 months. (Figure3)

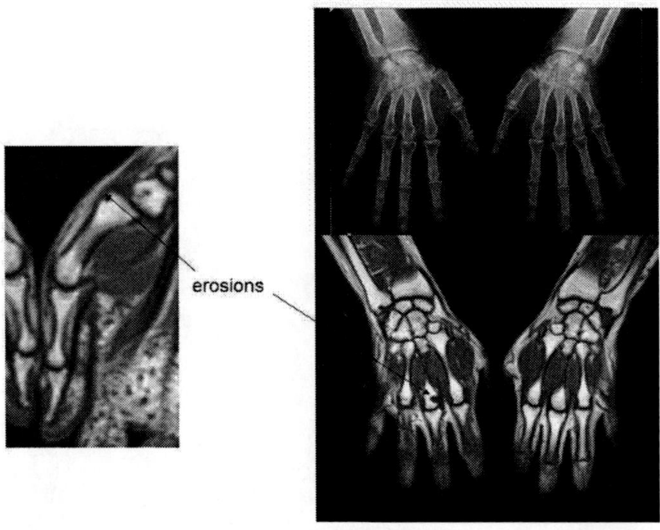

Figure 3.

She was diagnosed having early RA and treated with methotrexate (MTX) and adalimumab; ADA (anti-TNF-alpha monoclonal antibody).

Final diagnosis: early RA

Case 2. A 67-year-old Female, stage II RA, disappearance of erosion by etanercept

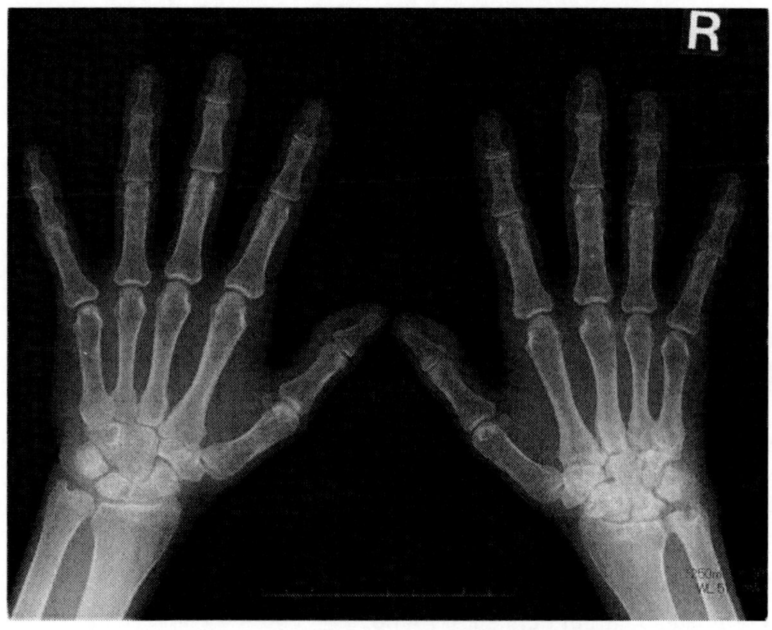

Figure 4. Pain at hands and MCP joints, morning stiffness, and swelling of right hand.

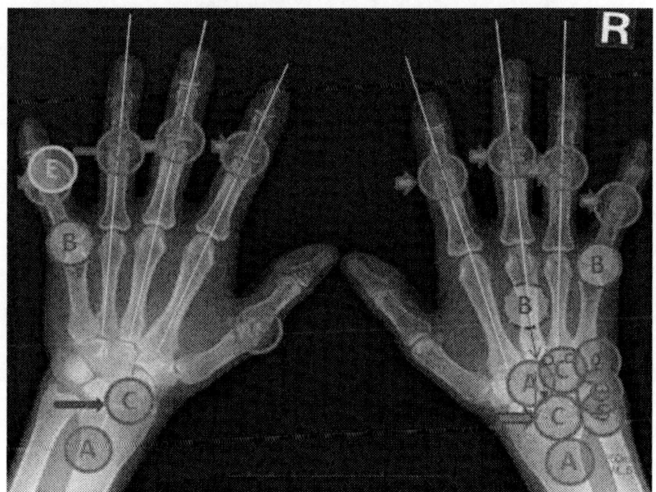

Figure 5.

   A. fingers: maintained
  RC joints: radial deviation, mild
   Loss of height of rt. Carpals: positive
   Rt. Carpal collapse (scaphoid, trapezium, trapezoid and capitate)
   lt. carpals: maintained

B. mineralization:
        II metacarpal   borderline
        possible periarticular osteoporosis at bil. 5MCPs

C. joint spaces: DIP, PIP, MCP: maintained
        except lt.1MCP
        carpals: rt. narrowing as a unit
        RCs: narrowing

   erosions: DIP, PIP, MCP: none
        rt. carpals: erosions
        rt. 4,5 CMC
        Head of ulna
        Styloid process of ulna

  osteophytes: none
  calcification: none

D. bil. PIPs, bil. MCPs, bil. Carpals (rt.>lt.)

E. distal soft tissues: normal
    lt. 5PIP swelling

G. diagnosis: RA (stage II)

Although the changes of arthritis are relatively stronger in right hand, symmetrical changes of PIP joints and carpal bones are found.

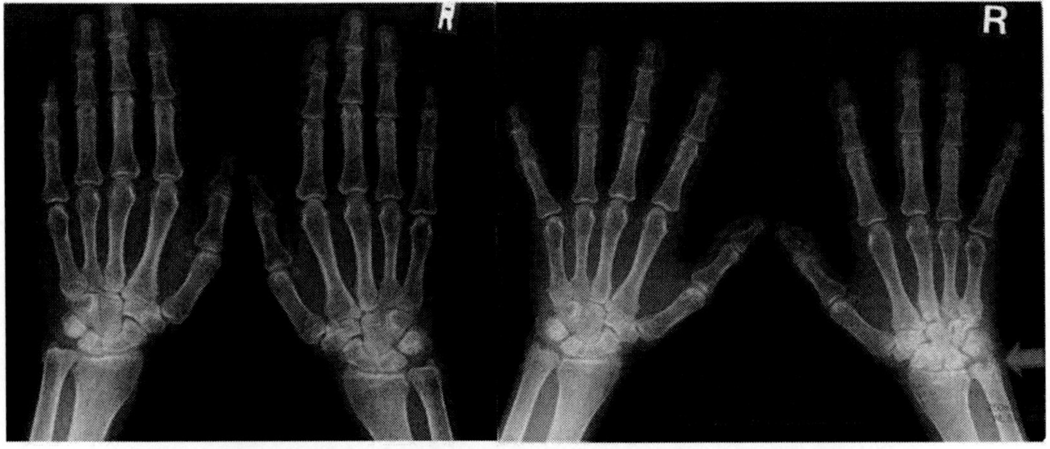

Figure 6. Posteroanterior hand radiographs.

For 3 years, joint space narrowing and multiple erosion has been established, the patient has been treated with etanercept from 2008.

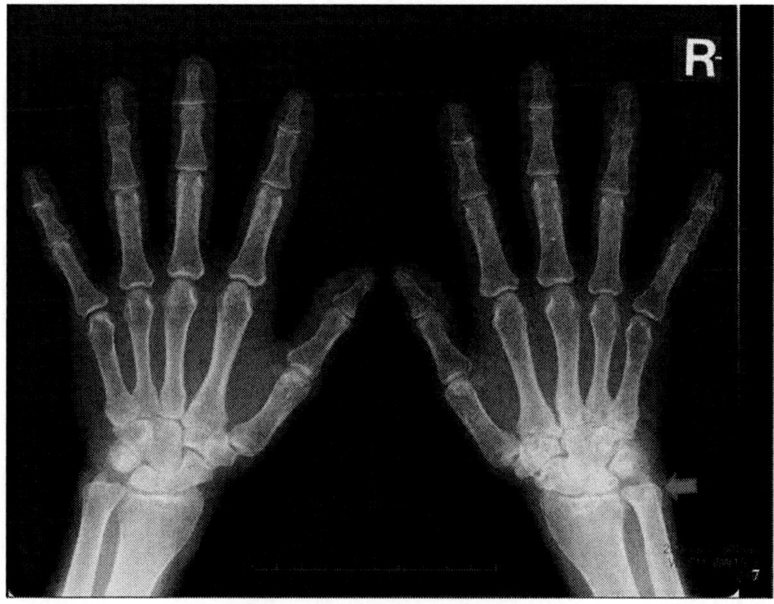

Figure 7. Posteroanterior hand radiograph.

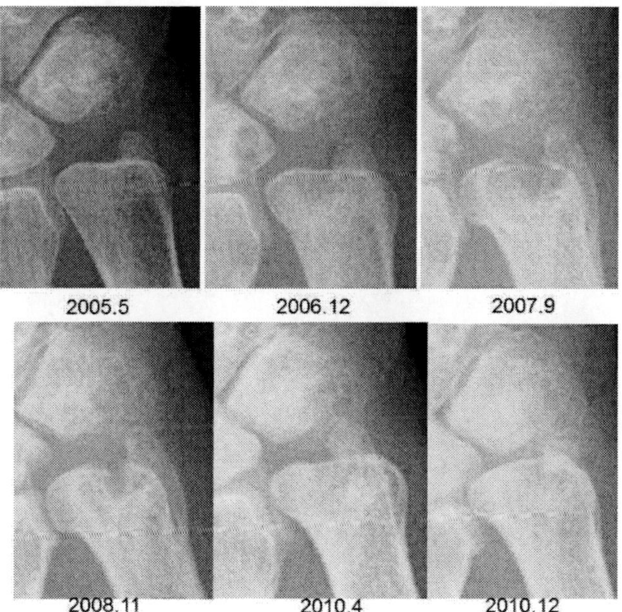

Figure 8. Progress erosion from 2005 to 2008 (Before biological) and Repair of Erosion after treatment with etanercept (2010).
2010 (69-year-old). Disappeareance of erosion at head of ulna.

Case 3. A 29-year-old Female, stage III RA

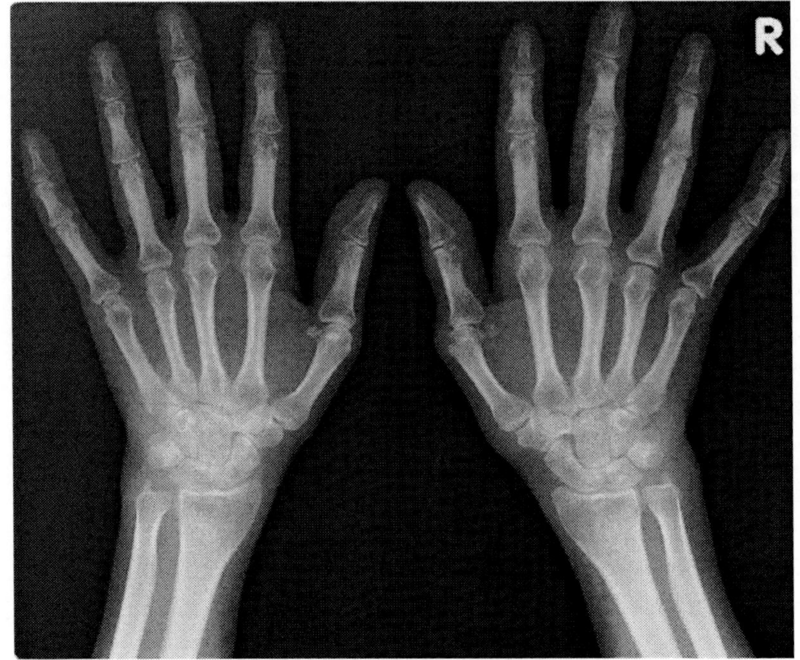

Figure 9. Polyarthralgia.

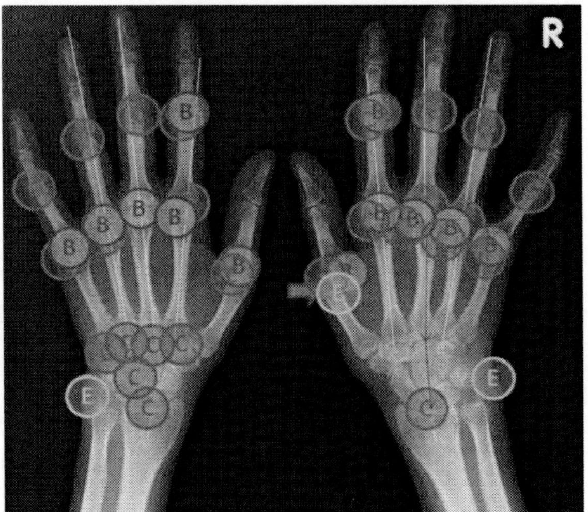

Figure 10.

    A.   fingers: slightly ulnar deviation in the MCP joints
           subluxation at rt 1 MCP
           RC joints: maintained
           Loss of height of Carpals: none
           Carpal collapse: none

B. mineralization:
II metacarpal: normal
periarticular osteoporosis at bil. All MCPs and 2PIPs

C. joint spaces: PIPs, MCPs: narrowing
lt. carpals: narrowing
RCs: narrowing
erosions: rt. 1MCP (marginal)
osteophytes: none
calcification: none

D. bil. PIPs, bil. MCPs, bil. Carpals

E. distal soft tissues: normal
rt. 1MCP, bil wrist: swelling

G. diagnosis: RA (Stage III)
Symmetrical changes of PIP, MCP and carpal joints with marginal erosion are typical for RA.

Case 4. A 30-year-old female, stage III RA, treated with Infliximab

CC: polyarthralgia
Case History:
2002.   1. left hip pain
3. morning stiffness, pain and swelling of bilateral hands
4. arthralgia at bilateral wrists and knees
She visited our office. She was diagnosed having early RA and treated with MTX.

2004.1. However, the RA was progressive, stage III, class 2, and then infliximab (anti-TNF-alpha monoclonal antibody) started.

MTX	8 mg/week	Other DMARDs	none
NSS	+	PSL	0 mg/day
Tender joints (28 joints)	13	Swelling joints (28 joints)	20
CRP	1.41 mg/dl	VAS	75 mm
MMP-3	156 ng/ml	DAS28 (CRP)	6.26 (high)
Morning stiffness	24 hours		Stage III
symptoms	Severe polyarthralgia		Class 2

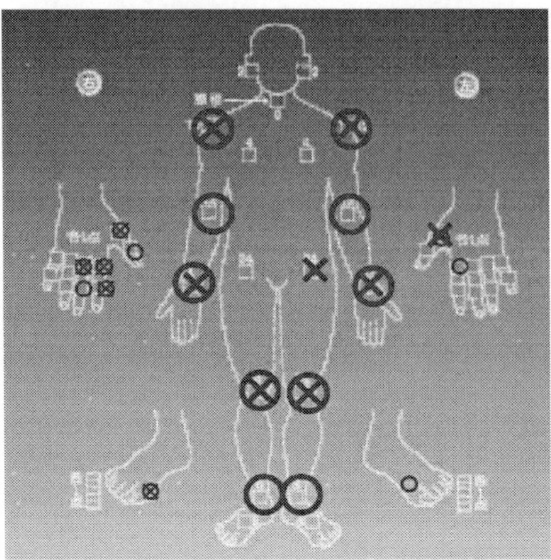

Figure 11.

Tender joints 13
Swelling joints 20
VAS 75mm

CRP   1.41 mg/dl
RF   108 IU/ml
MMP-3   156 ng/ml
Autoantibody to galactose deficient IgG (CARF)   196 AU/ml

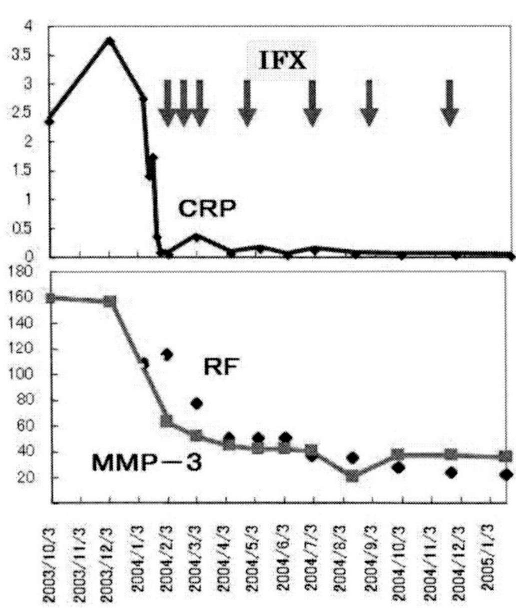

Figure 12. Clinical Course.

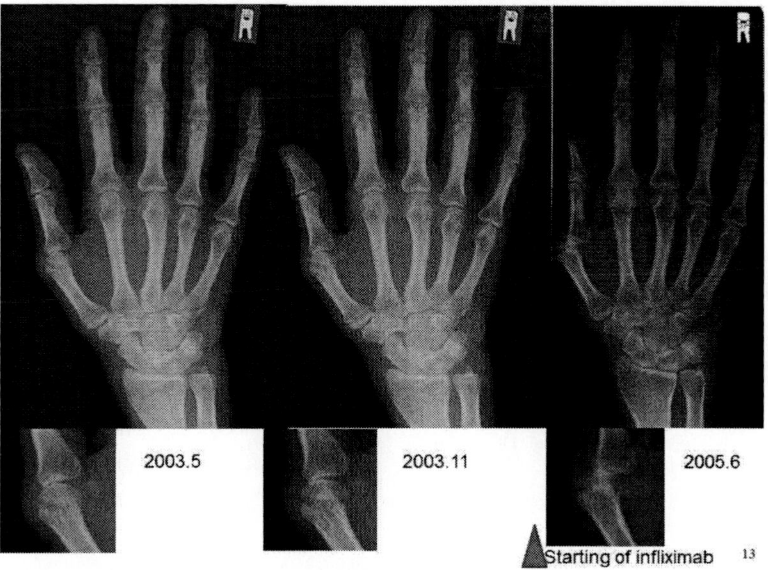

Figure 13. Clinical Course.

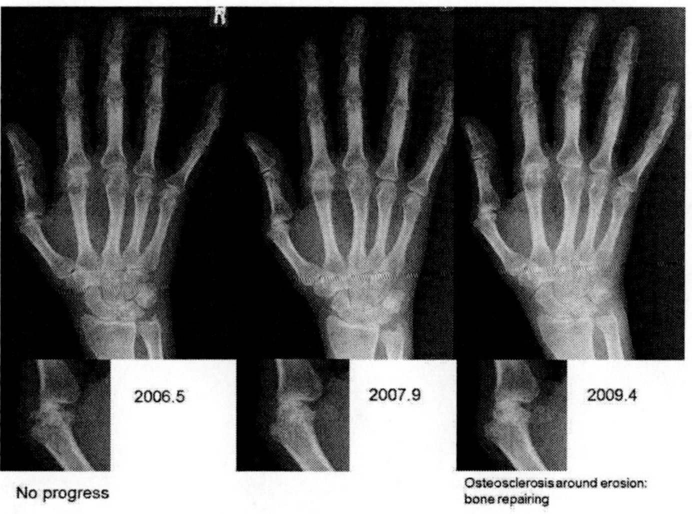

Figure 14. Clinical Course.

2004. 1. Infliximab (3mg/kg) started
→on the day, shoulder pain disappeared
the next day, other arthritis improving
2004. 2 CRP(-), decreased RF level and normal range of MMP-3
Entering remission

During 6 years, she has been treated with infliximab followed by etanercept.
In this period, there is no progress of arthropathy in radiography.

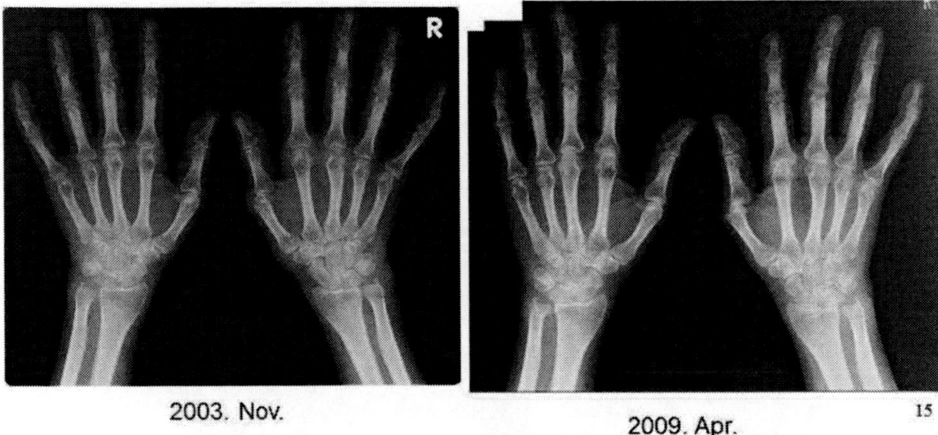

Figure 15.

Case 5. A 52-year-old Male; stage I, early RA, Biological (IFX) free remission

Biologics-free remission in early RA
Radiographies at the visiting our office.

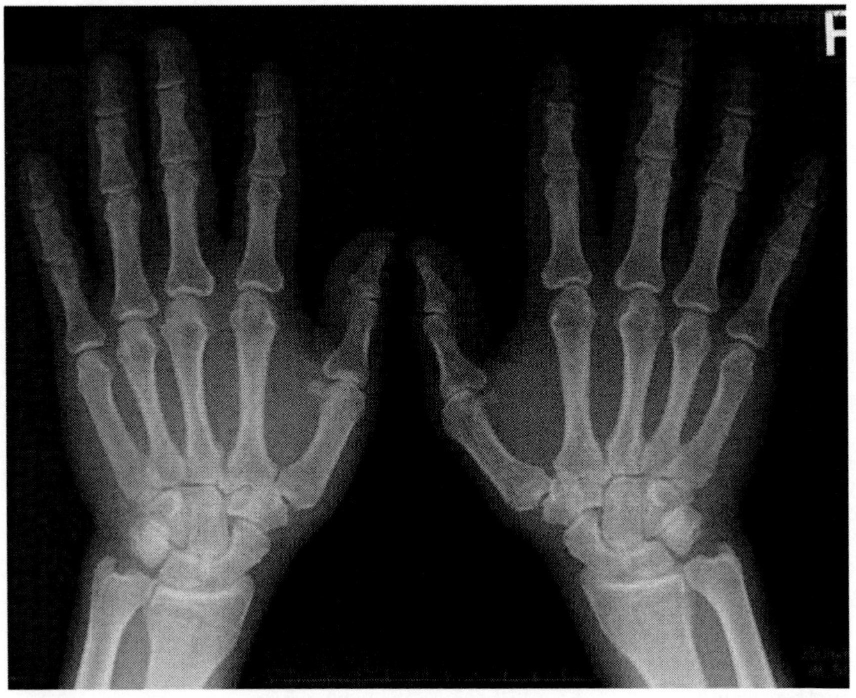

Figure 16. Normal hand radiography

CC: polyarthralgia
Case History:
2009. 9. (49 y.o.) polyarthralgia

10. visitied our office

 morning stiffness, pain and swelling of bilateral hands

 anti-CCP Ab(+), CRP+

 plain radiography: normal but in MRI, early erosions

He was diagnosed having early RA and treated with MTX.

2010. 2. His arthritis continued and then infliximab (anti-TNF-alpha monoclonal antibody, 3 mg/kg) and PSL 5-7.5mg/day started. Despite of intensive treatment with MTX+IFX+PSL, his symptoms were not resolved. After the dose escalation of IFX from 3 mg/kg to 6 mg/kg, his arthritis improved and stopped medication of PSL. After the maintaining of remission for 6 months, IFX stopped. His remission maintained for 2 years by bio-free.

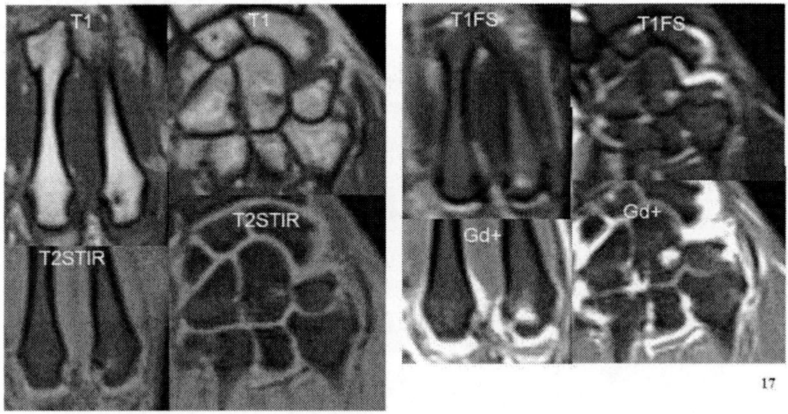

Figure 17. MRI: bone erosions and osteitis.

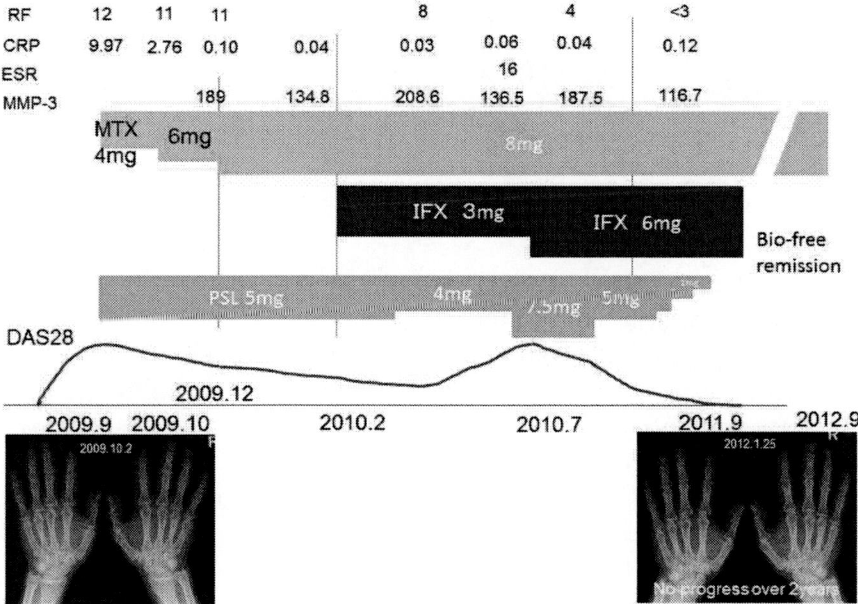

Figure 18. Clinical Course.

MTX	8 mg/week	Other DMARDs	none
NSAIDS	(-)	PSL	0 mg/day
Tender joints (28 joints)	0	Swelling joints (28 joints)	1
CRP	0.20 mg/dl	VAS	22 mm
MMP-3	62 ng/ml	DAS28 (CRP)	1.94 (remission)
Morning stiffness	0		Stage I Class 1
symptoms	free		

Case 6. A 48-year-old Female with advanced RA – biologics-free remission even in advanced RA

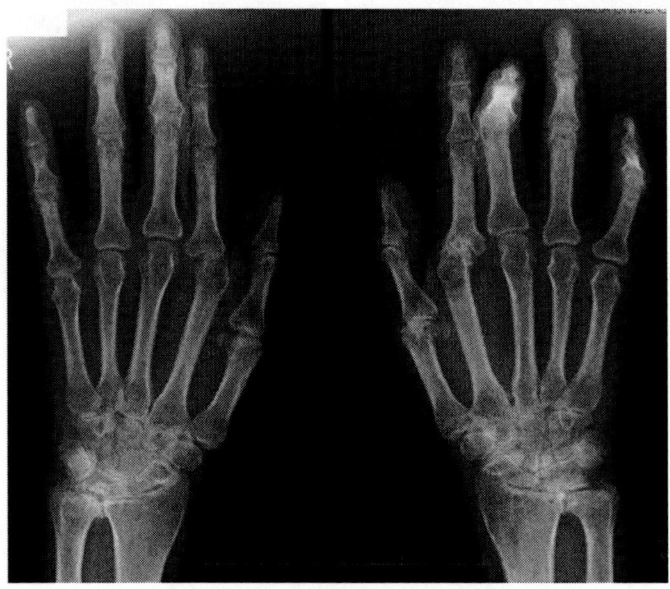

Figure 19.

CC: polyarthralgia
Case History:
1985 (21 y.o.) RA
        active arthritis for long time
2010. 11.   The patient visited our office to ask using biologics for her RA
        because severe joint pain
        at this time, severe arthritis and stageIV
        CRP 0.57, MMP-3 67.7, RF 28
        DAS28-ESR 7.44, DAS28-CRP 6.01 (high disease activity)
        within a week, introduced IFX (3mg/kg)
gradually, her symptoms improved and enter remmision for 1 year
2012. 12. finished IFX and maintain remission by bio-free

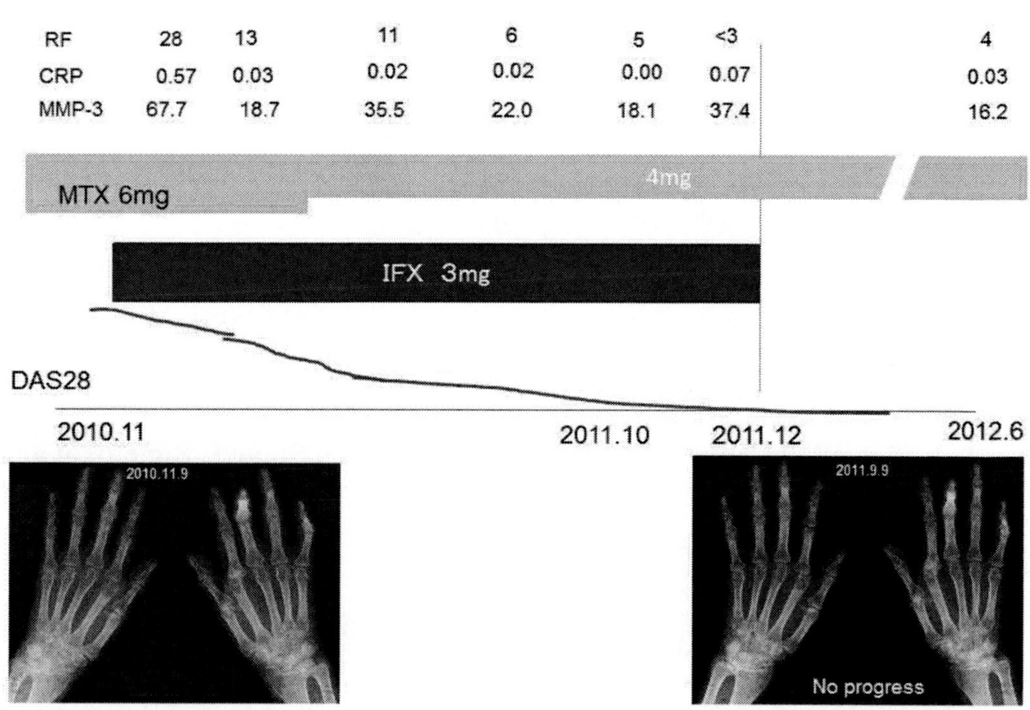

Figure 20. Clinical Course.

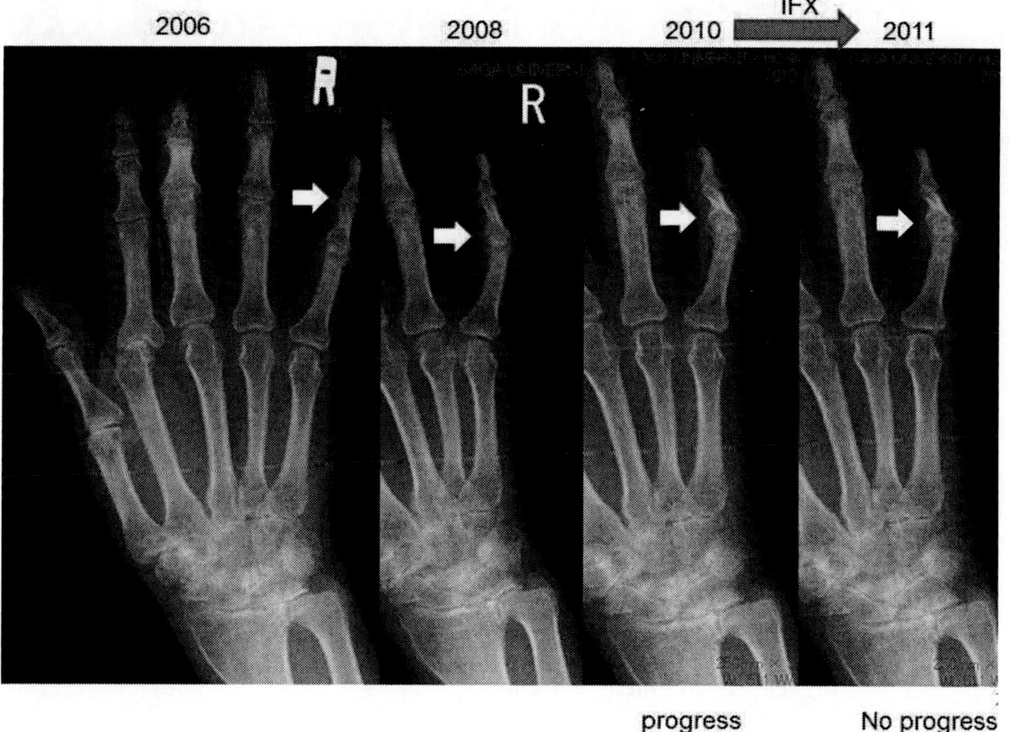

Figure 21. Clinical Course.

MTX	4 mg/week	Other DMARDs	none
NSAIDS	(-)	PSL	0 mg/day
Tender joints (28 joints)	2	Swelling joints (28 joints)	0
CRP	0.03 mg/dl	VAS	13 mm
MMP-3	16.2 ng/ml	DAS28(CRP)	2.03(remission)
Morning stiffness	0		Stage IV Class 2
symptoms	Mild pain at wrists		

Case 7. A 25-year-old Female - Severe polyarthralgia. Stage I, Biologival and DMARDs free remission

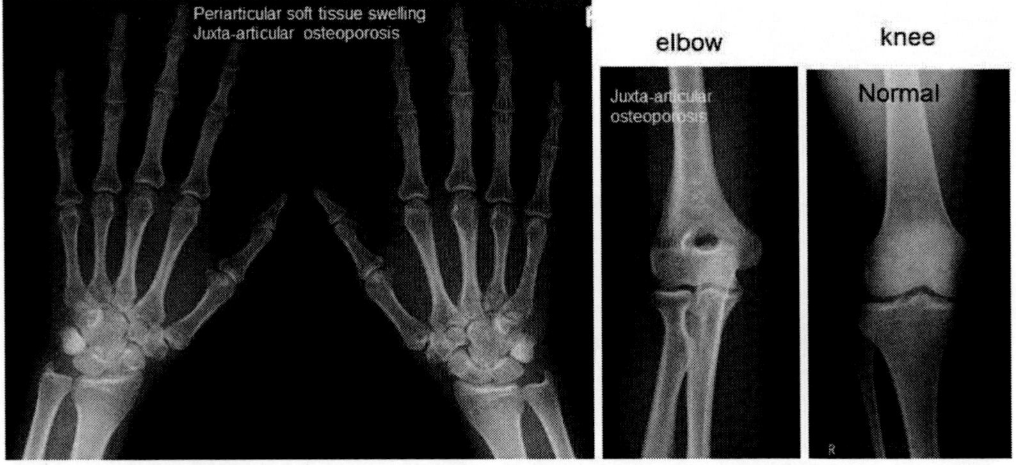

Figure 22. Hoping drug free by early intervention of biologics.

CC: polyarthralgia

Case History:

2011. 1. mild polyarthralgia

2011. 2. marriage

    4. severe pain of multiple joints

        The patient visited our office

        She was diagnosed having early RA

        However, she hoped to become pregnant in the state of drug-free starting MTX

    8. immediate medication of infliximab

    11. achieve complete remission

2012. 7. stopping IFX

    9. stopping MTX.

Her remission maintained for months by drug-free.

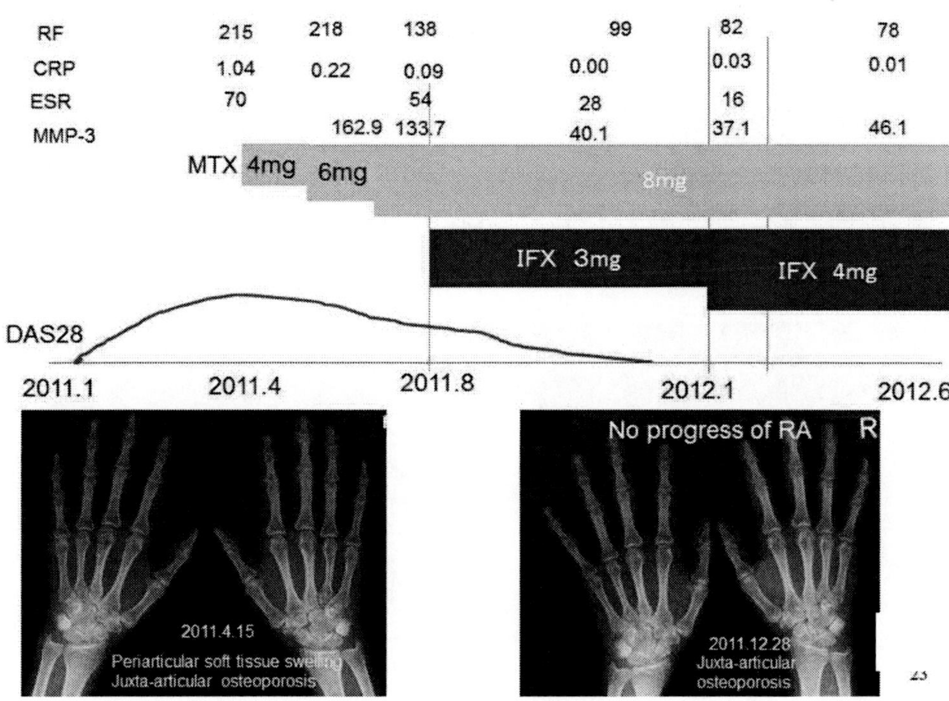

Figure 23. Clinical Course.

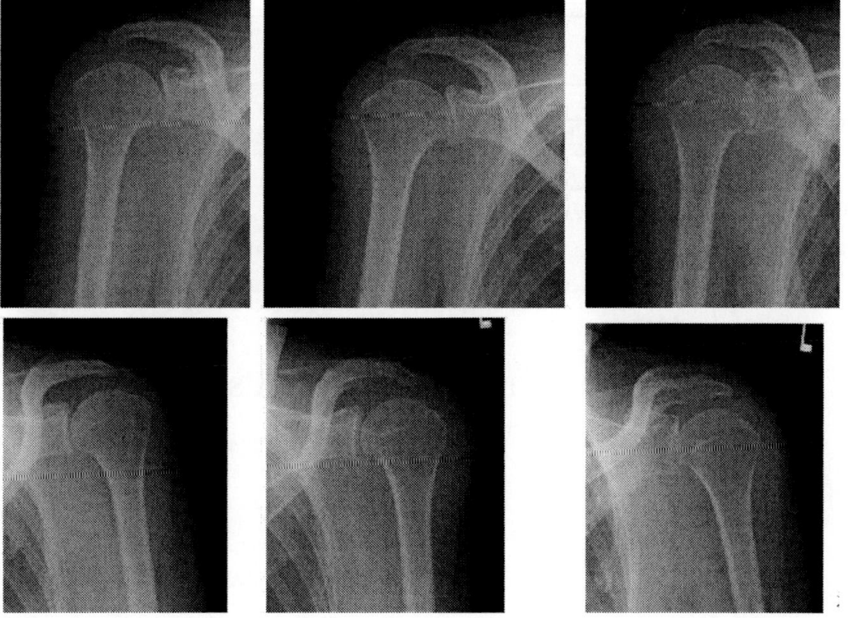

Figure 24. Clinical Course; Shoulders.

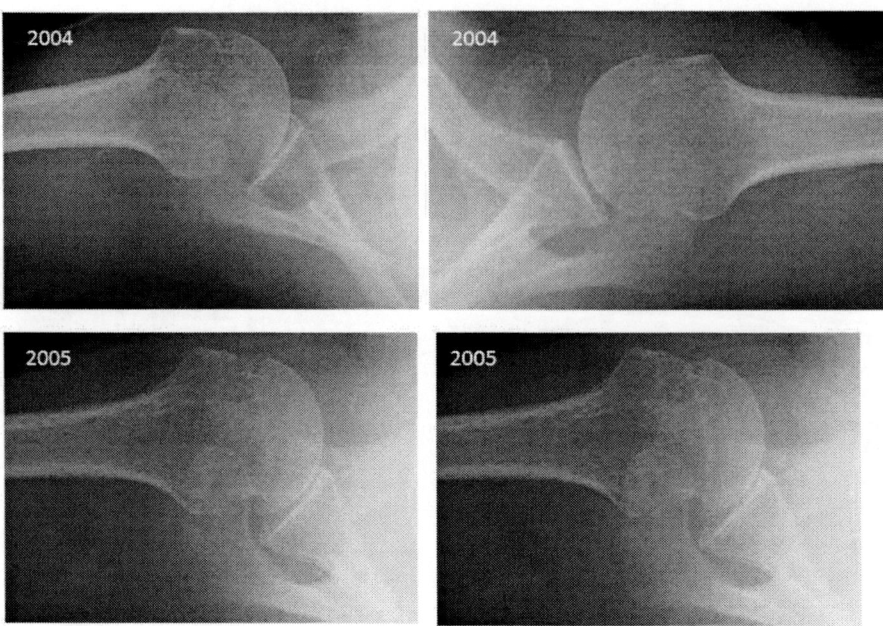

Figure 25. Clinical Course; Shoulders.

MTX	8mg/week	DMARDS	(-)
NSAIDS	(-)	PSL	0 mg/day
Tender joints(28)	0	Swelling joints (28)	0
CRP	0.01 mg/dl	VAS	9 mm
MMP-3	46.1 ng/ml	DAS28(CRP)	1.12(remission)
Morning stiffness	0	Clinical data	stageI
symptoms	None		Class1 RF 78 KL-6 258

PSORIATIC ARTHRITIS (PsA)

Wrists, hand, feet, ankles
Sacroileum
Spine: rare

Difference between RA and PsA
    Usually, non-symmetrical
    DIPs not MCPs
    Juxta-articular osteoporosis; unusual
    Sublaxation; unusual
    Ankyrosis +

Case 8. A 72-year-old Female: Polyarthralgia

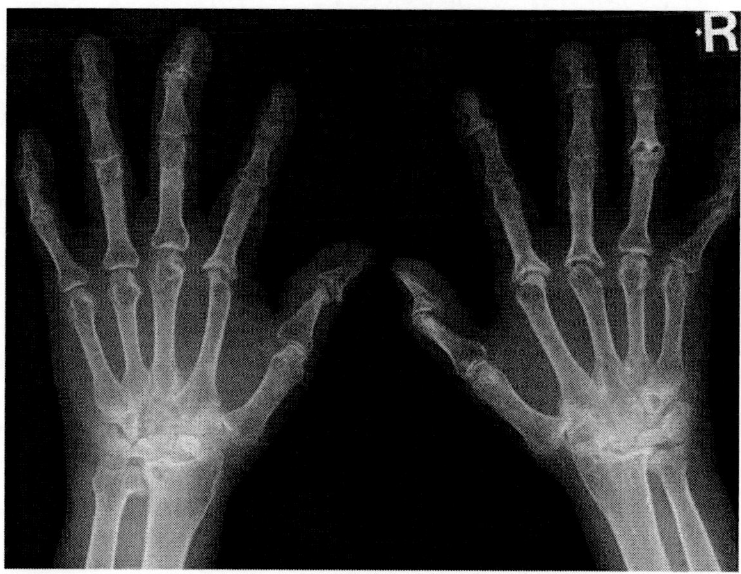

Figure 26. Polyarthralgia.

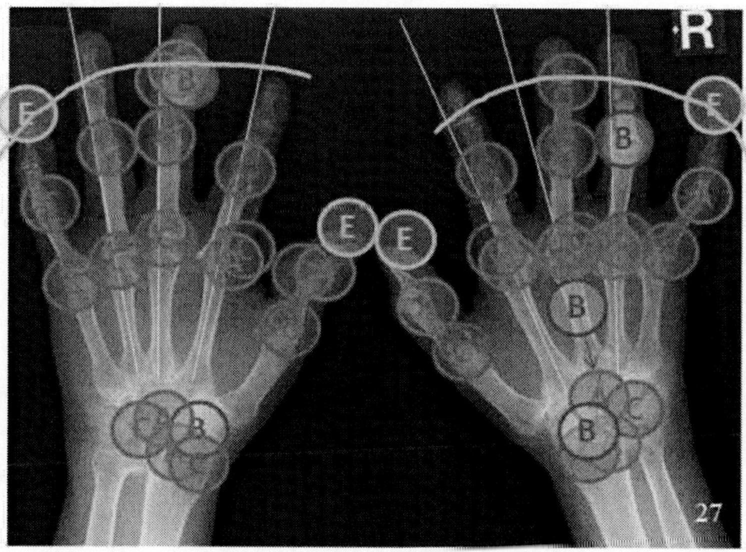

Figure 27.

A   fingers: ulnar deviation at the rt. 1,2,3 and lt 2 MCP joints
         radial subluxation at rt 5 PIPs and lt.3 DIP
         RC joints: radial deviation
         Loss of height of Carpals: positive
         Carpal collapse: positive
B   mineralization:
         II metacarpal: osteopenia
         periarticular osteoporosis: none

          subchondral osteosclerosis: lt. 3 DIPs, rt. 4 PIP and bil. carpals

C   joint spaces: PIPs, MCPs: narrowing except rt. 2,3 MCPs

          rt. 2, 3 MCPs: widening

          carpals: narrowing

          RCs: narrowing

erosions: generalized erosions at rt. 3, lt.3 DIPs lt. IPs and rt. 4,5, lt. 5 PIPs

pencil and cup erosion: rt. 2,3 and lt 2 MCPs

osteophytes: lt. 3DIP, rt. 4,5 lt. 5 PIP, rt. 2,3 lt. 2 MCPs and bil. IPs , possibly rt. RC

calcification: none

D   DIPs, PIPs, Ips, carpals and RCs

E   calcification: none

    distal soft tissues: normal

    fingers: swelling like as a hot-dog

F   nails: psoriatic lesion+

G   Psoriatic arthritis (PsA)

    Generalized osteoporosis

Distribution may be compatible for RA with OA. However, periarticular osteoporosis can not be found. Several DIP and PIP joints have osteophyte and osteosclerosis. Several joints show pencil in cup deformity. These findings srtongly suggest PsA.

Case 9. A 65-year-old Female, PsA

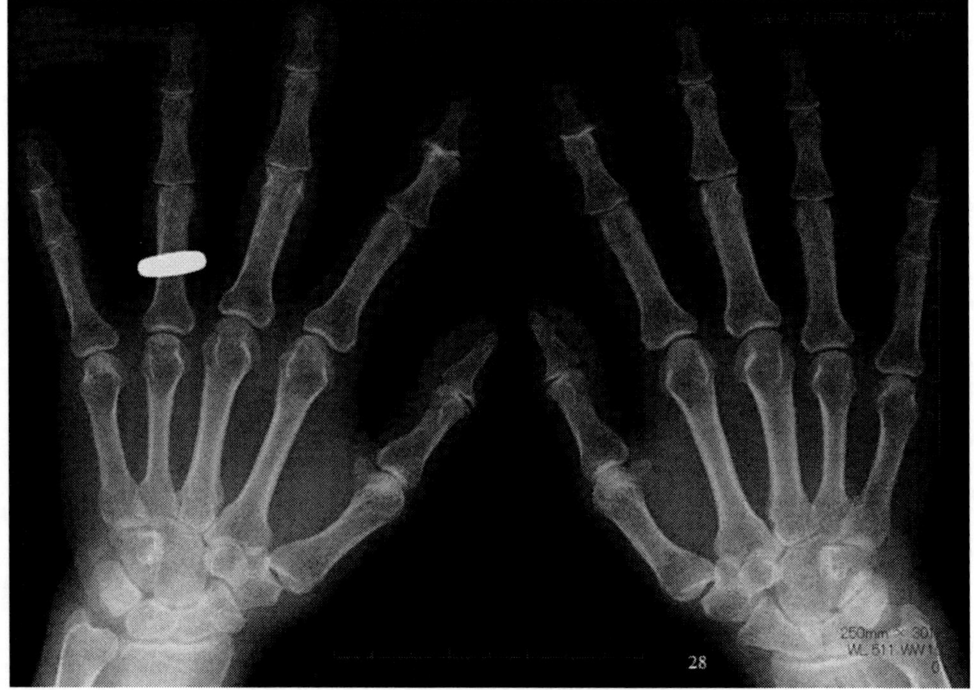

Figure 28. Polyarthralgia.

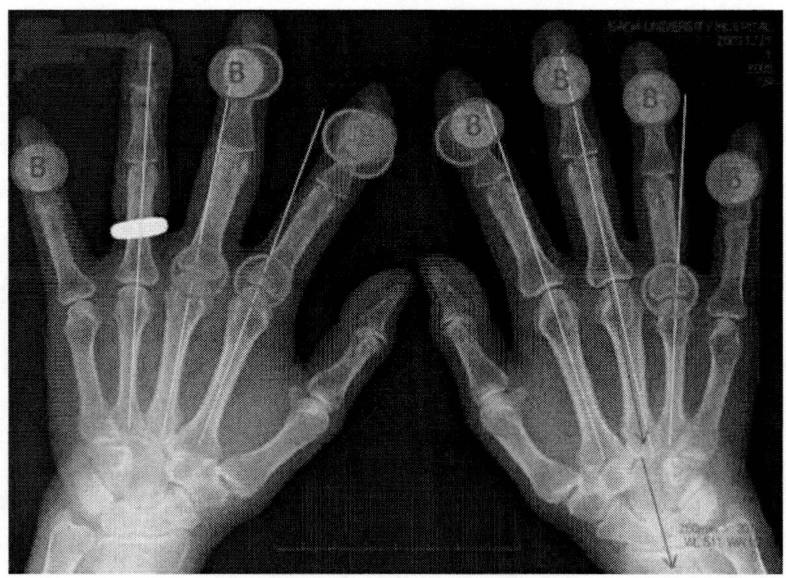

Figure 29.

A   fingers: slightly radial deviation at the several MCP joints, and ulnar deviation at the lt. 2, 3 DIP joints.
RC joints: maintained
Loss of height of Carpals: none
Carpal collapse: none

B   mineralization:
        II metacarpal: normal
        periarticular osteoporosis: none
        osteosclerosis: DIP joints

C   joint spaces: bil. 2,4,5 DIPs: narrowing
        MCPs, carpals: maintained
        RCs: maintained
erosions: bil 2 DIPs, generalized
osteophytes: none
calcification: lt. 2 DIP

D   bil. DIPs and MCPs

E   distal soft tissues: normal
calcification: lt 2 DIP

F   skin eruption at bil. Knees

G   diagnosis: PsA

Symmetrical changes of DIPs with osteosclerosis and joint space narrowing. Extensive survey of skin lesions and hisoty taking including family history are important to diagnose PsA.

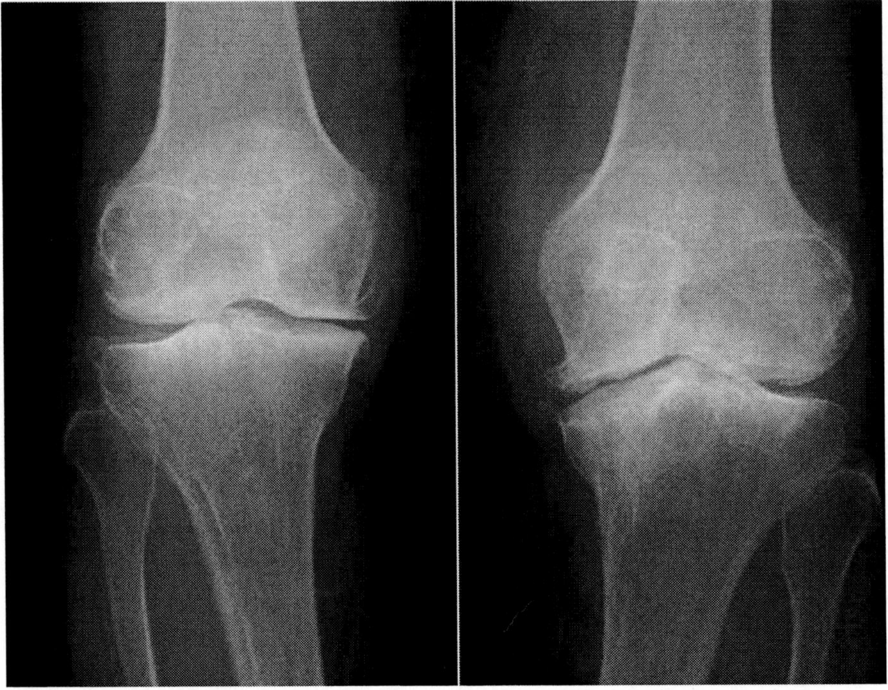

Figure 30. The knees.

Case 10. A 79-year-old Female. PsA + CPPD

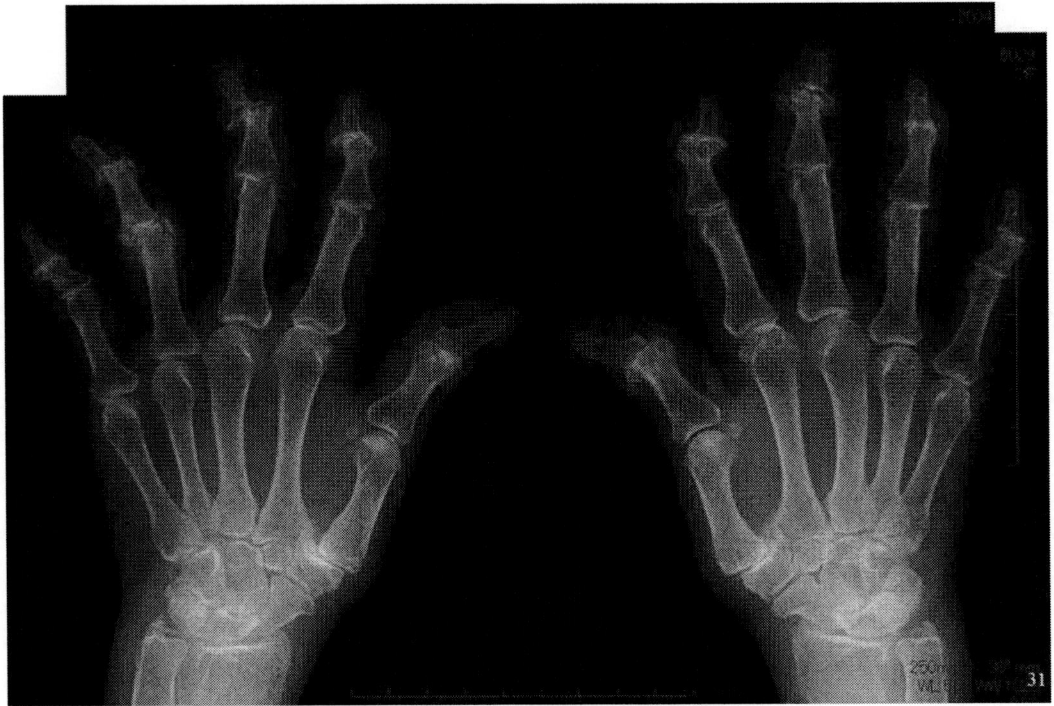

Figure 31. Polyarthralgia of hands.

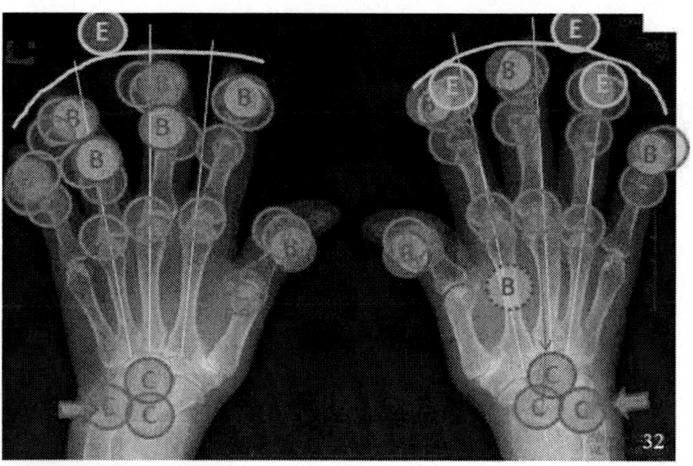

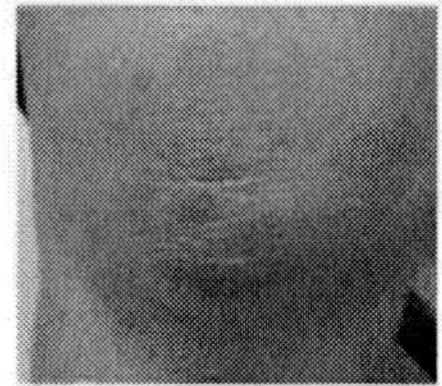

Figure 32.

A   fingers: radial deviation at the MCP joints
         ulnar subluxation at DIPs and severe bone destruction
         RC joints: maintained
         Loss of height of Carpals: none
         Carpal collapse: none

B   mineralization:
         II metacarpal: osteopenia
         periarticular osteoporosis: none
         subchondral osteosclerosis: bil. DIPs and several PIPs

C   joint spaces: DIPs, PIPs, IPs: narrowing
         MCP: maintained except lt.1MCP
         carpals: slightly narrowing
         RCs: slightly narrowing
         erosions: generalized erosions at DIPs and PIPs
         osteophytes: DIPs, several PIPs
         calcification: bil. triangular cartilage

D   bil DIPs and PIP, carpals with calcification

E   calcification at rt. 2DIP and lt. 4PIP
         distal soft tissues: normal
         fingers: swelling

F   skin eruption

G. diagnosis: PsA
         CPPD
Symmetrical severe disalignments of DIP and PIP joints with osteophyte and osteoscletosis are found in PsA.
Carpal change with calcification suggests CPPD.

OSTEOARTHRITIS (OA)

In women over the age of 45 years
Primary osteoarthritis
     No other causative factors for the generative forms
     Aside from a genetic disposition

The proximal and distal interphalangeal joints
Interphalangeal osteoarthritis is usually painless
Morning stiffness and decreased grip strength exist
Joint function is usually maintained
Handedness and mechanical loading by overuse influence distribution and severity of degenerative changes in joints

Case 11. A 60-year-old Female (OA)

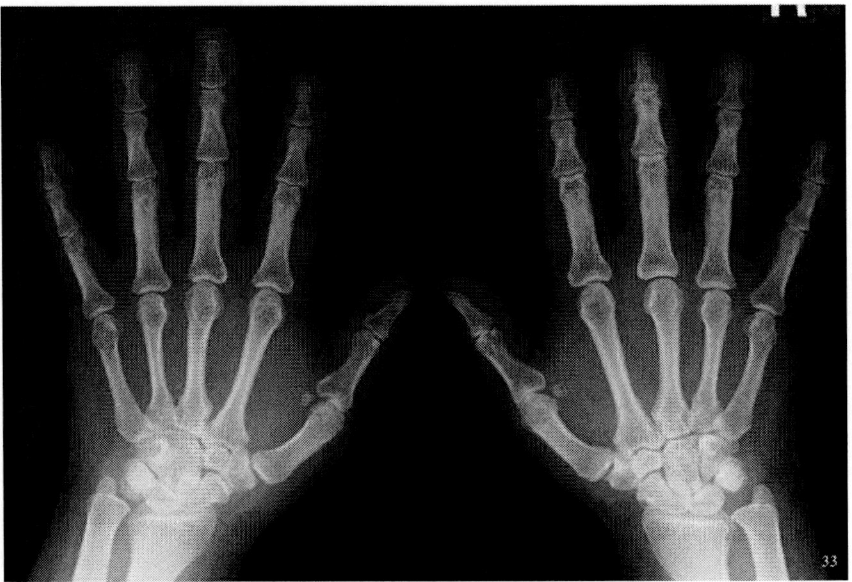

Figure 33. Swelling of hands.

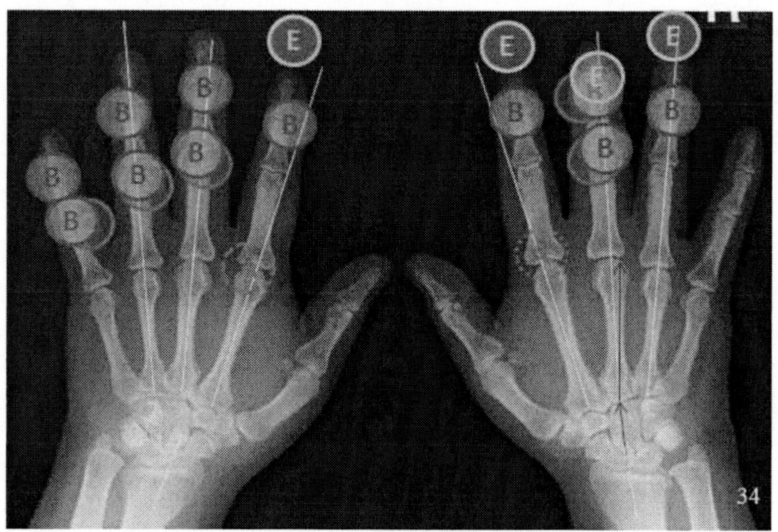

Figure 34.

A   fingers: slightly ulnar deviation at bil. 2MCP joints
RC joints: maintained
 Loss of height of Carpals: none
Carpal collapse: none

B   mineralization:
II metacarpal: normal
periarticular osteoporosis: none
subchondral osteosclerosis: mildly, bil. DIPs and several PIPs

C   joint spaces:
       rt. 3DIPs, rt. 3 and lt. 3,4,5 PIPs: narrowing
       MCP: maintained
       carpals: almost maintained
       RCs: maintained
erosions: none
osteophytes: rt. 3DIP
calcification: bil. triangular cartilage: none
       MCPs: none

D   mainly bil. DIPs and PIPs

E   calcification: none
distal soft tissues: normal
fingers: rt. 2, 4 and lt 2: swelling
 joint: swelling: rt. 3DIP

RF(-), ANA(-), no skin eruption

G　diagnosis: OA

Symmetrical degenerative changes at DIP and PIP joints with osteophyte and osteosclerosis.

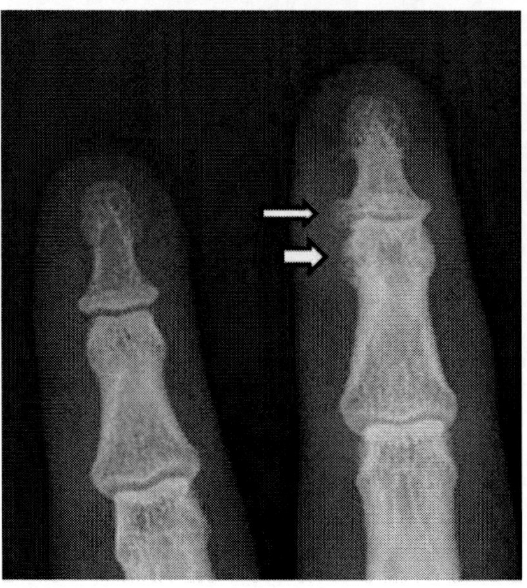

Figure 35. Heberden's node.

Case 12. A 67-year-old Female (Erosive OA) (EOA)

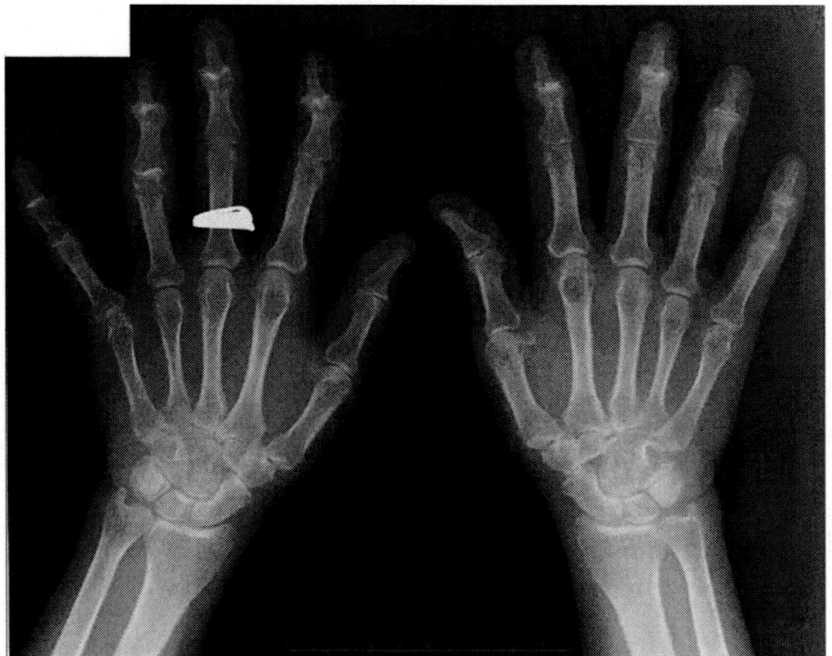

Figure 36. Arthralgia and stiffness of finger joints.

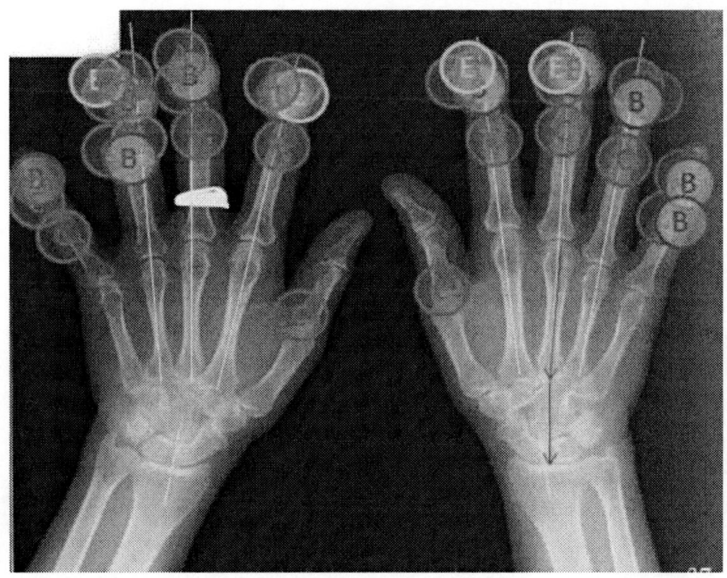

Figure 37.

    A. fingers: randomly, ulnar or radial deviation at the rt. 2 DIP, 4PIP and lt. 2,3, 4DIP joints
        RC joints: maintained
        Loss of height of carpals: none
        Carpal collapse: none

    B. mineralization:
        II metacarpal: maintained
        periarticular osteoporosis: none
        osteosclerosis: all DIPs and several PIP joints

    C. joint spaces:
        DIPs: severely narrowing
        PIPs and 1MCPs: narrowing
        2-5MCPs, carpals: relatively maintained
        RCs: maintained
        erosions: bil. 3DIPs: central erosions "seagull sign"
                other DIPs. generalized
        osteophytes: rt. 2-5 and lt 2-4 DIPs
        calcification: none

    D. bil. DIPs, PIPs, and 1MCPs

    E. distal soft tissues: normal
        joint swelling: bil. DIPs
        calcification: none

F.   not particular

G.   diagnosis: erosive OA (EOA)

Osteogenerative changes of mainly DIP joints with osteosclerosis and osteophyte formations with central erosions, typical for EOA. MCPs and carpal bones are spared.

Case 13. A 65-year-old Female (EOA)

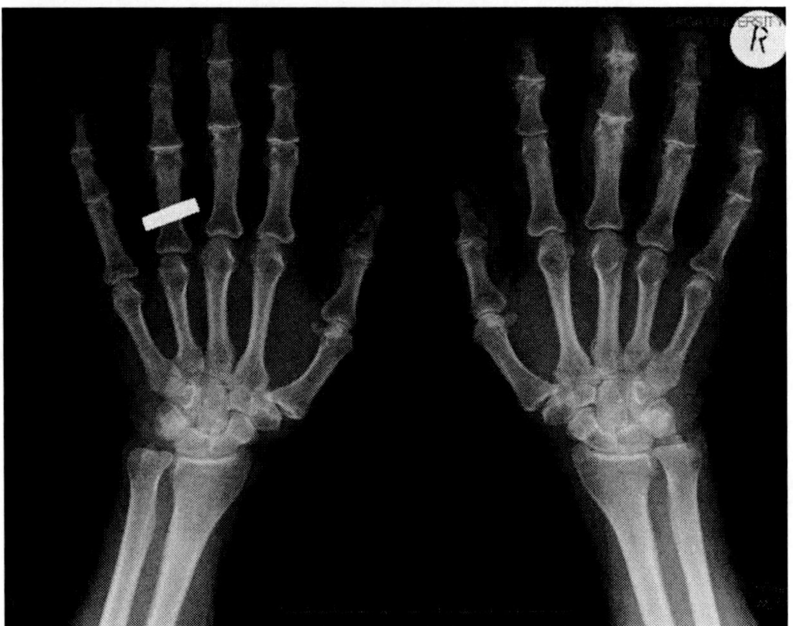

Figure 38. Arthralgia of hands.

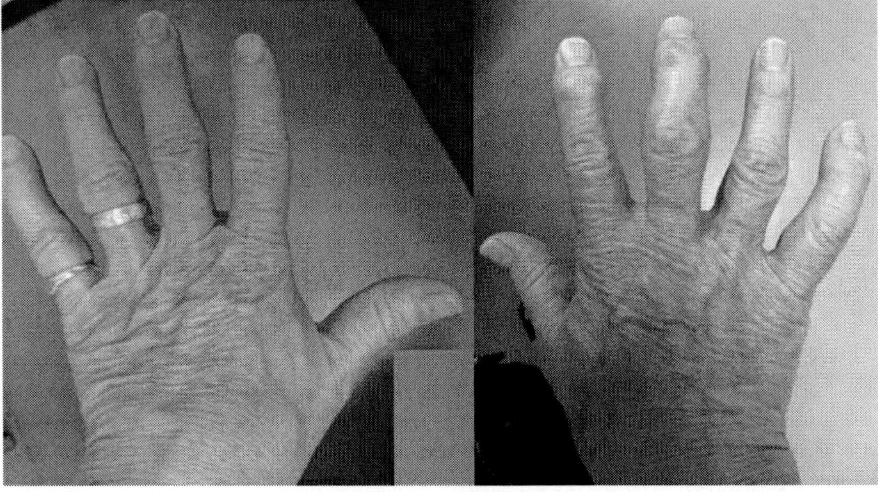

Figure 39. Picture of hands.

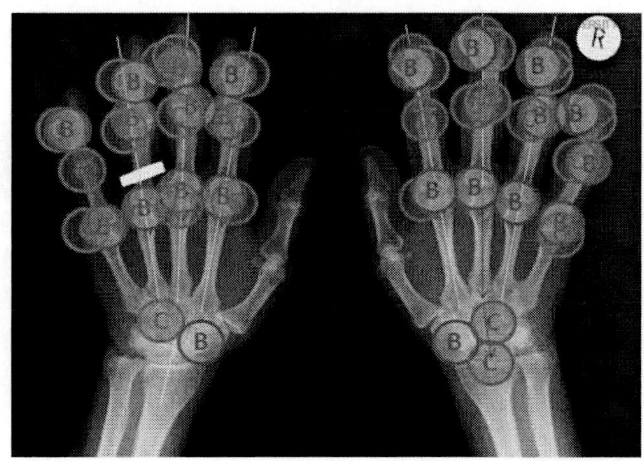

Figure 40.

A. fingers: randomly, ulnar or radial deviation at the rt. 2-5 and lt.5 DIP, rt. 3PIP joints
MCP joints: RC joints: maintained
Loss of height of carpals: positive
Carpal collapse: none

B. mineralization:
II metacarpal: maintained
periarticular osteoporosis: bil. MCPs and carpals
osteosclerosis: all DIPs and several PIPs

C. joint spaces:
DIPs and PIPs: severely narrowing
several MCPs, carpals: narrowing
RCs: narrowing
erosions: rt. 2,3,5 DIPs: generalized, bil. MCPs and carpals
osteophytes: rt. 2,3 DIPs
               rt. 3 and lt. 2,3,4 PIPs
calcification: none

D. bil. DIPs, PIPs, MCPs, and carpals

E. distal soft tissues: normal
joint swelling: bil. DIPs and DIPs
calcification: none

F. RF(+)

G. diagnosis EOA + RA

Osteogenerative changes of DIP and PIP joints with osteosclerosis and osteophyte formations shows OA changes. Moreover, MCPs and carpal bones are affected with osteoporosis and suggestive RA erosions. Both changes make combined complex distribution of affected joints.

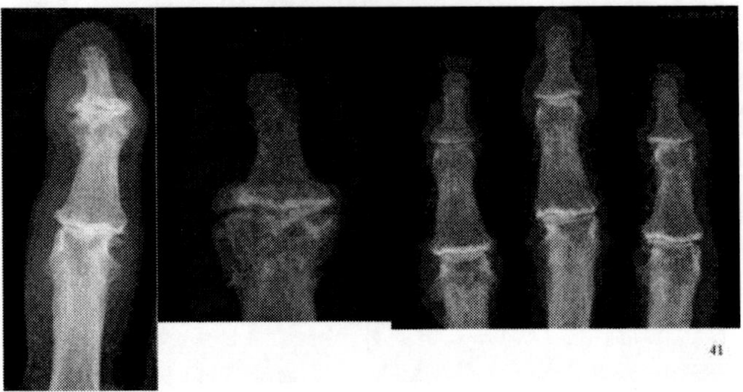

Figure 41. Osteophyte formation at DIPs and PIPs.

ADULT ONSET STILL'S DISEASE (AOSD)

Case 14. A 25-year-old Female. Bilateral wrist pain. (AOSD)

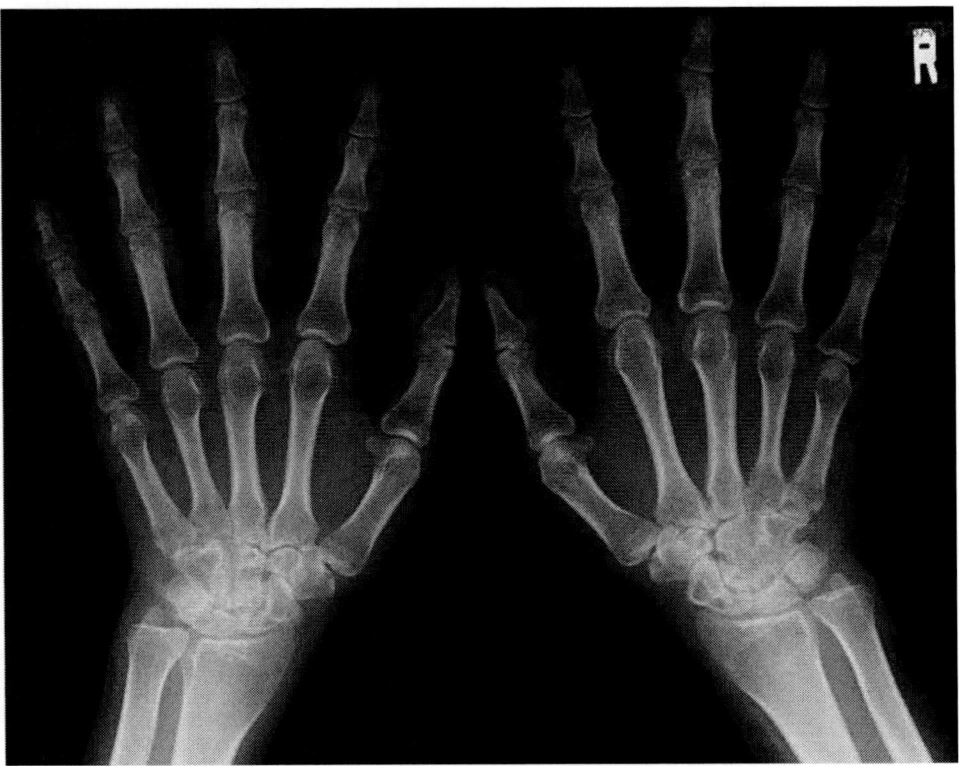

Figure 42. MRI of the hands.

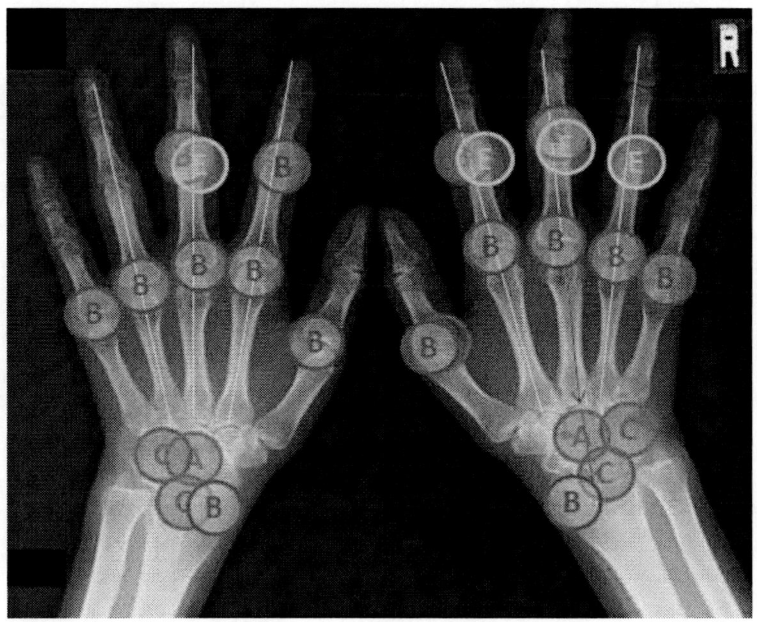

Figure 43.

    A.   fingers: maintained
         RC joints: maintained
         Loss of height of Carpals: positive
         Carpal collapse: positive

    B.   mineralization:
         II metacarpal: maintained
         periarticular osteoporosis: bil. MCPs, PIPs and radius
         osteosclerosis: none

    C.   joint spaces:
         DIPs, PIPs and MCPs: maintaianed
         carpals: narrowing (especially, around capitate)
         RCs: narrowing
         erosions: rt. 2,3,5 DIPs: generalized
         osteophytes: rt. 1 MCP, bil. carpals
         calcification: none

    D.   bil. DIPs, PIPs, MCPs, and carpals

    E.   distal soft tissues: normal
         joint swelling: rt. 2, 3, 4 and lt. 3, 4 PIPs
         calcification: none

    F.   RF(-), ANA(-)

G. diagnosis AOSD

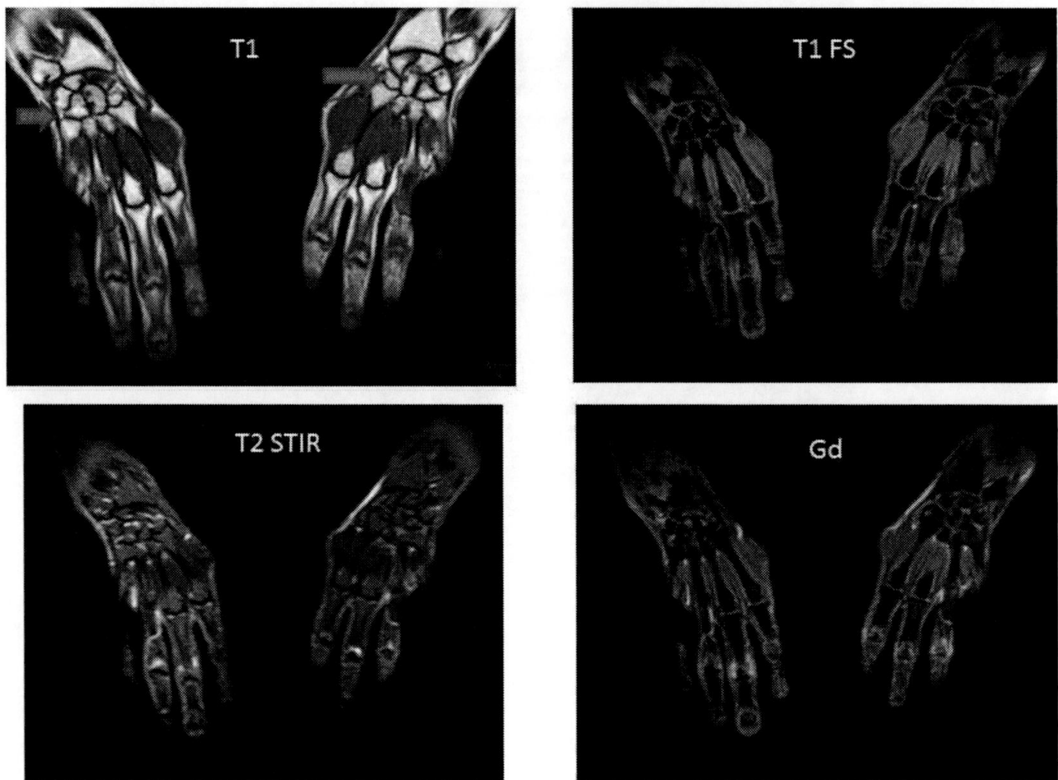

Figure 44.

In AOSD, sometimes arthritis makes wrist ankylosis. In this patient, progressive changes at carpal bones are prominet compared to finger joints.

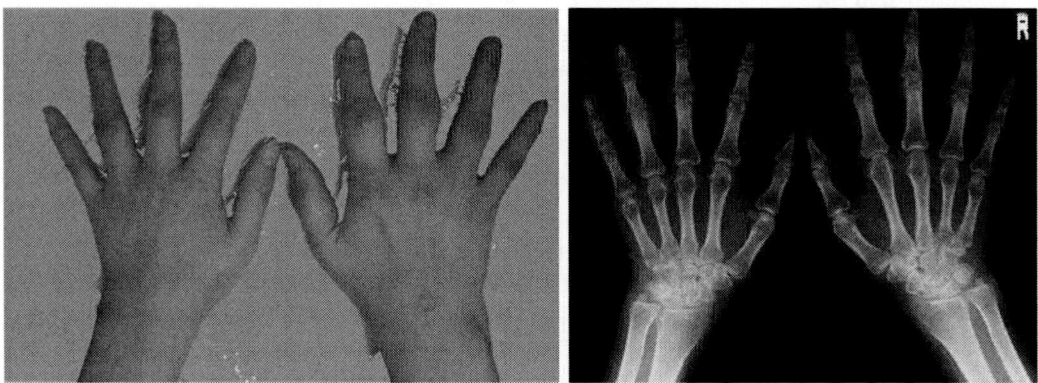

Figure 45. The swelling of finger joints.

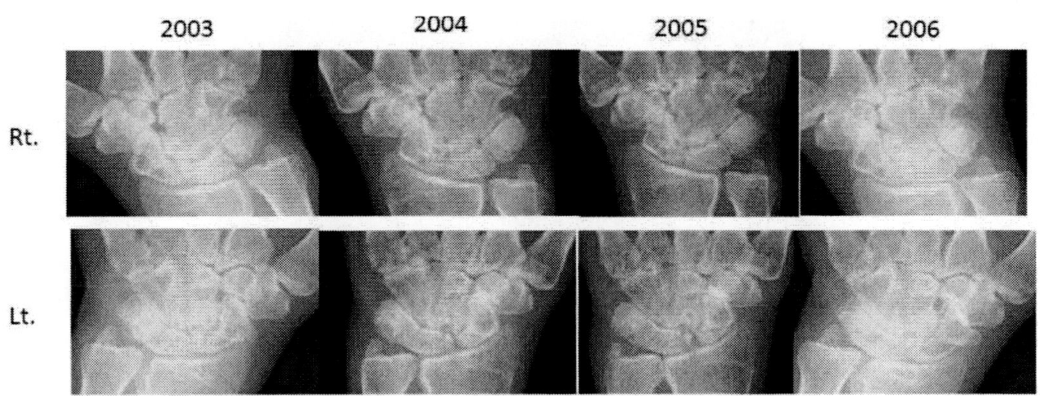

Figure 46. Progressive Changes of Carpal bones.

GOUT

Case 15. A 60-year-old Female, Gout

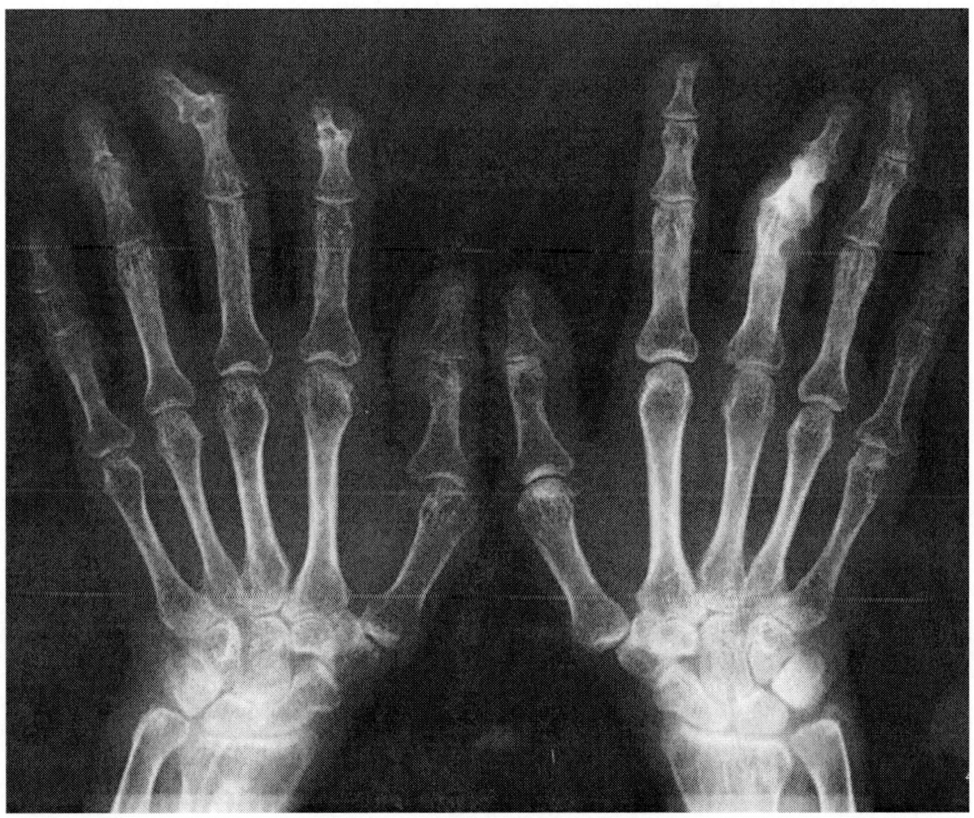

Figure 47. Polyarthralgia.

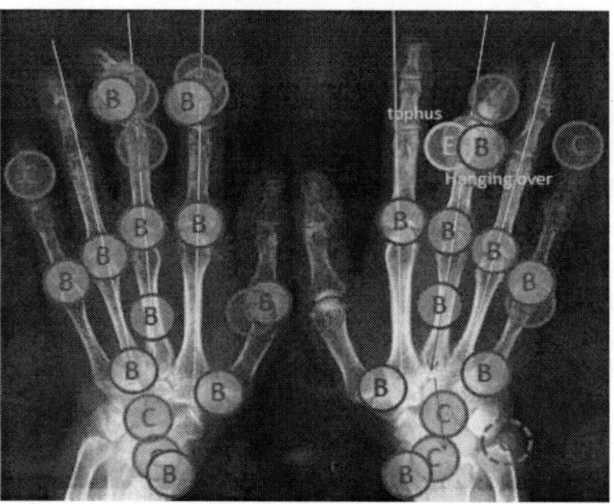

Figure 48.

A. fingers: rt. 3PIP, lt. 2, 3 DIPs: ulnar deviation
    RC joints: maintained
    Loss of height of Carpals: none
    Carpal collapse: none
B. mineralization:
    II metacarpal: normal, III: osteoporotic
    periarticular osteoporosis: bil. MCPs, CMCs and radius
    osteosclerosis: rt. 3 PIP, lt. 2, 3 DIPs
C. joint spaces:
    narrowing at
    rt. 3,5 and lt. 2,3,5 DIPs
    bil. 3 PIPs
    rt. 5 and lt. 1 MCPs
    carpals: narrowing
    RCs: narrowing
    erosions:
    lt. 2, 3 DIPs
    rt. 3 (hanging over) and lt. 3 PIPs
    rt. 5 and lt. 1 MCP
    osteophytes: rt. 3 DIP
    calcification: rt. wrist suspected
D. asymmetrical and non-specific distribution
E. distal soft tissues: normal
    joint swelling: rt. 3 PIP (tophus)
    calcification: none
F. UA 9.8 (high)
G. diagnosis gout

Hanging over type erosion strongly suggests gout and high level UA supports the diagnosis.

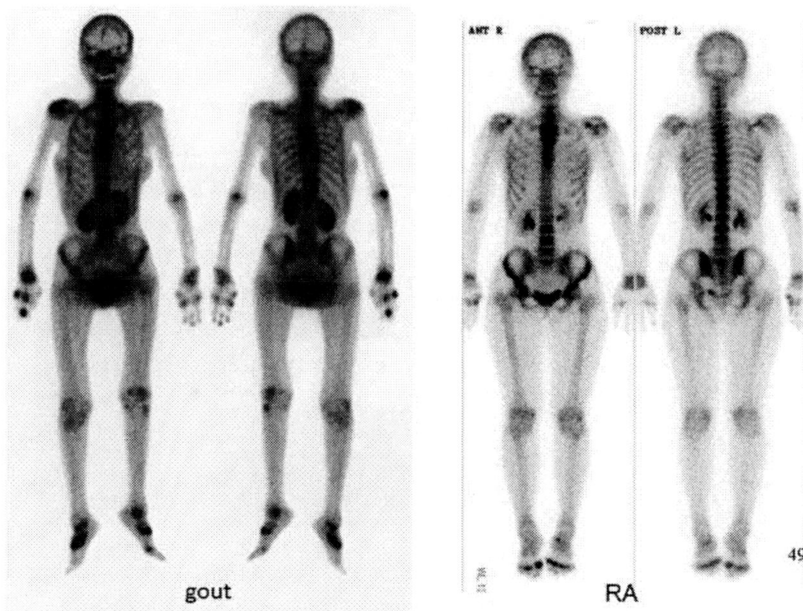

Figure 49. Bone scintigraphy.

Compared symmetrical and peripheral distribution in a RA patient, larger joints are affected in an asymmetrical pattern.

PSEUDO-GOUT (CPPD)

Case 16. A 70-year-old Female, CPPD=OA-Osteoporosis, Crownded dens Syndrome

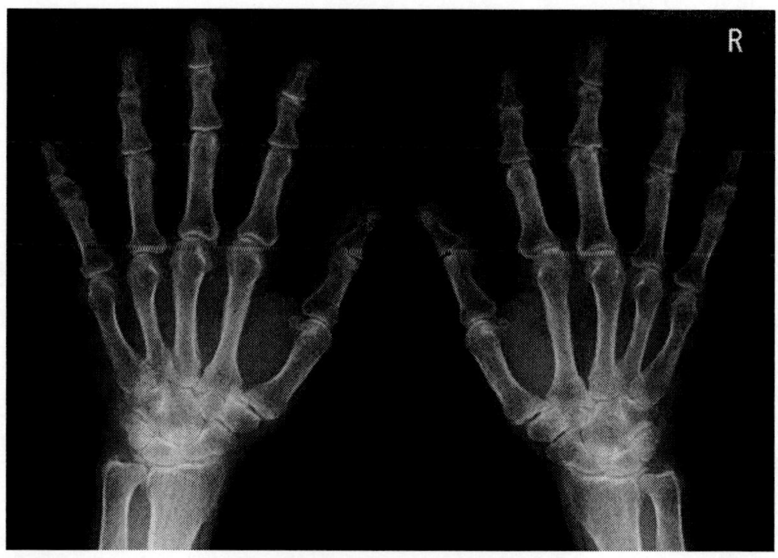

Figure 50. Sudden-onset arthralgia of fingers and wrist.

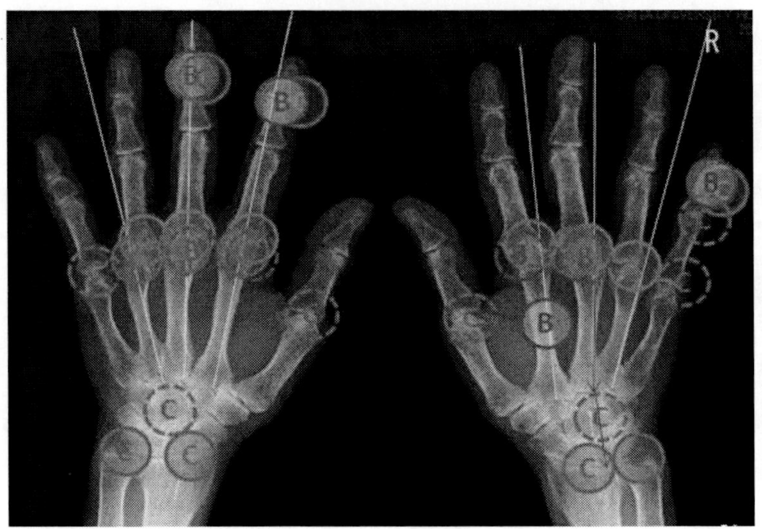

Figure 51.

A. fingers: bil. 2,3, 4 MCPs: radial deviation
RC joints: maintained
Loss of height of Carpals: none (B/A>0.54)
Carpal collapse: none
B. mineralization:
II metacarpal: osteoporotic
periarticular osteoporosis: bil. 2,3 MCPs suspected
osteosclerosis: rt. 5 and lt. 2, 3 DIPs
C. joint spaces:
narrowing at
rt. 5 and lt. 2,3 DIPs
rt. 5 PIP (slightly)
bil. 1,5 MCPs (slightly)
carpals: narrowing (slightly)
RCs: narrowing
erosions: rt. IP possible
osteophytes: none
calcification: in the triangular fibrocartilage of the wrists.
rt. 3 and lt. 2,3,4 MCPs
D. DIPs: osteogenetic
MCPs+carpals: inframmatory
E. distal soft tissues: normal
joint swelling: none
calcification: none
F. calcification in other joints
G CPPD
OA
Osteoporosis

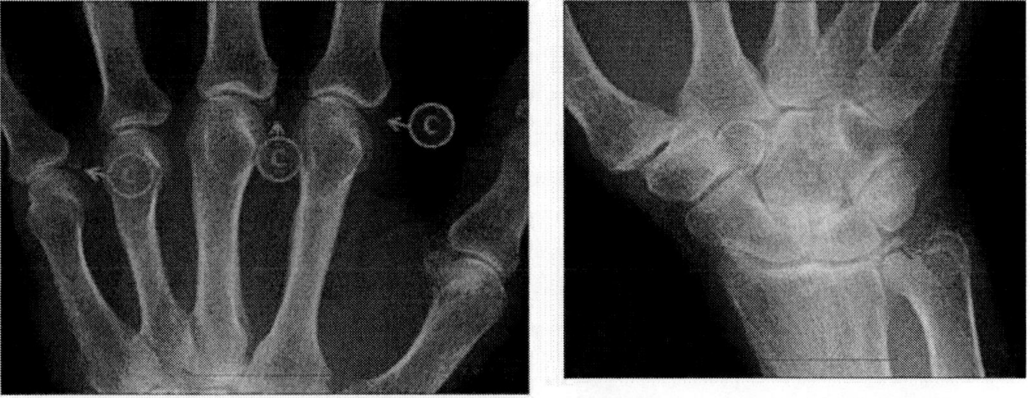

Figure 52. Calcification of the MCP joints.

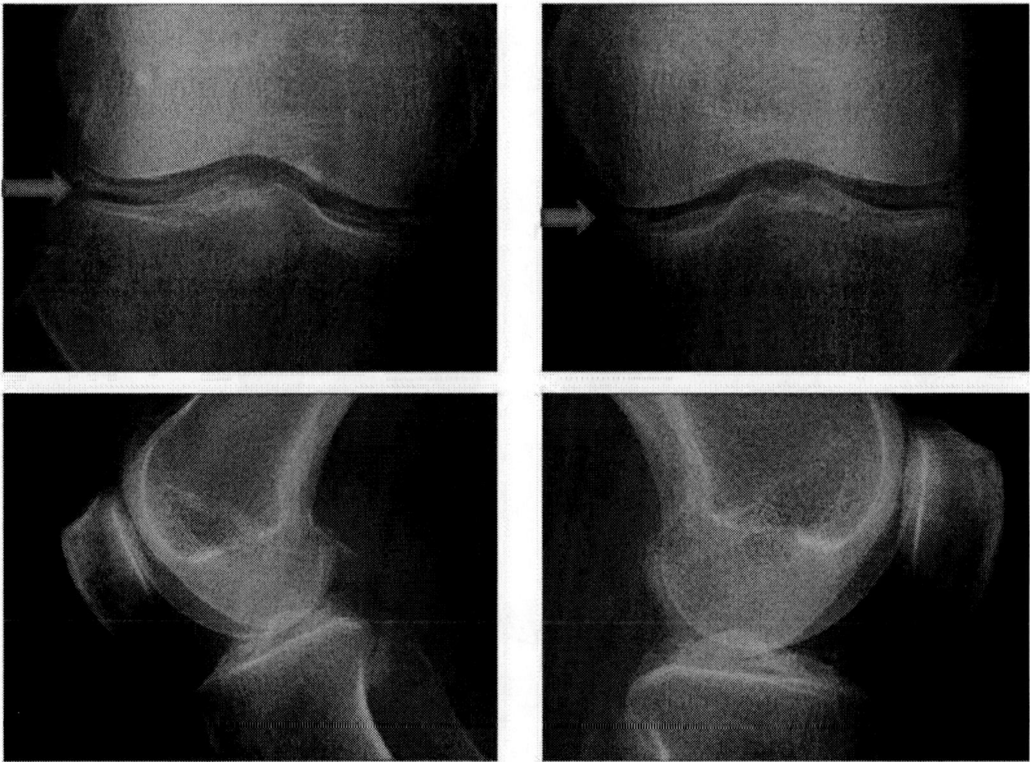

Figure 53. Calcification of the knees in the same patient.

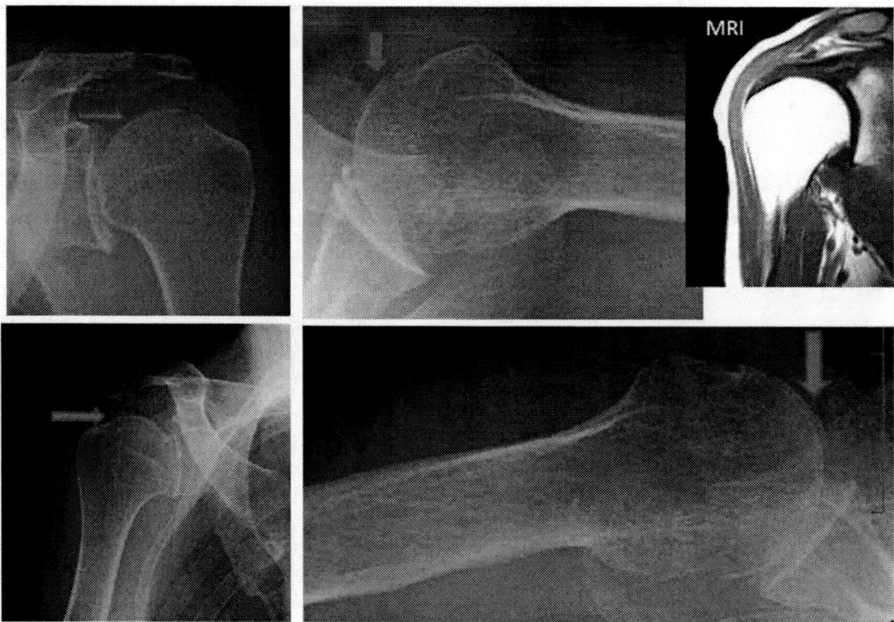

Figure 54. Calcification of the shoulders in the same patient.

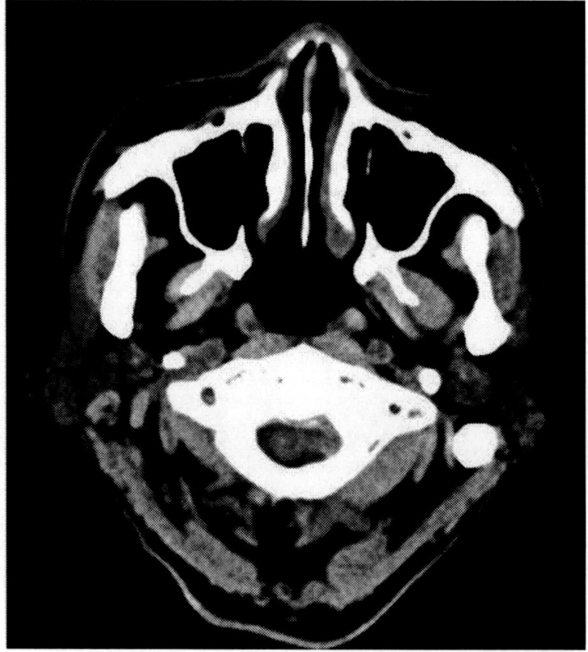

Figure 55. A 84-year-old Male. The patient with sudden onset severe headache transferred to ER.

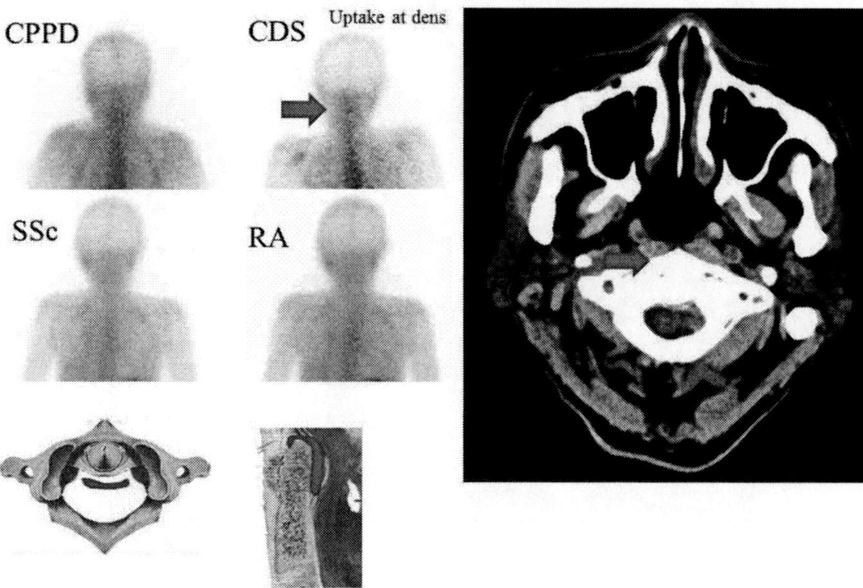

Figure 56. Crowned dens syndrome.

Sudden onset occipital headache

CT image shows calcification surrounding the dens. This may cause headache located at the back of the head suddenly in an elder person.

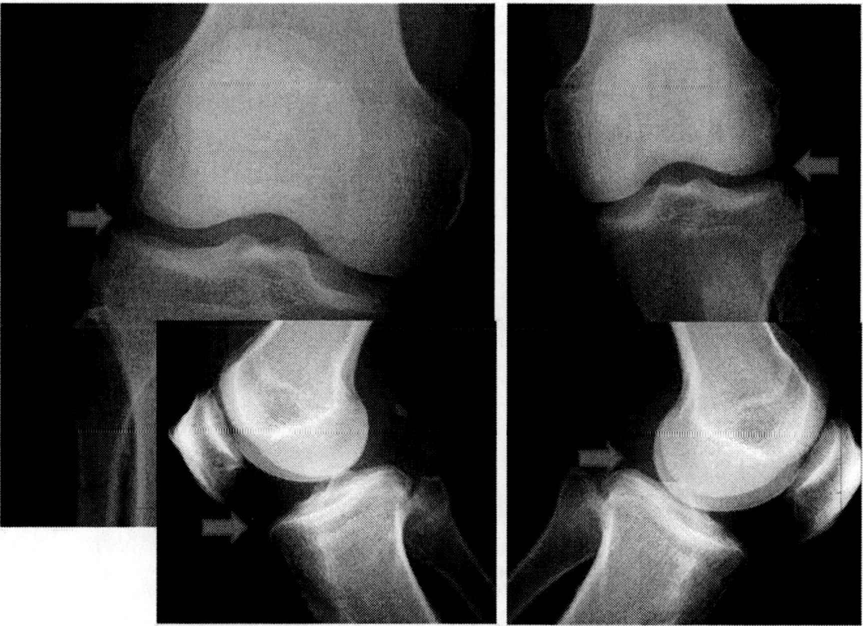

Figure 57. Chondrocalcinosis is present (arrows) in CPPD crystal deposition disease in the knees of the same patient.

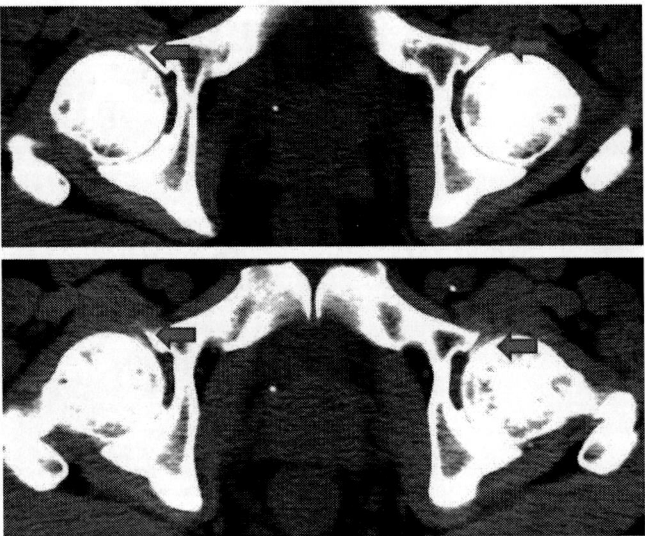

Figure 58. Chondrocalcinosis is present (arrows) in CPPD crystal deposition disease in the hip joints in the same patient.

HYDROXYAPATITE DEPOSITION DISEASE(HADD)

HADD is relatively common
Calcium hydroxyapatite deposition disease
deposits in muscles, capsules, bursae, and tendon sheaths
showing periarticular disease with tendinitis or bursitis
Occasionally, it induces articular disorders
However, articular disease: rare

Case 17. A 84-year-old Female (HADD)

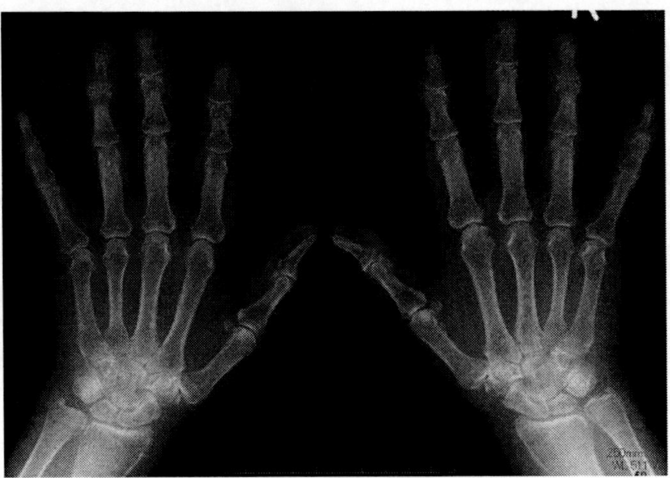

Figure 59. Polyarthralgia, including right shoulder and hands.

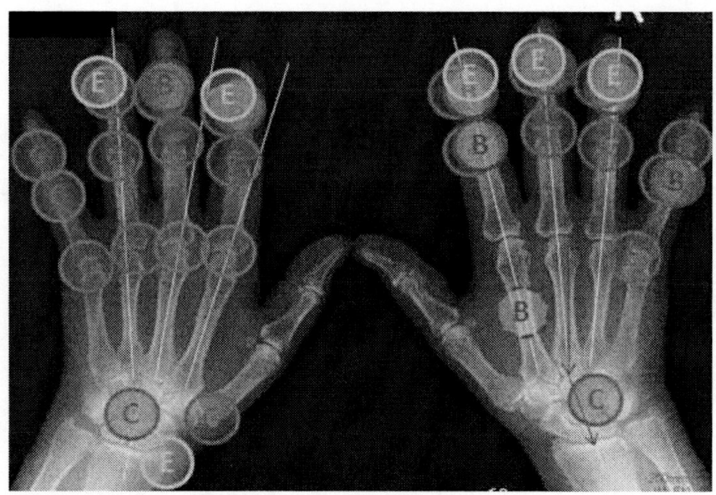

Figure 60.

    A. fingers: slightly ulnar deviation at the lt. 2,3MCP joints
        RC joints: maintained
        Loss of height of carpals: none
        Carpal collapse: none

    B. mineralization:
        II metacarpal: low
        periarticular osteoporosis: none
        osteosclerosis: mild at DIP, PIP joints

    C. joint spaces: DIPs, PIPs: narrowing
        MCPs, carpals: slightly narrowing
        RCs: narrowing
        erosions: lt. 1CMC?
        osteophytes:5MCP
        calcification: none

    D. bil. PIPs, bil. MCPs, bil. Carpals

    E. distal soft tissues: normal
        calcification: DIPs and lt. wrist

    F. Calcification and arthritis in other joints were checked by various modality including
        plain radiography, CT, MRI and scintigraphies

Pre G. Tentative diagnosis: calcification at various joints

    G. final diagnosis HADD and CPPD
            mild OA
            osteoporosis

Symmetrical changes of DIP, PIP and carpals with osteosclerosis are typical for OA but it is mild change. Calcification is due to HADD, and overlapped CPPD.

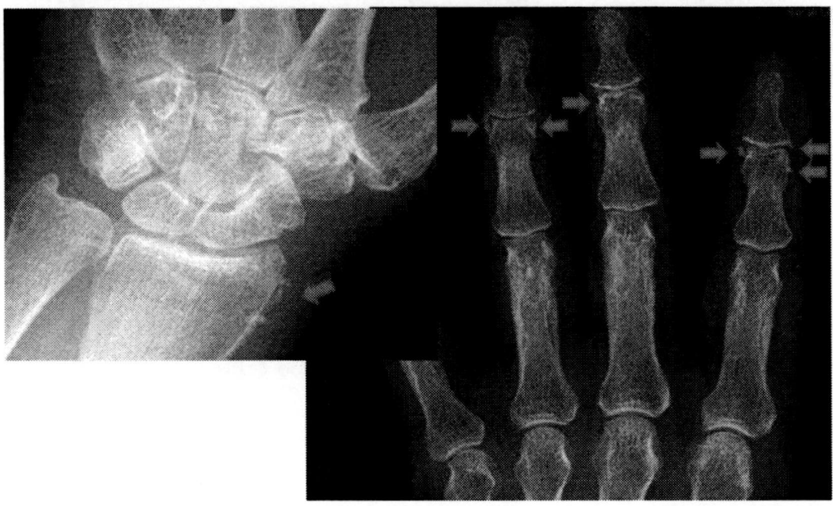

Figure 61. Hydroxyapatite crystals in the wrist (left) Hydroxyapatite crystals in the capsule of the distal interphalangeal joints. Mild OA change but spare JCN (right).

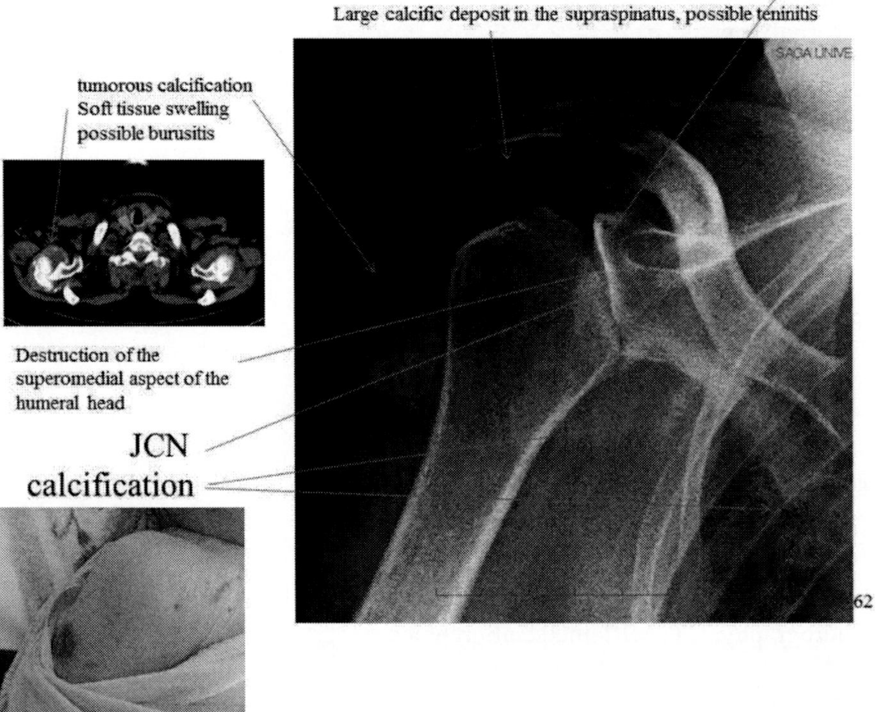

Figure 62. Shoulder: Mainly periarticular calcification.

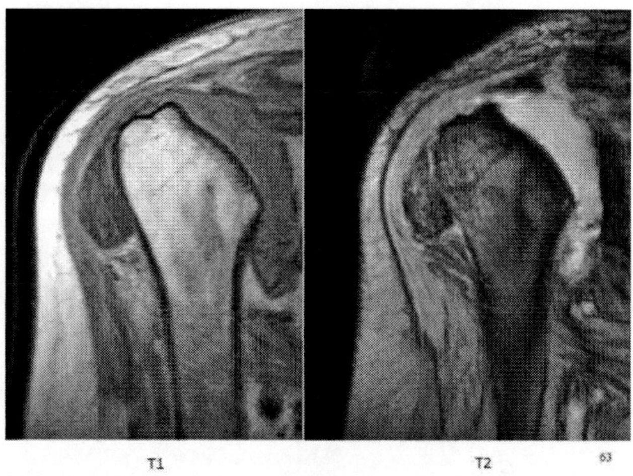

Figure 63. MRI.

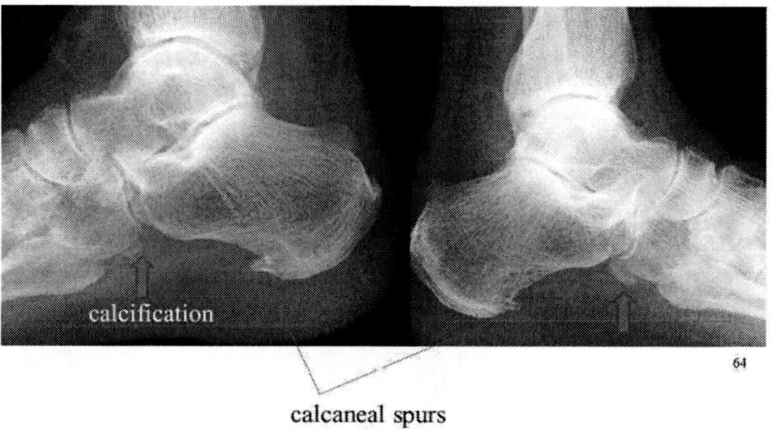

Figure 64. Calcaneal spurs and calcification.

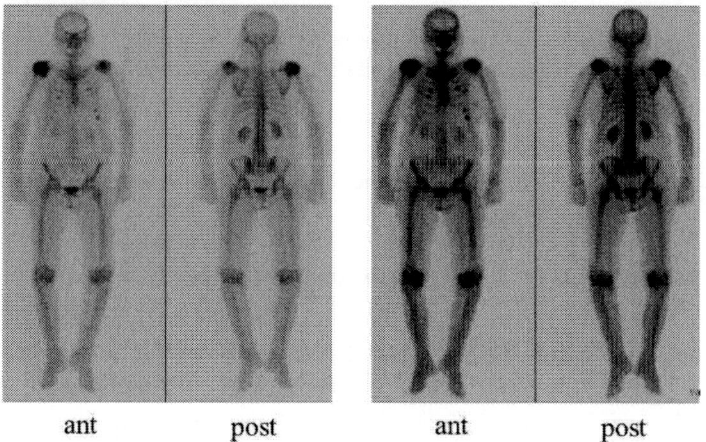

Figure 65. Bone scintigraphy.

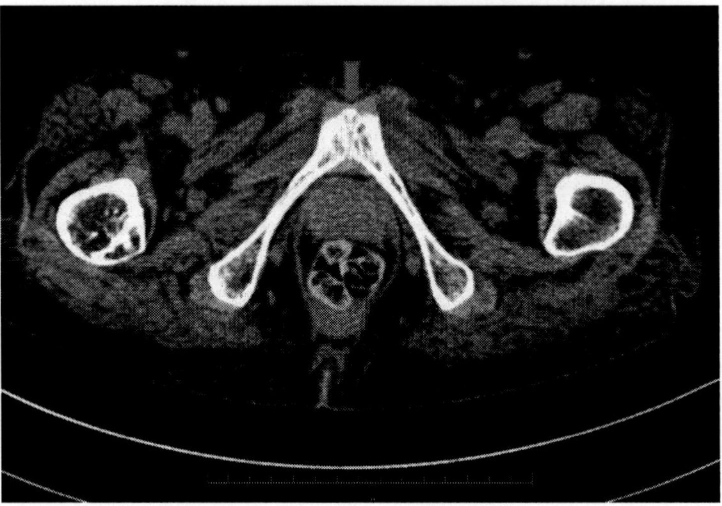

Figure 66. Calcification of pubic symphysis.

Although HADD may deposit in the joints, true articular disease is very rare. HADD sometimes accompanies with CPPD. Usually, HADD affects mainly soft tissue around joint, muscles, capsules, bursae, and tendon sheaths. Severe secondary OA is probably caused by CPPD.

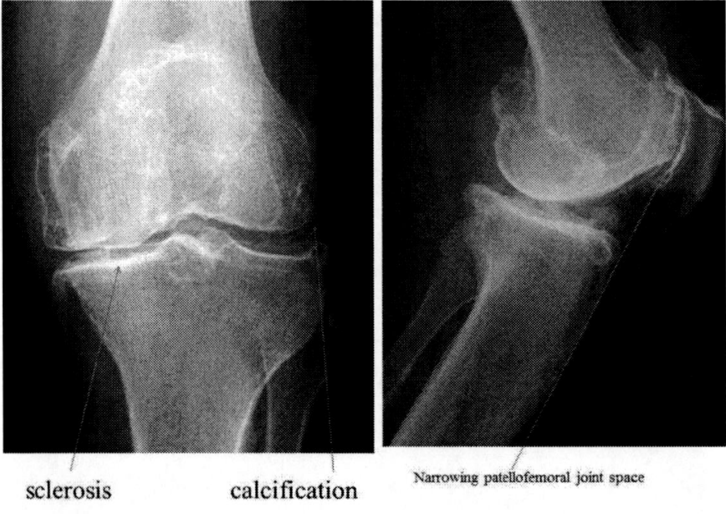

Figure 67. HADD accompanied with CPPD presenting secondary severe OA.

SYSTEMIC LUPUS ERYTHEMATOSUS (SLE)

Systemic lupus erythematous (SLE) is common and chronic, inflammatory, autoimmune multi-systemic disorder with autoantibody-production showing extremely diverse manifestations. The etiology of the disease is still unknown. It is believed that genetic, hormonal, and environmental factors play important roles in the pathophysiology in SLE. Multiple genes show genetic susceptibility to SLE. Environmental factors including ultraviolet light, viral infections, female gender, and exposure to estrogen-containing medications may induce SLE.

A

Posteroanterior (PA) view of both hands

Jaccoud's Arthritis: the hallmark of SLE

A deforming nonerosive arthritis is seen most commonly in the hands and wrists

Severe subluxations or dislocations without erosive disease are present.

PA view of the same hand shows very small mal-alignment of fingers, especially at MCP joint of the second finger, when the fingers are rigidly positioned.

Because the subluxations are reducible, plain PA view, positioning the digits properly, do not show evident deformity. Therefore, four views of the hand show subluxation of the MCP joints in SLE patients. To know the deformity and deviation of fingers, these views are helpful occasionally.

Subluxations and dislocations

Four views of the hand: subluxation of the MCP joints in SLE patients

However, only minor subluxation of the MCP and PIP joints of the fingers is found in normal plain hand XP even in the same hand

Deformity of nonerosive arthritis may exist in the knee and/or the shoulder with difficulty of finding by radiograph.

B

Osteoporosis may be present.

Posteroanterior (PA) view of both hands in a patient with SLE shows osteoporosis.

Juxta-articular osteoporosis

Juxta-articular osteoporosis is present that eventually becomes diffuse osteoporosis.

Osteonecrosis

The first radiographic change may be increased smudgy density, which represents either dead bone that appears dense in comparison to the surrounding osteoporosis or reparative bone.

C

No joint space loss

No erosions

When not distorted by subluxation or dislocation, the joint space appears preserved.

D

hand and wrist, hip, knee, and shoulder

Bilateral and symmetrical

MCP joints in the hands: deformity

Osteonecrosis
Usually, bilateral and asymmetrical
the lunates, the scaphoids, and the metacarpal and metatarsal heads
MTP joints: in the heads of metatarsals

The most common sites of osteonecrosis in SLE
The femoral heads, the humeral heads, the femoral condyles, the tibial plateaus, and the tali
In femoral head, a combination of osteoporosis and osteosclerosis is found.

E
Soft tissue swelling
Early in the course of the disease, soft tissue swelling is seen, with eventual soft tissue atrophy.

Calcification
Calcification in the subcutaneous tissue
    linear and streaky
    no association with the deforming nonerosive arthritis or with the osteonecrosis
    isolated finding of calcification is difficult to differentiate from other rheumatic diseases.

F
Woman of child-bearing age
Female: male ratio = 10:1
Genetic predisposition DR3
Symptoms and examinations
Skin   Butterfly erythema
Raynaud's
musculoskeletal system
digestive system
Lung
Circulation Myocarditis
Kidney   Lupus nephritis

Nervous system

Complications

ANA
autoantibodies
Chest X-ray

G
Diagnosis: ACR criteria
Treatment: immunosuppressive therapy

Case 18. A 63-year-old Female; SE (Jaccoud's arthritis)

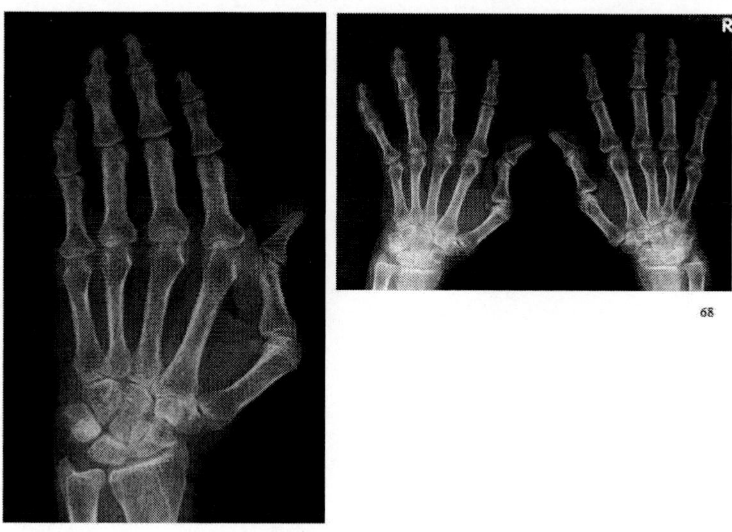

Figure 68. Deformity of the hands and Raynaud's.

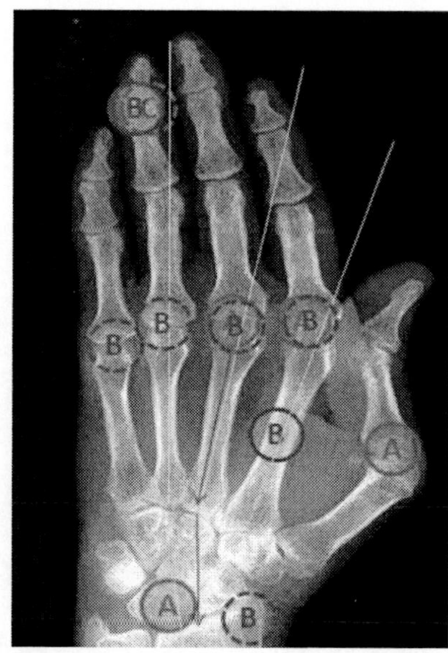

Figure 69. PA view of the hand in a patient with SLE.

    A.   fingers: extremely ulnar deviation at the lt. 2,3MCP joints.
It can be reducible in another position
deformity at 1st MCP joint
RC joints: radial deviation
Loss of height of carpals: none
Carpal collapse: none

B. mineraliation II metacarpal: osteoporotic
    Possible periarticular osteopenia of the MCP and RC joints
    osteosclerosis: mild at DIP joints

C. joint spaces: DIPs, PIPs, MCPs, carpals and RCs: maintained
    erosions: none
    osteophytes: possible 4 DIP
    calcification: none

D. MCPs and RC joint having only deformity
    DIP

E. distal soft tissues: normal
    calcification: none

F. ANA+
    anti-dsDNA antibodies +
    PSL medication

G. diagnosis
    SLE (Jaccoud's arthritis)
    Osteoporosis due to corticosteroids
    OA

Reversible deformity without evident joint destruction

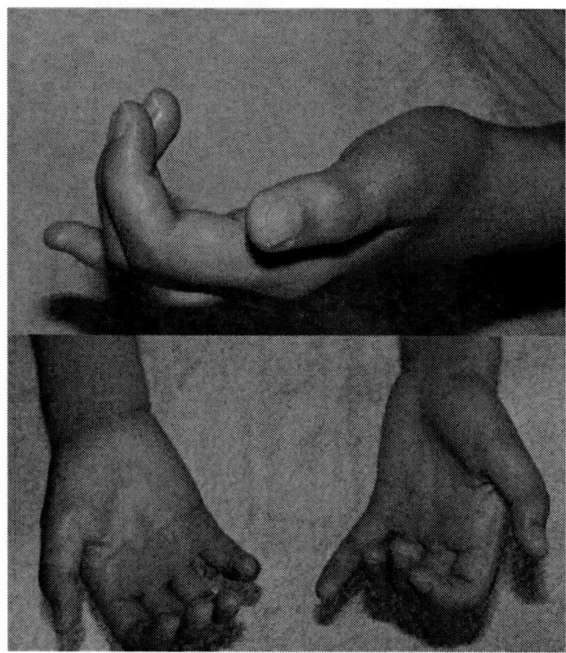

Figure 70. Tenosynovitis in SLE.

SYSTEMIC SCLEROSIS

Case 19. A 43-year-old Female. Calcification of Skin in Systemix Sclerosis (CREST)

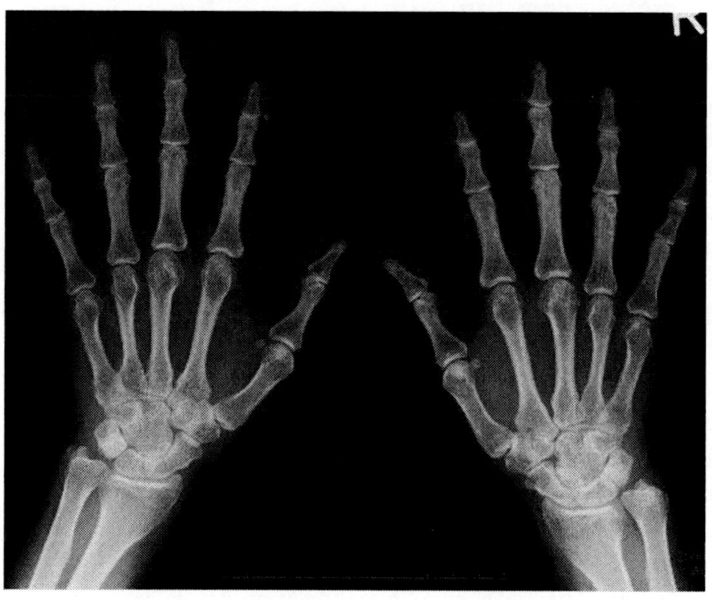

Figure 71. Raynaud's phenomena.

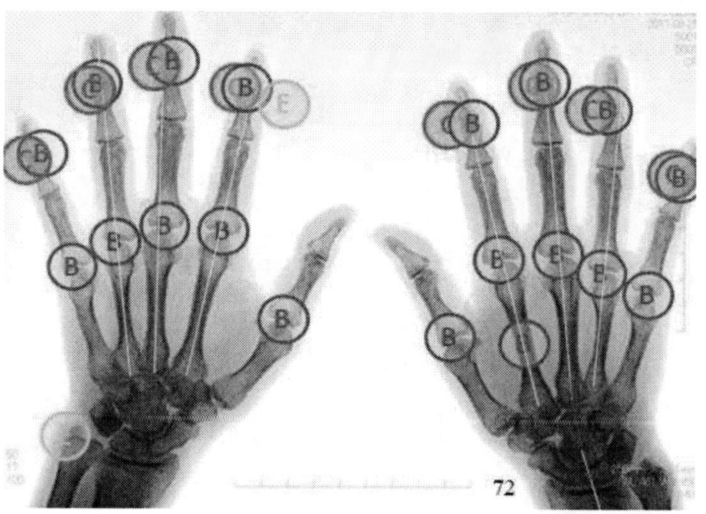

Figure 72.

A. fingers: maintained
    RC joints: maintained
    Loss of height of.carpals: none
    B/A>0.54
    Carpal collapse: none

B. mineralization:
    II metacarpal: osteoporosis
    periarticular osteoporosis: all MCPs
    osteosclerosis: all DIPs
C. joint spaces: DIPs: narrowing
    PIPs, MCPs, carpals and RCs: maintained
    erosions: none
    osteophytes: none
    calcification: none in joints
D. bil. DIPs: mild osteosclerosis and JSN
E. distal soft tissues: normal
    calcification: lt. 2nd finger and lt. wrist
F. ANA(+)
    anti-centromere antibodies(+)
    scleroderma (+)
    gastroesophageal reflux disease; GERD(+)
    PSL medication
G. Calcification of skin in systemic sclerosis (CREST)
    Osteoporosis
    Possible early OA (mild)

CREST— calcinosis, Rlynaud's, esophageal dysmotility, sclerodactyly, telengectasia.

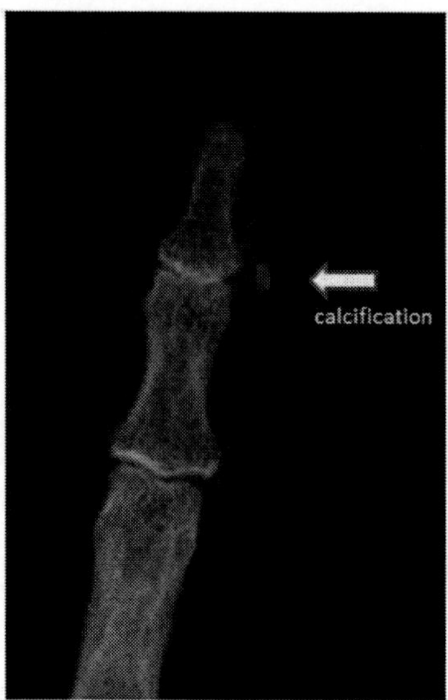

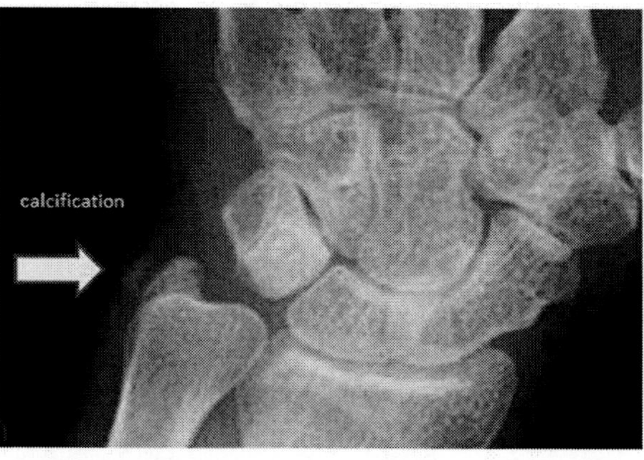

Figure 73. Calcification at the knee in the same patient with Scleroderma.

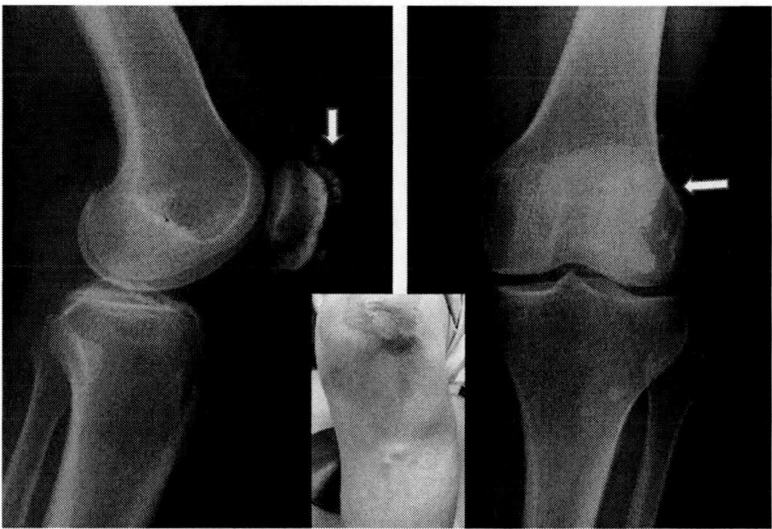

Figure 74. There is amorphous calcification in the soft tissues at the knee (arrow).

Figure calcification is proved in histology of the skin.

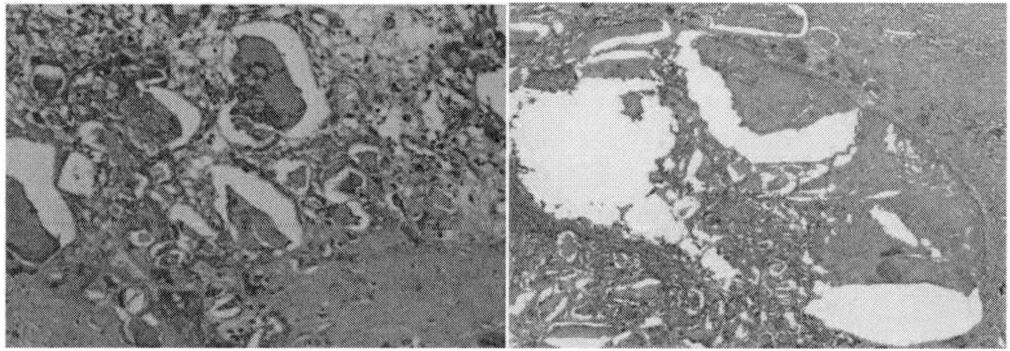

Figure 75. Histology of the skin.

IgG4 Related Disease (IgG4-RD)

Case 20. A 66-year-old male, Retroperitoneal Fibrosis

IgG4   901mg/dl

History
He visited a doctor due to fatigue.
In laboratory findings, renal dysfunction was pointed out.
The abdomen CT revealed hydronephrosis with swelling of soft tissue around the ureter.

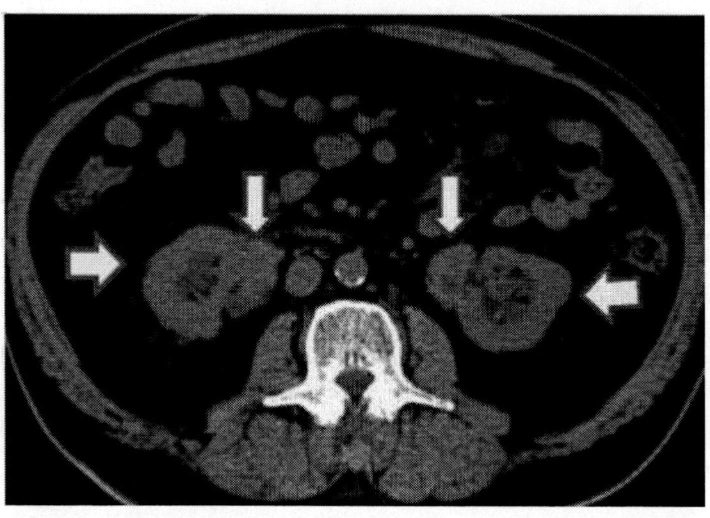

Figure 76. Abdomen CT.

Laboratory findings

CBC
WBC   9060 /μl
  neut 62.96%
  Ly   20.9
  Mo   5.7
  Eo   9.9
  Ba   0.9
Hb   11.6 g/dl
PLT   22.3 X 10₄/μl

Blood chemistry
TP   8.5 g/dl
Alb   4.1 g/dl
AST   17 I/U
ALT   15 I/U
LDH   197 I/U
Cr   3.93 mg/dl

u.Protein (+-)
u.RBC   (-)

IgG subclass

IgG1	1010	mg/dl	(320-748)	32.86 %
IgG2	1050		(208-754)	34.16 %
IgG3	113		(6.6-88.3)	3.68 %
IgG4	901		(4.8-105)	29.31 %

CRP   4.99 mg/dl
ESR   72 mm/hr

ANA   40x
Anti-SSA   (-)
Anti-SS-B   (-)
Anti-Ds-DNA   (-)
C3   122 mg/dl
C4   27 mg/dl
CH50   46.1 CH50U/ml

77

Figure 77. Laboratory findings.

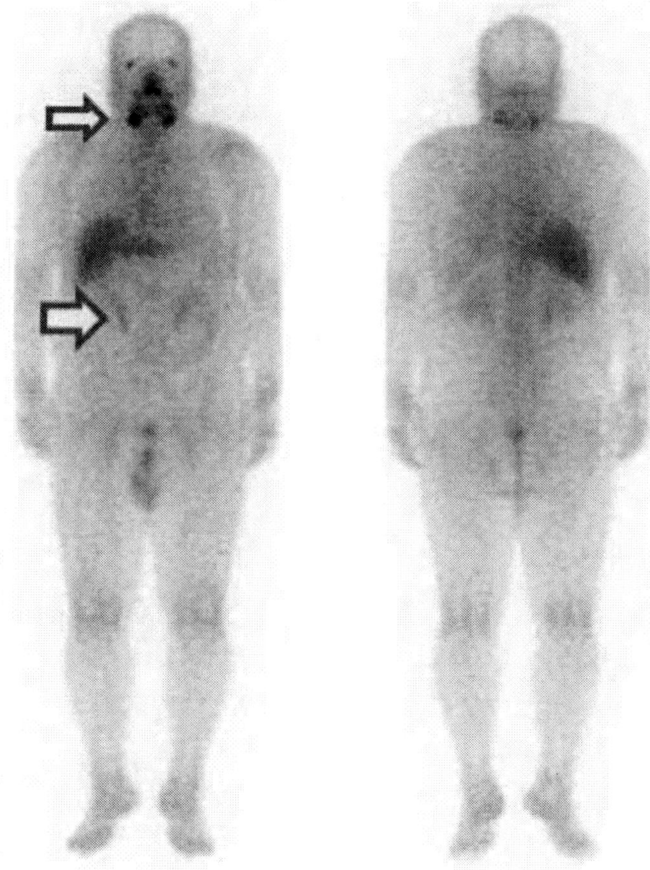

Figure 78. In Gallium scintigraphy showed the uptakes of bilateral submandibular glands, kidney, and periureteral tissue. Biopsy of the left renal pelvis proved dense inflammatory cell infiltration with fibrosis.

Possible IgG4-RD

Promptly, Oral PSL 30 mg /day improved renal function and dissappeared the tumor-like lesions.

Case 21. A 53-year-old male. Retroperitoneal fibrosis

IgG4   403mg/dl

History
H24.3.12 lumbago

 Syuichi Koarada and Yoshifumi Tada

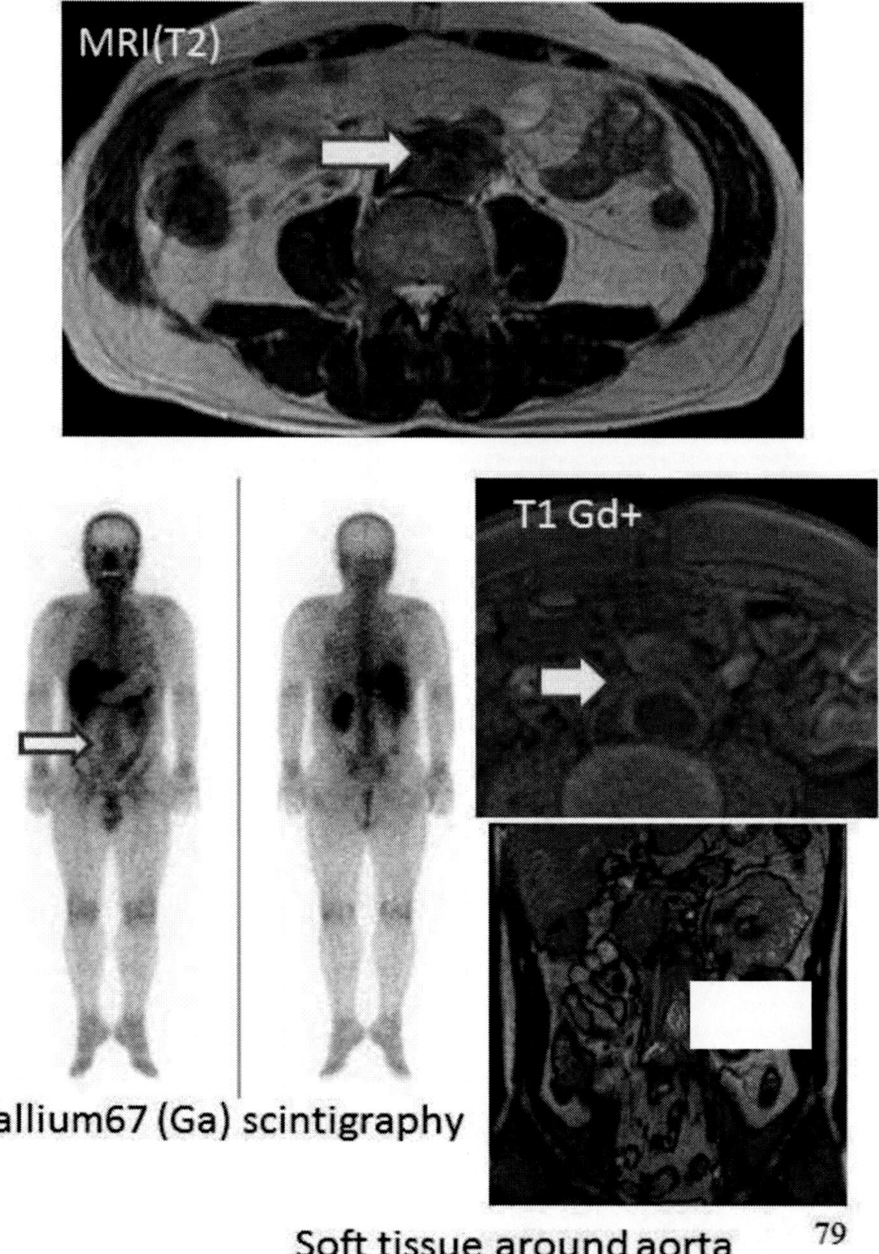

Figure 79. He visited a doctor and the abdomen CT showed hydronephrosis.

MRI showed soft tissue swelling and the high level of IgG4 was found.

Laboratory findings

CBC
WBC   11400 /µl
  neut 64.4 %
  Ly   28.1
  Mo   5.8
  Eo   1.3
  Ba   0.4
Hb   13.1 g/dl
PLT   32.3 x104/µl

Blood chemistry
TP   8.6 g/dl
Alb   4.1 g/dl
AST   16 I/U
ALT   16 I/U
LDH   150 I/U
BUN   19.5 mg/dl
Cr   1.26 mg/dl
eGFR   48.2 ml/min

u.Protein (-)
  Blood   (-)

CRP   3.54 mg/dl
ESR   60 mm/hr
C3   151 mg/dl
C4   41 mg/dl
CH50   72 CH50/ml
IgG   1985 mg/dl
IgG4   403 mg/dl
IgA   358 mg/dl
IgM   45 mg/dl

ANA   <40x
RF   6 IU/ml
sIL-2R   372 U/ml
Anti-dsDNA <10 IU/ml
PR3-ANCA   <10 EU
MPO-ANCA   <10 EU
QFT-3G   (-)

80

Figure 80. Laboratory findings. Oral PSL 30mg/day improved his symptoms promptly.

Case 22. A 38-year-old male. Interfollicular plasmacytosis

IgG4   619mg/dl

History
2011.10. In the office of family doctor, hypergammaglobulinemia was pointed out (IgG 5049mg/dl).
Whole body CT showed lymphadenopathy.
In our hospital, lymph node biopsy was performed.
Physical examination

BT 35.6°C P 80/min R 12/min BP 108/68mmHg
Chest and abdomen: normal
Skin eruption: free
Right inguinal: 2 LNs (2cm and 1cm)
Left inguinal: 1 LN (2cm)

Laboratory findings

CBC
WBC   6900 /μl
  neut 63.5 %
  Ly   24.5
  Mo   8.0
  Eo   3.5
  Ba   0.5
  Hb   13.1 g/dl
PLT   35.1 x104/μl

Blood chemistry
TP   10.8 g/dl
Alb   2.8 g/dl
AST   13 I/U
ALT   9 I/U
LDH   104 I/U
BUN   9.2 mg/dl
Cr   0.85 mg/dl
eGFR 81.6 ml/min

u.Protein (-)
  blood   (1+)

u.sed
  RBC   5-9/HPF
  WBC   (-)
  cast (-)

Beta2-MG   5.59 ug/ml
NAG   25.5 IU/g/Cr

Blood culture x2   (-)
Urine culture   (-)
Sputum culture   (-)

CRP   5.99 mg/dl
C3   122 mg/dl
C4   39 mg/dl
CH50   67 CH50/ml
IgG   5048 mg/dl
IgG4   619 mg/dl
IgA   629 mg/dl
IgM   157 mg/dl
IgE   2907 IU/ml

ANA   40x
RF   19 IU/ml
sIL-2R   1294 U/ml
Anti-dsDNA   <10 IU/ml
Anti-SS-A/Ro <7.0 u/ml
Anti-SS-B/La <7.0 u/ml
Anti-GBM   <10 EU
PR3-ANCA   <10 EU
MPO-ANCA   <10 EU
HIV   Ag(-) Ab(-)
EB-anti-VC (IgG, IgM)   (-)
HTLV-1-PA   (-)
Cytomegalovirus IgM   (-)
QFT-3G   (-)

Figure 81. Laboratory findings.

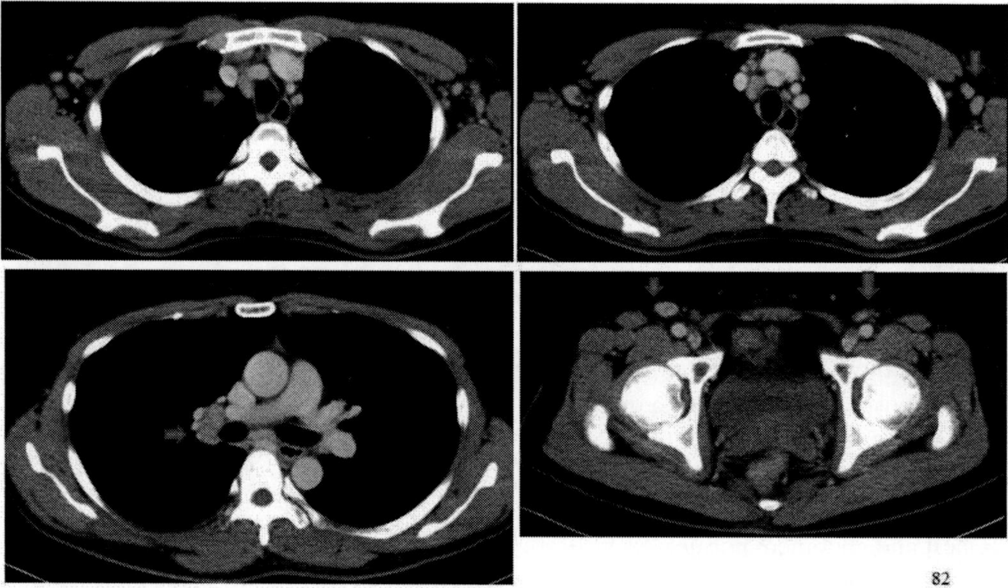

Figure 82. Lymphadenopathy in CT.

Histology of Lymph Node (Figure 83)

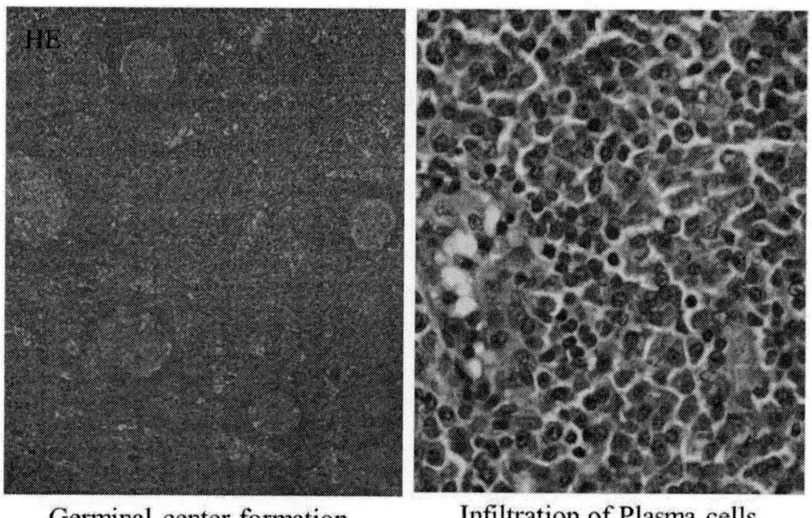

Figure 83. Follicular hyperplasia.

Immunohistochemistry

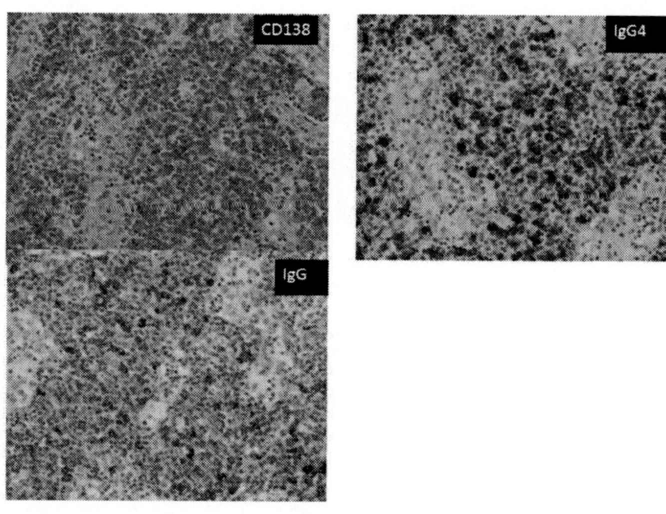

CD138+
IgG4+/IgG=50%

Figure 84. IgG4-related interfollicular plasmacytosis.

REFERENCES

Arnett FC, Edworthy SM, Bloch DA, McShane DJ, Fries JF, Cooper NS, et al. The American Rheumatism Association 1987 revised criteria for the classification of rheumatoid arthritis. *Arthritis Rheum.* 1988;31:315–24.

Agudelo CA, Wise CM. Gout: diagnosis, pathogenesis, and clinical manifestations. *Curr Opin Rheumatol.* 2001;13:234–9.

Barth WF. Office evaluation of the patient with musculoskeletal complaints. *Am J Med.* 1997;102(1A):3S–10S.

Brower AC and Flemming DJ. *Arthritis in Black and White Saunders* 2012.

De Smet AA, Radiographic projections for the diagnosis of arthritis of the hands and wrists. *Radiology,* 139, 577-581, 1981.

El-Gabalawy HS, Duray P, Goldbach-Mansky R. Evaluating patients with arthritis of recent onset: studies in pathogenesis and prognosis. *JAMA.* 2000;284:2368–73.

Gladman DD. Clinical aspects of the spondyloarthropathies. *Am J Med Sci.* 1998;316:234–8.

Hadler NM, Franck WA, Bress NM, Robinson DR. Acute polyarticular gout. *Am J Med.* 1974;56:715–9.

Klinkhoff A. Rheumatology: 5. Diagnosis and management of inflammatory polyarthritis. *CMAJ.* 2000;162:1833–8.

Klippel JH, Weyand CM, Crofford LJ, Stone JH, eds. Primer on the rheumatic diseases. 12th ed. Atlanta: *Arthritis Foundation,* 2001: 140–3.

Koarada S, Tada Y, Ushiyama O, Morito F, Suzuki N, Ohta A, Miyake K, Kimoto M, Nagasawa K. B cells lacking RP105, a novel B cell antigen, in systemic lupus erythematosus. *Arthritis Rheum.* 1999; 42: 2593-600.

Koarada S, Wu Y, Ridgway WM. Increased entry into the IFN-gamma effector pathway by CD4+ T cells selected by I-Ag7 on a nonobese diabetic versus C57BL/6 genetic background. *J Immunol.* 2001 1; 167:1693-702.

McGonagle D, Gibbon W, Emery P. Classification of inflammatory arthritis by enthesitis. *Lancet.* 1998;352:1137–40.

Reilly PA. The differential diagnosis of generalized pain. *Baillieres Best Pract Res Clin Rheumatol.* 1999;13:391–401.

Richie AM and Francis ML. Diagnostic Approach to Polyarticular Joint Pain. *Am Fam Physician.* 2003 Sep 15;68(6):1151-1160.

Sangha O. Epidemiology of rheumatic diseases. *Rheumatology* [Oxford]. 2000;39(suppl 2): 3–12.

Schmitt R, Ulrich, Lanz U, Herzberger AB. *Diagnostic Imaging of the Hand.* George Thieme Verlag 2008

Sood A, Panush RS, Pinals RS. Case management study: polyarthritis with fever. *Bull Rheum Dis.* 1998;47(3):1–4.

INDEX